Constitutional Medicine in the East

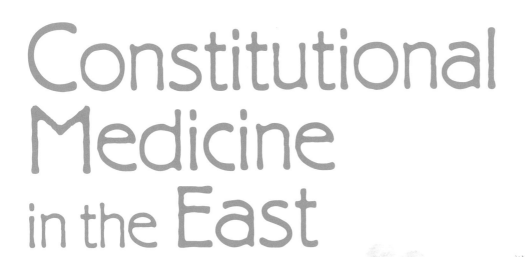

Writen by
Lee Je-ma

Translated by
Choi Seung-hoon

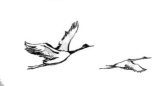

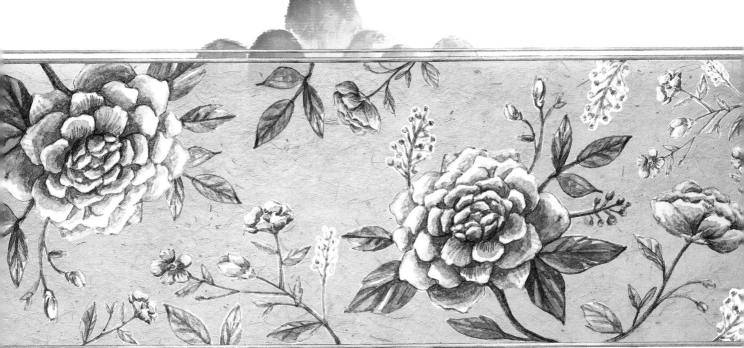

| 東醫壽世保元 |

Constitutional Medicine in the East

1st Print : 2021-06-25
1st Publication : 2021-07-05

Written by Lee Je-ma, and translated by Choi Seung-hoon
Editor | Do-sung Kim
Text Designer | Won-bae Cho
Cover Designer | Jae-wook Kim

Published by Koonja Publishing Inc.
338 Hwadong-gil, Pajoo-si, Gyeonggi-do, Republic of Korea
https://www.koonja.co.kr

ISBN 979-11-5955-731-6
USD 70.00

Constitutional Medicine in the East

| 東醫壽世保元 |

Dedicated to my wife, Sung-hye,
and our children, Suon and Kyuha,
and to all those who share Lee Je-ma's dreams.

"When the Taoism meets

the Confucianism in Medicine"

It has been 25 years since 『Longevity and Life Preservation in Oriental Medicine』, the first English translation of 『*Dongui Suse Bowon* (東醫壽世保元)』. At that time, I was obsessed with the mission to realize the prophecy of Lee Je-ma 100 years ago. Fortunately, with many colleague's help, I was able to achieve that. Ten years later, while working at the World Health Organization (WHO), based on the achievements of 『WHO International Standard Terminologies on Traditional Medicine in the Western Pacific Region (WHO-IST)』, which I had promoted, I released the 2nd edition called 『Longevity and Life Preservation in Eastern Medicine』.

Another 12 years later, 『Constitutional Medicine in the East』 is published. Although the contents are not very different, the reader was added to the convenience in the form of English-Chinese contrast. Here, the support of Koonja, a leading medical publishing company in Korea, was very helpful. Now, the prophecy of Lee Je-ma has become more feasible.

I think Sasang Constitutional Medicine (SCM) is not the ultimate destination of medicine and will play an important role in the process of getting there. The incorporation of Confucianism into ancient Chinese medicine in the background of the Taoism has enabled a holistic approach to humans, linking them to clinical practice, providing insights that humans are all different. The four humors theory of Hippocrates or Ayurvedic Medicine of India, which have completely different historical and cultural and philosophical backgrounds, draw similar pictures for constitutions. It can be evidence that SCM is universal.

After the 『Longevity and Life Preservation in Oriental Medicine』 came out, although SCM was known internationally, it still has a long way to go. Now, by combining modern cutting-edge science and technology such as artificial intelligence and genetic engineering, SCM will be realized and globalized.

During the COVID-19 outbreaks, the body's immune capacity has emerged as an important issue. Constitution refers to the various tendencies of each person's immunity. Hence it will still be an important factor for prevention and treatment no matter what diseases including pandemic occur in the future, and SCM will exert its value even more. This book also seeks to contribute to the advancement of medicine by providing readers with better readability of 『*Dongui Suse Bowon*』.

2021. 7. 1

Translator's Note

The 『*Dongui Suse Bowon*』 consists of two parts: basic theory and clinical studies. Lee Je-ma opens his basic theory by defining the environments that surround man and the body itself using a quarternary paradigm. This paradigm is an extension of the Confucian tradition in employing the number four.

The terminology, which Lee Je-ma employs, is quite hard to understand as his philosophical ideas are of his own development based on neo-Confucianism (新儒學). Even widely experienced Oriental medical doctors find it hard to comprehend, which has resulted in many doctors exhibiting interest only in the clinical aspects. However, understanding his philosophical attitude is required prior to studying his Sasang Constitutional Medicine.

Additionally, a thorough understanding of the 『*Shanghanlun*』(傷寒論: "Treatise on Cold-induced Diseases") written by Zhang Zhongjing (張仲景) is a prerequisite to understanding Lee Je-ma's clinical studies. As a translator, I have tried to translate the terminology literally and avoided including my own interpretations, so as to allow the readers to understand Lee Je-ma's original words.

The terminology used in the translation, such as stomach and blood, which can be translated into English without much difficulty, does not necessarily denote the stomach and blood as understood in western medicine. Those words having no equivalents in English, except for the already widely known terms such as 'qi' and 'yin-yang', have been inscribed phonetically in italic letters. Some of the terms newly employed in this translation are provided with explanations or footnotes in brackets.

The names of traditional Chinese prescriptions were written in Chinese pronunciation while the names of newly formulated prescriptions by Lee Je-ma were written in Korean pronunciation. To prevent confusion, all titles of books are written in italic letters inside the punctuation marks 『 』.

The following table of the pinyin phonetic alphabet shows pronunciations with approximate English equivalents. In parentheses are the corresponding letters in the Wade-Giles system.

Pronunciation Guide

a (a) as in *father*

b (b) as in *book*

c (ts', tz') like *ts* in *its*

ch (ch) as in *church*, strongly aspirated

d (t) as in *door*

e (e) as in *her*

f (f) as in *finger*

g (k) as in *go*

h (h) as in *her*, strongly aspirated

i (i) like the vowel sound in *eat* or the *i* in *sir*

j (ch) as in *jeep*

k (k') as in *kite*, strongly aspirated

l (l) as in *love*

m (m) as in *me*

n (n) as in *no*

o (o) like the vowel sound in *law*

p (p') as in *park*, strongly aspirated

q (ch') like the *ch* in *cheese*

r (r) as in *red*

s (s, ss, sz) as in *sister*

sh (sh) as in *show*

t (t') as in *tough*, strongly aspirated

u (u) as in *too* also in the French *tu*

w (w) semi-vowel in syllables beginning with *u* when not preceded by consonants, pronounced
   as in *want*

x (hs) like *sh* in *sheety*

y semi-vowel in syllables beginning with *i* or *u* when not preceded by consonants, pronounced
   as in *yes*

z (ts, tz) as in *zone*

zh (ch) like the first consonant in *jump*

ai like *ie* in *pie*

ao like *ow* in *how*

ei like *ay* in *day*

ie like *ie* in *experience*

ou like *oe* in *toe*

Acknowledgements

In 1989, I was fortunate to be the first visiting professor from Korea to teach at China Medical College, currently China Medical University in Taiwan. There, I had an opportunity to teach a graduate course in English about the 『*Dongui Suse Bowon*』(東醫壽世保元). That opportunity laid the foundation, which inspired me to further my study of Lee Je-ma and to launch this task, one of the most meaningful endeavors in my life. I wish to express my gratitude to China Medical College and its graduate students. This work is a product of the many people who volunteered their time, energies and talents in countless ways.

Professor Moon Joon-jeon, who showed me the joys of scholastic pursuit, and Professor Kim Young-oak, who taught me how to be a true scholar. Chancellor Choue Young-seek, the founder of Kyung Hee University, who, early on, suggested the birth of a third medicine through the development of an East-West Cooperative Medicine, and who gave both financial and moral support to this task. And the patrons organized by Chancellor Choue, Professor Song Il-byung, Professor Goh Byung-hee of Kyung Hee University, and other scholars of the Sasang Medical Society whose input during our group discussions was truly invaluable.

My assistants and students: Dr. Shim Bum-sang, Dr. Park Gyeong-mo, Dr. Lee Neung-ki, Dr. Lee Hang-jae, Dr. Kim Sung-woo, and Dr. Jang Hwan-sun and Sun-woo in Los Angeles. Their energies and efforts in all the tasks – big and small – I assigned, kept the project alive. Professor Fred J. Seligson of Hankuk University of Foreign Studies, who since my college days has been my big brother in heart and spirit to Professor Kim Nam-hee of Chung-ang Sangha College, Andy Douglas of Iowa State University, and especially my student, David Rhee from the University of Chicago, all of whom helped the project to take shape.

There were many others who were truly unsparing with their assistances to the completion of this task. I regret I could not name them all.

Finally, I thank the Lord, who sent the great man, Lee Je-ma, to our nation, Korea, and who also allowed me to bring Lee Je-ma's dream to fruition by opening the doors of Sasang Constitutional Medicine to the world.

1996. 12. 5

Introduction

Traditional Chinese medicine (TCM) regards the human body as a black box, and diagnoses the condition of the internal organs by their external manifestations. Every individual's face, shape and temperament are different. TCM understands that each human being has a different internal structure, as do the main organs. TCM also recognizes that those differences can be categorized as certain types. For example, in the 『*Lingshu*』(靈樞: "Miraculous Pivot"), the bible of TCM, the discourses of the '*Tongtian*' (通天: "Communication with Heaven") and the '*Yinyang Ershewuren*' (陰陽二十五人: "Yin-yang with Twenty Five Types of People") present very sophisticated theories using yin-yang and five phases ideas as categorizing guidelines.

Confucianism (儒家) and Taoism (道家) have traditionally dominated Chinese thought. While Confucianism has become the root and trunk of the philosophy applied to political, social and moral problems, Taoism represents Chinese natural science. This includes TCM, which, from the beginning, has been totally rooted in Taoist thought. In ancient times, the natural environment directly affected living conditions, but as human science and civilization developed, the relationship between man and nature became less important than the relationship between man and his social environment. The incidence of mental or psychological problems from social relationships increased relative to that of physical diseases from the natural environment.

TCM doctors, who had been mostly concerned with the physical universe (the Taoist mind), gradually realized the importance of our mental and moral natures, which are the main objects of Confucian philosophy. Consequently, Confucianism and Taoism became unified under the auspices of Sasang (four types) Constitutional Medicine (SCM).

The influence of TCM had made human beings passive by putting more emphasis on the natural environment rather than on themselves. However, the theories of SCM tell us that men can control both their physical and mental condition through their own efforts. In this way, we are presented with a method of treating people that does more than just eliminate the pathogen (邪氣) as in TCM focusing on man's relationship with natural influences. This new medicine can do that and also transforms what we are at our core. Even though SCM is an encounter between Taoist and Confucian thought, it essentially adopts a TCM view of pathogenesis. This includes the concept that healthy qi (正氣) is the first consideration in promoting health and treating disease. TCM states that disease occurs when the pathogen is stronger than the healthy qi. Therefore, the primary treatment principle is the cultivation and preservation of healthy qi. However, the compositions of quantity and quality of healthy qi are different in each individual. There are some people with more yang qi, while others have more yin blood. While the 『*Huangdi Neijing*』 (黃帝內經: "Yellow Emperor's Canon of Internal Medicine") and Chinese medical doctors had a vague concept of constitution and only touched upon constitutional problems superficially, SCM has extensively and systematically resolved this issue. SCM focuses on the different constitutional manifestations of the individual's nature and emotions. A person's nature and emotions drive the ascending and descending of qi in the body, and this dynamic of the qi's ascent and descent shapes the different types of structures, functions and temperaments.

The ideas of the 『*Huangdi Neijing*』, 『*Shanghanlun*』 and Confucianism have existed for a long time, but each took a different path. The prototypes of the four constitutional types (greater yang, lesser yang, greater yin and lesser yin) were brought forth in the discourses of the '*Tongtian*' in the 『*Huangdi Neijing*』, and the treatment principle of each constitutional type is rooted in the 『*Shanghanlun*』. For the Confucianist element, the 『*Zhongyong*』 (中庸: "The Doctrine of the Mean") discusses in depth the four emotions: sorrow, anger, joy and pleasure.

Taoism and Confucianism finally meet in SCM. This has allowed the physical and mental planes of human beings to actually meet and become one. At the same time, it is also a successful unification of philosophy and science. Herein lies the greatness of SCM.

It is an interesting question as to how SCM bore fruit in Korea, and not in China where Confucianism, Taoism and TCM originated. Since the two countries have the same Taoist tradition, we cannot find any further clues in the Taoistic field. Therefore, we need to compare the two countries' Confucianist history. During the Song dynasty (宋代), through the neo-Confucianist Zhu Xi (朱熹: 1130-1200), Confucianism underwent a huge revival and spread throughout large areas of Asia, including the Joseon (朝鮮) kingdom. At that time, China and Joseon held a common Confucian tradition. However, after that period, China passed on to the metaphysics of the Ming (明) and Qing (清) dynasties and continued changing and evolving with the doctrines of Wang Yangming (王陽明) and the bibliographical study of Chinese classics. This trend did not take hold in Joseon. During the Joseon dynasty, the country was absolutely controlled by the neo-Confucianist philosophy for hundreds of years. The rigidness and absoluteness of authority favored by neo-Confucianism brought much hardship to the people and stifled the gradual development of new ideas. However, towards the end of Joseon, centuries of repressed creativity and suffering led to an explosion. In contrast, China did not experience such a revolution, but rather underwent a gradual change from one new system to another. As modern western science sprang out from the long, dark Middle Ages, the new revolutionary Confucianist mind, which gave birth to SCM was able to spring out of these difficult times at the end of the Joseon dynasty. This was the climate into which SCM's founder Lee Je-ma – a Confucianist doctor - was born.

Just before his death, Lee Je-ma predicted that SCM would become a universal medicine in one hundred years. In recent decades, TCM has disclosed its long-held medical secrets and made significant inroads in the West. As an advanced type of TCM, still following the essence of TCM and its techniques, SCM, now presented in English, can move on to world-wide renown and application.

Life Story of Lee Je-ma

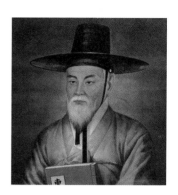

Lee Je-ma was born in 1836, during the reign of King Heonjong (憲宗), in the Joseon dynasty. His birthplace was Cheonseo Township (川西面), Hamheung County (咸興郡), Hamgyeong Province (咸鏡道), in northern Korea. He lived for 64 years and died in 1900. The period in which he lived was chaotic, with extreme political confusion mainly caused by party strife. There were serious economic difficulties, and the people were dissatisfied with the seemingly endless internal and external problems. The Joseon dynasty finally collapsed in 1910.

The founder of the Joseon dynasty was King Taejo (太祖), who was born in Yeongheung County (永興郡) in Hamgyeong Province. He did not like the temperament of the northern people and began a tradition that lasted for more than 500 years: no one from the north, not even a man of talent, would be appointed to a high-ranking official post. Because of this, none of Lee Je-ma's family in the past 20 generations had been given a government post. Finally, his father, Lee Ban-o (李攀五), passed the civil - and military - service exams, and became a noble in the northern part of the nation.

There is an interesting story about the birth of Lee Je-ma. One day, Je-ma's father was coming home from the school where he was studying Confucian philosophy. On the road he ran into some of his friends, who were drinking at a tavern. An older barmaid lived there with her daughter, still single but made unmarriageable by age. The daughter was not very attractive, being gifted with neither beauty nor intelligence. Because of this, the barmaid realized that it would be difficult to find a husband for her daughter.

Ban-o was not accustomed to drinking, but on that evening, his friends persuaded him to join them. He soon lost consciousness and remained in the tavern sleeping. At twilight, his friends left, asking the barmaid to take care of him. The barmaid thought that this was a good opportunity to try to bring her daughter and the young nobleman together, so she made a bed for him and sent her daughter in to warm it.

One day, ten months later at dawn, Ban-o's father was asleep and having a marvelous dream. He was given a charming colt by a mysterious person and told, "This colt is from Jeju (濟州) Island. No one claims it. I am giving it to you. Please feed it and take good care of it." The person tied the colt to a stake and disappeared. Ban-o's father looked at the colt and found it lovely and attractive. He was patting the colt on its back when he woke up.

Ban-o's father was pondering his wonderful dream when he heard someone calling from the gate. His servant opened the gate and brought the guests to him. The lady said, "This is your son's baby. Please accept him."

Ban-o's father called his son and asked him how this could have happened. Even though the younger Lee had been drunk, he was able to remember everything and told his father the truth. On any other day, the new grandfather might have been angry, but recalling his special dream, he decided that it was a good omen. The baby and the mother were taken in. Grandfather Lee named the baby Je-ma, after his dream's Jeju Island and Ma (meaning 'horse'). The elder Lee thus had always expected his grandson to become a great man, and showered the child with love.

Since Ban-o had not as yet sired any children, he was able to enter Je-ma's name into the family register as legitimate offspring. However, the feudalistic society did not accept Je-ma. His birth from unmarried parents left him with physical and mental barriers to overcome.

By nature, Je-ma was a very cheerful and brave boy. Moreover, his grandfather's heartfelt love nourished and supported him. Because of this, in later years, Je-ma left a will to his descendants, which declared that his grandfather was to be considered the founder of their line.

When Je-ma turned seven, he was sent to be taught by his uncle. He studied one to ten pages every day. There was, at first, concern that he seldom reviewed his lessons but the next morning, Je-ma would always recite what he had learned the previous day.

During childhood, Je-ma was more fond of the military arts than of reading or writing. When young Je-ma played outside, he always chose a sword or a bow and arrow. Je-ma wanted to be a military commander when he grew up.

One day, while studying the 『Tongshi』 (通史: "Introduction to History"), young Je-ma came upon a sentence, which read, "… Warrior Xiang Yu (項羽) committed suicide at Niao River (烏江) …." He closed the book. The legendary hero Xiang Yu had incredible strength and was strong enough to move a mountain, but life had been harsh, and he suffered a miserable fate. Je-ma sighed, "Alas! It is so sad" and cried. His family and teachers were astonished at how a seven-year-old boy could experience such mature insight.

When Je-ma was thirteen years old, his uncle gave a poetry examination to all the young scholars. While all of the scholars were concentrating on their exam, Je-ma came in and got a piece of paper. He quickly wrote something on it and left. When Je-ma's writing won first place, all the scholars were surprised, and they began to admire Je-ma.

Because of Je-ma's illegitimate birth, he was discriminated against by many of the towns-people. This affected his temperament, and he found that he could not control his anger. It was during this same time that Joseon society was experiencing instability. Je-ma could not bear these burdens in his hometown, so he left home at the age of thirteen.

For many long years, between the ages of fourteen and forty, Je-ma led a wandering life. Many of the details of this period, including those of his whereabouts, are unknown, but it is clear that this period had a great influence on his knowledge and writing. What is known is that this period was spent seeking the ultimate truth.

According to various scholars' research, at thirty, Lee Je-ma had the rare opportunity to read the 『*Myeongseonlok*』 (明善錄: "Book of Illuminating Goodness") written by Han Seok-ji (韓錫地). This book criticized the metaphysics of the Joseon dynasty, overburdened with academic discussion. The 『*Myeongseonlok*』 made brave assertions for that era and contained very original thinking. Joseon Confucianists who followed the government's philosophy would have deemed this book politically harmful. For this reason, Han Seok-ji had requested that his descendants withhold the book from the public. Je-ma stayed at the home of Han's descendants for a while during the time of his search for the truth. This is how he had the opportunity to read this book, which was unpublished at the time. Later, the 『*Myeongseonlok*』 was to become an important book in Korean academic society. Je-ma was inspired to systematize Han's thoughts. Je-ma acknowledged Han's work from then on, and wrote books to spread Han's thoughts to the world. As a result, he became the target of criticism.

Je-ma studied for three years with Gi Jeong-jin (奇正鎭), who developed a creative type of metaphysics. Je-ma suffered from *jieyi* (generalized fatigue and lassitude) disease, which inspired Gi Jeong-jin to tell him that he was a genius, but one who needed to learn humility and control his quick temper. Je-ma followed Gi's directions and his health improved.

Je-ma's thought was influenced by the ideas of Han Seok-ji and Gi Jeong-jin. At the end of the 19th century, in eastern Asia, in the small town of Joseon, the foundation of Sasang Constitutional Medicine came to maturity through the insightful teachings of his talented mentors.

Je-ma was ill for a long period of time. This illness enabled him to discover SCM. Je-ma suffered from generalized fatigue and lassitude, *yege* (dysphagia) and *fanwei* (regurgitation of food from stomach). He knew that these diseases tend to affect a greater yang person. Generalized fatigue and lassitude results in restriction of movement to the upper body, preventing the lower limbs from functioning properly, but it is neither a paralysis nor is it accompanied by swelling or pain. According to the 『*Neijing*』 (內經: "Canon of Internal Medicine"), generalized fatigue and lassitude appears as weakness, but in reality is not. Moreover, the symptoms resemble those of sthenia. It is also mistaken for a coldness disease or a febrile disease. It was, in a word, very hard to identify.

Je-ma's Liver and Kidney meridians were depleted the *chi* (cubit) pulse was slow and choppy. Heat stagnating in the middle-*jiao* caused the slow pulse. The choppy pulse was caused by collapse of the blood. These symptoms rarely happen to the greater yin type or the lesser yin type. When they do, it is as a complication of another disease.

Lumbar vertebral disease affecting the greater yang type causes the lower limbs to be too weak to walk. The Kidney is located in the lumbar region. These symptoms occur when someone is in deep sorrow. Symptoms of dysphagia and regurgitation of food from the stomach are different, but the causes are identical. The small intestine qi is blocked. Dysphagia creates difficulty in swallowing (gagging), or results in vomiting soon after the food is swallowed. Regurgitation of food from the stomach is milder than dysphagia, with the person vomiting in the evening whatever he ate in the morning, and vice versa. A person with this disease should not eat greasy food. He should also avoid anger and sorrow. According to the 『Neijing』, at certain times, yin qi should predominate, but does not at other times, yang qi should predominate, but does not.

Je-ma suffered from the above-mentioned diseases. He had been treated with traditional medicine, but never had been cured. Je-ma became aware that each individual's constitution is different, and that the symptoms and treatment of disease depend on the individual's constitution. At this point, Je-ma devoted his life to research the constitutional types. After a long period, he was finally cured, but people were frightened of him because he acted like an insane man trying to refine his theories on SCM.

For example, one day, a lady came in with a severe illness. Je-ma had a difficult time defining which constitutional type she belonged to. The lady was shy and did not express any emotion, which he needed to observe in order to make a proper diagnosis. Je-ma decided to use a trick and asked the other people to leave the room. When he was alone with the lady, he asked her to take off her clothes one piece at a time. She could not disobey him, because in those days, one always did as the doctor asked, but she felt ashamed. When the patient was left wearing only her undergarments, Je-ma asked her to take off everything. She was about to stand up, when Je-ma tugged on her underwear. The lady was astonished at his dishonorable attitude and she screamed, thinking that he was trying to rape her. In this display of emotion, he was able to figure out her original nature. She was then asked to put her clothes back on. He decided that her constitution was of the lesser yang type, and he used the proper medication to cure her. This sort of medical subterfuge was resorted to many times during the process of his research.

Choi Lin (崔麟) wrote in his autobiography, "When I was ill, I went to see Je-ma to be treated by him. In order for him to know my constitutional type, he analyzed my handwriting and palpated my arms and legs. Later, he took me to a detached room, reserved for men only, and asked me to carry firewood, which I did three times. This was to see my movements and complete the diagnosis. He figured out that I was of the lesser yin type and prescribed medication that cured me." This type of diagnostic method was common with Lee Je-ma.

Je-ma was a philosopher as well as a doctor, writing several books, including the 『Cheonyucho』 (闡幽抄: "Writings of Elucidations"), 『Jejung Sinpyeon』 (濟衆新編: "New Compilation for Relieving People"), 『Gwangjeseol』 (廣濟說: "Discourse on General Health Maintenance"), 『Gyeok-chigo』 (格致藁: "Draft on an Inquiry into the Properties of Things") and 『Dongui Suse Bowon』 (東醫壽世保元). The 『Cheonyucho』 was only two or three pages long, but its denotation is so profound that it is difficult to comprehend the contents. The purpose of these works was to provide lessons to his disciples he did not intend them to be handed down to posterity.

The 『Gwangjeseol』 teaches about the care of the health and states: "Therefore, being jealous of the wise and able is the most prevalent disease in the world. Respecting the wise and practicing virtue is the greatest medicine in the world. "In order for us to live a long and healthy life, we should distinguish right from wrong and be ethical in all our actions. The 『Gwangjeseol』 was added while the 『Dongui Suse Bowon』 was in the process of being edited. The 『Jejung Sinpyeon』 was written on ethics and attached to the 「*Gyeokchigo*」 as an appendix.

Je-ma began writing the 「*Gyeokchigo*」 at the age of forty four. It took him thirteen years to complete the book. It progressed intermittently, showing us the development of his thoughts. The ideas of this book are a completion of Confucianism and, at the same time, helped open up a new path for Joseon philosophy.

While Je-ma was writing the 「*Jejung Sinpyeon*」, he passed the special military service examination and was appointed head of the Jinhae District (鎭海縣). He was fifty years old at the time and interested in medical research. He completed the 「*Gyeokchigo*」 seven years later in 1893, and began work on the 「*Dongui Suse Bowon*」. This book is a continuation of the 「*Gyeokchigo*」's philosophy, and is an achievement of Joseon Confucianism. It opened up new academic possibilities during the Joseon dynasty.

Neither in the East nor in the West did most of the medical world recognize the specific characteristics of an individual's constitution, as human beings and specific diseases were all considered to have the same nature. This thinking has been an obstacle in preventing effective treatment, and also had led to less than desirable results. The internal organs are different because of the individual's constitution if recovery from disease depends on the patient's reaction to the medicine, then prevention, treatment principles and prescriptions ought to be different for each different type. In the 「*Dongui Suse Bowon*」, Je-ma classified the constitutional types of human beings into greater yang type, lesser yang type, greater yin type and lesser yin type, thus introducing SCM as a new accomplishment presenting constitutional physiology, pathology and its treatment.

After he finished writing the 「*Dongui Suse Bowon*」, Je-ma returned to his hometown. He quelled a rebellion, which occurred in Gangwon Province (江原道), and was appointed to be the acting provincial governor of Hamheung for his meritorious deed. He retired from his government position at the age of 62 in 1898. Later, he opened a private clinic, named Bowon-guk (保元局: Clinic for Life Preservation) in the city of Hamheung.

Je-ma again devoted himself to medical research and revised the 「*Dongui Suse Bowon*」. He revised the discourses from the 'Origin of Eastern Medicine' to the 'Lesser Yin Person's Disease', although the discourse on the 'Greater Yang Person's Disease' was never touched and has remained in its original form.

In Je-ma's later years, he offered treatment to the poor. When he was recompensed, he only accepted a small amount of hulled millet. He did not want to exchange money for treatment, and was not preoccupied with worldly gain. His second son, Yong-su (龍水), took over Je-ma's clinic after he died.

One day, Je-ma went to his hometown with his disciples to choose his own grave. He selected a place, which looked wonderful. However, when the disciples took a good look, they saw that, in *fengshui* (風水) terms, there was a white tiger on the right side, but no blue dragon on the left. The disciples pointed this out to him. Then Je-ma responded, "It is only temporary the water dragon will come by and by", and decided on that place. The disciples were doubtful as to the auspiciousness of this location, but in the year he died, a reservoir was built, creating the missing water dragon. The disciples were astonished at his foresight.

Lee Je-ma died at the age of 64 in 1900. He left a will that states as follows: "One hundred years after I die, Sasang Constitutional Medicine will be in the spotlight around the world."

Chronological Table of Lee Je-ma's Life

Age	Year	Historical Events	Personal History	Academic Works	Medical Works
1	1837		Born in Hamheung City (Mar.9)		
7	1843		Began to study under his uncle		
13	1849		Took first place in regional exam., left home		
14 - 29	1850- 1865		Details of his where-abouts are unknown		
30	1866	The invasion of Kangwha Island by a French Fleet		Read 『Myeongseonlok』	
39	1875				Administered Liuwei Dihuang Tang to a *mangyin* patient
44	1880			Began to write 『Gyeokchigo』	
46	1882	The Military Revolt			
50	1886		Passed the special military exam., appointed in charge of the Jinhae District and its army		
57	1893			Finished writing 『Gyeokchigo』	Began to write 『Dongui Suse Bowon』 (Jul.13)
58	1894	Donghak Revolution			Finished writing 『Dongui Suse Bowon』 (Apr.13)
59	1895		Returned to his hometown	Began to write 『Jejung Sinpyeon』 (Nov. 24)	
60	1896	Choi Moon-hwan's Revolution	Supressed Choi-Moon-hwan's Revolution and appointed in charge of Gowon County		
61	1897	Korean Empire began		Finished writing 『Jejung Sinpyeon』	
62	1898		Resigned from public life and opened his private clinic		Administered Jingfang Dihuang Tang to a *mangyin* patient. Revised and modified 『Dongui Suse Bowon』
64	1900	Opening of the Kyungin Railway	Died (Sep.21)		

CONTENTS

"When the Taoism meets the Confucianism in Medicine"
Translator's Note
Acknowledgements

Introduction
Life Story of Lee Je-ma

PART I

PART II

PART III

PART IV

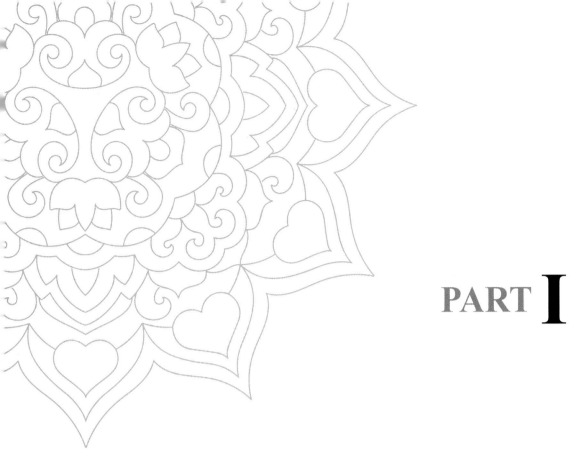

PART I

Constitutional Medicine in the East

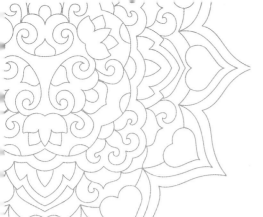

01

Discourse
on Nature and Order

性命論

1 There are four environmental frames: locality, human relationships, social relationships, and times of heaven.

天機有四一曰地方二曰人倫三曰世會四曰天時

2 There are four human affairs: living quarters, clanships, social acquaintances and appointed roles.

人事有四一曰居處二曰黨與三曰交遇四曰事務

3 The ears are capable of hearing times of heaven. The eyes are capable of seeing social relationships. The nose is capable of smelling human relationships. The mouth is capable of tasting locality.

耳聽天時目視世會鼻嗅人倫口味地方

4 Times of heaven are extremely variable. Social relationships are extremely extensive. Human relationships are extremely wide. Locality is extremely diverse.

天時極蕩也世會極大也人倫極廣也地方極邈也

5 The Lung executes appointed roles well. The Spleen harmonizes social acquaintances. The Liver establishes clanships. The Kidney determines living quarters.

肺達事務脾合交遇肝立黨與腎定居處

6 Appointed roles should be well developed. Social acquaintances should be well arranged. Clanships should be well organized. Living quarters should be well managed.

事務克修也交遇克成也黨與克整也居處克治也

7 There is cleverness in the jaw. There is administration in the chest. There is moderation in the navel. There is generosity in the abdomen.

頷有籌策臆有經綸臍有行檢腹有度量

8 Cleverness should not be arrogant. Administration should not be overconfident. Moderation should not be too domineering. Generosity should not be excessive.

籌策不可驕也經綸不可矜也行檢不可伐也度量不可夸也

9 There is discernment in the head. There is nobility in the shoulders. There is resourcefulness in the waist. There is method in the hips.

頭有識見肩有威儀腰有材幹臀有方略

10 Discernment should not be deprived. Nobility should not be extravagant. Resourcefulness should not be idle. Method should not include pilfering.

識見必無奪也威儀必無侈也材幹必無懶也方畧必無竊也

11 The ears, eyes, nose and mouth perceive the environment. The Lung, Spleen, Liver and Kidney are established among human affairs. The jaw, chest, navel and abdomen actualize wisdom. The head, shoulders, waist and hips add conduct to action.

耳目鼻口觀於天也肺脾肝腎立於人也頷臆臍腹行其知也頭肩腰臀行其行也

Environmental frames (Sensory Organ)	Times of heaven	Social relationships	Human relationships	Locality
	Ears	Eyes	Nose	Mouth
Human affairs (Organ)	Appointed roles	Social acquaintances	Clanships	Living quarters
	Lung	Spleen	Liver	Kidney
Wisdom (Body)	Cleverness	Administration	Moderation	Generosity
	Jaw	Chest	Navel	Abdomen
Action (Body)	Discernment	Nobility	Resourcefulness	Method
	Head	Shoulders	Waist	Hips

12 Times of heaven are universal. Appointed roles are established individually. Social relationships are universal. Social acquaintances are established individually. Human relationships are universal. Clanships are established individually. Localities are universal. Living quarters are established individually.

天時大同也事務各立也世會大同也交遇各立也人倫大同也黨與各立也地方大同也居處各立也

13 Cleverness is universally accepted. Discernment is undertaken individually. Administration is universally accepted. Nobility is undertaken individually. Moderation is universally accepted. Resourcefulness is expressed individually. Generosity is universally accepted. Method is carried out individually.

籌策博通也識見獨行也經綸博通也威儀獨行也行檢博通也材幹獨行也度量博通也方略獨行也

14 The universally renowned is heaven. The individually established is human. The generally accepted is nature. The individually generated is order.

大同者天也各立者人也博通者性也獨行者命也

15 The ears are fond of pleasant sounds. The eyes are fond of beautiful colors. The nose is fond of sweet smells. The mouth is fond of good tastes.

耳好善聲目好善色鼻好善臭口好善味

16 Pleasant sounds please the ears. Beautiful colors please the eyes. Sweet smells please the nose. Good tastes please the mouth.

善聲順耳也善色順目也善臭順鼻也善味順口也

17 The Lung dislikes unpleasant sounds. The Spleen dislikes ugly colors. The Liver dislikes unpleasant odors. The Kidney dislikes bad-tasting foods.

肺惡惡聲脾惡惡色肝惡惡臭腎惡惡味

18 Unpleasant sounds displease the Lung. Ugly colors displease the Spleen. Unpleasant odors displease the Liver. Bad tastes displease the Kidney.

惡聲逆肺也惡色逆脾也惡臭逆肝也惡味逆腎也

19 There can be an arrogant mind in the jaw. There can be an overconfident mind in the chest. There can be a domineering mind in the navel. There can be a boastful mind in the abdomen.

頷有驕心臆有矜心臍有伐心腹有夸心

20 The arrogant mind is arrogant intention. The overconfident mind is confident thinking. The domineering mind is domineering resolution. The boastful mind is boastful will.

驕心驕意也矜心矜慮也伐心伐操也夸心夸志也

21 There is covetousness in the head. There is extravagance in the shoulders. There is idleness in the waist. There is greed in the hips.

頭有擅心肩有侈心腰有懶心臀有欲心

22 Covetousness has a tendency to deprive others of their share. Extravagance is prone to self-glorification. Idleness is inclined towards self-loathing. Greed is disposed to steal.

擅心奪利也侈心自尊也懶心自卑也欲心竊物也

23 There is nothing comparable to the fondness that human ears, eyes, nose and mouth have for the good, and the dislike that the Lung, Spleen, Liver and Kidney have for the bad. There is nothing comparable to the wickedness of the human jaw, chest, navel and abdomen, and the idleness of the human head, shoulders, waist and hips.

人之耳目鼻口好善無雙也人之肺脾肝腎惡惡無雙也人之頷臆臍腹邪心無雙也人之頭肩腰臀怠心無雙也

24 King Yao[1] and King Shun[2] reigned with perfect virtue 5,000 years ago, and to this day, people mention their names when it comes to virtue. This demonstrates that there is nothing comparable to the people's love for virtue. King Chieh[3] and King Chou[4] governed with tyranny 4,000 years ago, and everyone mentions their names when it comes to vice. This demonstrates that there is nothing comparable to the people's hatred for vice. Three thousand disciples studied under Confucius[5], but only Yen Hui did not stray from perfect virtue for three months. Among the rest, only 72 disciples did the same for only a few days to a month, but no longer were their hearts filled with joy in following Confucius. This demonstrates that there is nothing comparable to the people's wickedness. There was a king, Wen[6], to whom all virtue belonged, the virtue which prevailed for a hundred years. King Wu[7] and the Duke of Zhou succeeded Wen's achievements until virtue widely prevailed. Nevertheless, Kwan Shu and Chai Shu promoted a rebellion against their brother, the Duke of Zhou, so this demonstrates that there is nothing comparable to the people's idleness.

堯舜之行仁在於五千年前而至于今天下之稱善者皆曰堯舜則人之好善果無雙也桀紂之行暴在於四千年前而至于今天下之稱惡者皆曰桀紂則人之惡惡果無雙也以孔子之聖三千之徒受敎而惟顏子三月不違仁其餘日月至焉而心悅誠服者只有七十二人則人之邪心果無雙也以文王之德百年而後崩未洽於天下武王周公繼之然後大行而管叔蔡叔猶以至親作亂則人之怠行果無雙也

25 Therefore, through the ears, eyes, nose and mouth, everyone can become like King Yao and King Shun; but through the jaw, chest, navel and abdomen, not everyone can spontaneously become like Yao and Shun. Through the Lung, Spleen, Liver and Kidney, everyone can become Yao and Shun; but through the head, shoulders, waist and hips, not everyone can spontaneously be Yao and Shun.

耳目鼻口人皆可以爲堯舜頷臆臍腹人皆自不爲堯舜肺脾肝腎人皆可以爲堯舜頭肩腰臀人皆自不爲堯舜

26 When people's ears, eyes, nose and mouth love goodness, their minds are not inferior to Yao's and Shun's mind. When people's Lung, Spleen, Liver and Kidney detest vice, their minds are not inferior to Yao's and Shun's. So it follows that everyone can become like Yao and Shun. In the jaw, chest, waist and abdomen, frequently the tendencies to deceive others are hidden. They cannot become as wise as Yao and Shun, unless they preserve their minds and nourish their natures. In the head, shoulders, waist and hips, occasionally the tendencies to deceive others are covered in darkness. They cannot become like Yao and Shun, unless they cultivate their personal characters and establish their orders. The above-mentioned explain why not everyone can spontaneously become like Yao and Shun.

人之耳目鼻口好善之心以衆人耳目鼻口論之而堯舜未爲加一鞭也人之肺脾肝腎惡惡之心以堯舜肺脾肝腎論之而衆人未爲少一鞭也人皆可以爲堯舜者以此人之頷臆臍腹之中誣世之心每每隱伏也存其心養其性然後人皆可以爲堯舜之知也人之頭肩腰臀之下罔民之心種種暗藏也修其身立其命然後人皆可以爲堯舜之行也人皆自不爲堯舜者以此

27 The people on the street all agree upon righteousness, so the sentiment of ears, eyes, nose and mouth loves benevolence. Therefore, it is very natural and fair. Being fair means being unselfish. Even though people are together in the same room, they still stay selfish and only think about their own benefit, so the sentiment of the Lung, Spleen, Liver and Kidney detests evil. It is extremely unselfish. Unselfishness means extreme fairness. There is wisdom, ceaseless and like polished ivory, in the jaw, chest, navel and abdomen. If arrogance, overconfidence and a domineering or boastful mind suddenly appear, wisdom will spontaneously disappear and cannot be generally accepted. There is ceaseless glowing conduct in the head, shoulders, waist and hips; but if a covetous mind, extravagance, idleness or greed suddenly appear, consequently, conduct will be resigned and unable to act righteously.

耳目鼻口之情行路之人大同於協義故好善也好善之實極公也極公則亦極無私也肺脾肝腎之情同室之人各立於擅利故惡惡也惡惡之實極無私也極無私則亦極公也頷臆臍腹之中自有不息之知如切如磋而驕矜伐夸之私心卒然敗之則自棄其知而不能博通也頭肩腰臀之下自有不息之行赫兮咺兮而奪侈懶竊之慾心卒然陷之則自棄其行而不能正行也

28 All people's ears, eyes, nose, and mouth are extremely clever, while their jaw, chest, navel and abdomen are stupid. All people's Lung, Spleen, Liver and Kidney are wise, while their head, shoulders, waist and hips are unwise.

耳目鼻口人皆知也頷臆臍腹人皆愚也肺脾肝腎人皆賢也頭肩腰臀人皆不肖也

29 The ears, eyes, noses and mouths of human beings are connected to heaven, and heaven is perceptive. The Lung, Spleen, Liver and Kidney of human beings are related to man, and man is reflective. Our jaws, chests, navels and abdomens constitute our minds, but they are not free from stupidity. Being free from stupidity depends upon us. Our head, shoulders, waist and hips constitute our body, but they are not free from a lack of wisdom. Having wisdom depends upon us.

人之耳目鼻口天也天知也人之肺脾肝腎人也人賢也我之頷臆臍腹我自爲心而未免愚也我之免愚在我也我之頭肩腰臀我自爲身而未免不肖也我之免不肖在我也

30 Heaven created human beings and bestowed on to us good sense as a part of our nature. Good sense is necessary in order to live. Without it, one may die. Virtue originates from good sense.

天生萬民性以慧覺萬民之生也有慧覺則生無慧覺則死慧覺者德之所由生也

31 Heaven created human beings and bestowed on to us the means of livelihood that originates from heaven's order. The means of livelihood are necessary in order to live. Without it, one may die. The Tao originates from the means of livelihood.

天生萬民命以資業萬民之生也有資業則生無資業則死資業者道之所由生也

32 Every virtue - benevolence, righteousness, propriety, wisdom, loyalty, filial piety, friendship and fraternal love - originates from good sense. Every function - the scholar, the farmer, the craftsman, the merchant, fields, houses, countries and states - originates from the means of livelihood.

仁義禮智忠孝友悌諸般百善皆出於慧覺士農工商田宅邦國諸般百用皆出於資業

33 If one's good sense is used for service, then one can teach others. If one's means of livelihood is honest, one can receive merit. Despite an excellent nature, if one's good sense is selfish and trivial, and one is cunning like Cao Cao[8], one cannot teach others. Though a man is heroic, if his lifestyle is selfishly willful, and he is violent and ill-tempered like the first Emperor of Chin[9], he can receive no merit.

慧覺欲其兼人而有敎也資業欲其廉己而有功也慧覺私小者雖有其傑巧如曹操而不可爲敎也資業橫濫者雖有其雄猛如秦千而不可爲功也

34 If one appreciates the virtues of others and at the same time practices virtue, this is the ultimate nature of virtue. If one hates the vices of others and at the same time never has any vices himself, then this is the way of right order. If knowledge and deeds are accumulated, then this is the way and the virtuous. If the way and the virtuous are performed, this is the state of benevolence and sacredness. The way and the virtuous are just as good as the knowledge and the deeds, and the nature and the order are also just as good as the knowledge and the deeds.

好人之善而我亦知善者至性之德也惡人之惡而我必不行惡者正命之道也知行積則道德也道德成則仁聖也道德非他知行也性命非他知行也

35 Someone asked, "If it is possible to discourse on nature by referring to knowledge, then what is the meaning of the discourse on order by referring to deeds? " Order is a kind of destiny. If someone does good deeds, then his destiny will surely be glorious; but if he does bad deeds, his destiny will be surely ruined. We can understand this situation without divination. This has the same meaning as the verse "Always be studious in order to be in harmony with the ordinances of Heaven, and you will obtain much happiness," in the 『Shijing』10) ("Classic of Poetry").

或曰舉知而論性可也而舉行而論命何義耶曰命者命數也善行則命數自美也惡行則命數自惡也不待卜筮而可知也詩云永言配命自求多福卽此義也

36 Someone asked, "You said that the ears are capable of hearing times of heaven, the eyes are capable of seeing social relationships, the nose is capable of smelling human relationships, and the mouth is capable of tasting localities. That the ears are capable of hearing times of heaven, and the eyes are capable of seeing social relationships is acceptable, but how is it possible that the nose is capable of smelling human relationships, and the mouth is capable of tasting localities?" "Participating in human relationships - observing the outer appearances of others and trying to evaluate whether each individual's ability and conduct are wise or not - is what is meant by smelling. Living in a certain place - broadly experiencing the interests of human life - is what is meant by tasting."

或曰吾子之言曰耳聽天時目視世會鼻嗅人倫口味地方耳之聽天時目之視世會則可也而鼻何以嗅人倫口何以味地方乎曰處於人倫察人外表黙探各人才行之賢不肖者此非嗅耶處於地方均嘗各處人民生活之地利者此非味耶

37 To preserve one's mind, one must rebuke one's mind. It may seem that the mind is naturally clear. Actually, however, one must rebuke one's mind to make it clear; if not, the mind will be cloudy. The awakening mind of a horse is far quicker than that of a cow, because the mind of a horse is more self-rebuking and thus quicker than that of a cow. The mental vitality of the hawk is braver than that of the kite, because the self-rebuking mind of a hawk is far braver than that of the kite. From the above-mentioned, we can understand the clarity of mind and strength of mental vitality of animals. The same may be said of human beings. In human beings, the degrees of differences among individuals range from two to ten thousand fold. Then how can we say that the highest capacity is attainable without any efforts?

存其心者責其心也心體之明暗雖若自然而責之者清不責者濁馬之心覺黠於牛者馬之責心黠於牛也鷹之氣勢猛於鴟者鷹之責氣猛於鴟也心體之清濁氣宇之强弱在於牛馬鴟鷹者以理推之而猶然況於人乎或相倍蓰或相千萬者豈其生而輒得茫然不思居然自至而然哉

Notes

1) King Yao (堯)

Formally, in Chinese mythology, a legendary emperor of the golden age (c. 24th century B.C.) of antiquity, exalted by Confucius as an inspiration and perennial model of virtue and righteousness, and always mentioned with King Shun (舜王), his successor, to whom Yao gave his two daughters in marriage. Legends recount that after 70 years of Yao's rule, the sun and moon were as resplendent as jewels, the five planets shone like strung pearls, phoenixes nested in the palace courtyards, crystal springs flowed from the hills, pearl grass covered the countryside, rice crops were plentiful, two unicorns (omens of prosperity) appeared in the capital at Pingyang (平陽), and the wondrous calendar bean made its appearance, producing a pod a day for half a month before the 15 pods withered one by one on successive days. Two remarkable events marked Yao's reign: a rampaging flood was controlled by Da Yu (大禹); and Hou I (后羿), the Lord Archer, saved the world from destruction by shooting down nine of the ten suns burning up the earth. Like Fuhsi (伏犧), Shennong (神農), and Huangdi (黃帝) before him, Yao had special temples dedicated in his honor. He is said to have offered sacrifices and to have practiced divination. In choosing a successor, Yao bypassed his own less worthy son in favors of Shun and served as counselor to the new emperor.

2) King Shun (舜)

In Chinese mythology, a legendary emperor (c. 23rd century B.C.) of the golden age of antiquity, singled out by Confucius as a model of integrity and resplendent virtue. His name is invariably associated with that of Yao, his legendary predecessor. Though Shun's father repeatedly tried to murder him, the boy's filial piety never faltered. Because Heaven and Earth knew of his virtue, birds came to assist in weeding his paddies, and animals appeared from nowhere to drag the plow. Yao bypassed his own son in choosing Shun as the most worthy to rule. He likewise gave Shun his two daughters, Ohuang (娥皇) and Nuying (女英), in marriage. Shun offered sacrifice to the Six Honored Ones (whose identity is uncertain) and the springs of earth. He is credited with standardizing weights and measures, regulating waterways, and organizing the kingdom into 12 provinces. During his reign, marvelous phenomena occurred in the heavens and on earth.

3) King Chieh (桀)

The last king of the legendary Xia (夏) dynasty in ancient China. He is a typical despot who forms a striking contrast to King Yao and King Shun. The state of the Xia dynasty under his rule had already been so weakened that many feudal lords broke their relations with him. He was killed while trying to escape. The stories and dates attributed to him are unreliable, since they vary considerably in the Chinese and Western sources.

4) King Chou (紂)

Also called Ti Hsin (帝辛), last sovereign of the Shang (商), or Yin (殷) dynasty, who according to legend lost his empire because of his extreme debauchery. To please his concubine, Tachi (妲己), it is said that he built a lake of wine around which naked men and women were forced to chase one another. His cruelty was such that the nearby forests were littered with corpses. Moreover, he provoked the resentment of the people by levying taxes to build, over the course of seven years, the elaborate Deer Tower Palace (鹿臺). It was supposed to have been 600 feet high and a half mile in circumference, with doors and chambers constructed of precious stones. When King Wu, the founder of the succeeding Zhou (周) dynasty (1111 - 255 B.C.), overthrew the Shang, Chou set fire to his palace and committed suicide by leaping into the flames.

5) Confucius (孔子)

Original name Kung Chiu (孔丘), China's most famous teacher, philosopher, and political theorist whose ideas have influenced the civilizations of eastern Asia. A brief account of the life and works of Confucius follows. Although little reliable information exists on Confucius' ancestry and early life, his family was probably of the impoverished nobility. He was orphaned at an early age and grew up poor. He was largely self-educated, but apparently became the most learned man of his day. Learning, however, was not his greatest interest. Confucius was deeply disturbed by the political and social conditions of his times. Unable to obtain an official position in which he might affect his ideas of reform, he spent the greater part of his life educating a small group of disciples. Confucius was not a religious leader in the ordinary sense, for his teachings were essentially social ethics. Though his interest in books was secondary to his passion for reform, many ancient classics were attributed to his authorship and editorship. These books, interpreted in Confucian terms, were the basic curriculum of Chinese education for more than 2,000 years, and explain why Confucius must be counted among the most influential men of all time.

6) King Wen (文)

Father of King Wu, the founder of the Zhou dynasty and one of the sage rulers regarded by Confucian historians as a model king. Wen was a ruler of Zhou, one of the semi-barbaric states on the western frontier of China, a long-time battleground between the civilized Chinese and nomadic invaders. By 1144 B.C., he had begun to threaten the Shang dynasty and was captured and imprisoned by King Chou, the last Shang ruler. After King Wen returned to Chou, he spent the rest of his life remonstrating against the cruelty and corruption of his age. Upon his death, his son and successor, King Wu (武), destroyed the Shang and founded the Zhou dynasty.

7) King Wu (武)

The founder and the first ruler of the Zhou dynasty. Wu was respected by later Confucians as a wise king. He succeeded his father, the famous King Wen, as head of the semi-barbaric state of Zhou, located on the western border of China. Wu continued his father's work and formed a coalition with eight other border states, which defeated the last other evil border states and also defeated the evil ruler of the Shang. After establishing the Zhou dynasty, Wu, assisted by his brother, known as the Duke of Zhou (周公), consolidated his rule by establishing a feudalistic form of government, which parceled out territory to relatives and vassals willing to acknowledge Zhou sovereignty.

8) Cao Cao (曹操)

One of the greatest generals at the end of the Han (漢) dynasty. He was the adopted son of the chief eunuch of the imperial court, and wielded much influence in the last years of the Han. Cao rose to prominence as a general when he suppressed the Yellow Turban (黃巾賊) Rebellion, which threatened the last years of Han rule. The dynasty, however, was greatly weakened by the rebellion, and in the ensuing chaos, the country was divided among the major generals into three parts. Cao occupied the strategic northern section around the emperor's capital prerogatives. Cao's large armies and his skillful maneuvering have long been notorious in Chinese history. He was described by Confucian historians and in popular legends as the archetypal shrewd, bold and unscrupulous villain. He was portrayed in this role in the great 14th century historical novel, 『*Sanguo Yanyi*』 (三國演義: "Story of the Three Kingdoms"), and since then he has been one of the most popular figures of Chinese legend and folklore, with various evil magic powers ascribed to him. Modern historians tend to view Cao as a skillful general and pragmatic politician. After Cao's death, his son Cao Pi (曹丕) usurped the Han throne and proclaimed the Wei (魏) dynasty.

9) Emperor of Chin (秦始皇)

Shih Huangdi (始皇帝), creator of the first unified Chinese empire (259~210 B.C.) and emperor of the Chin (秦) dynasty. He was born while his father was being held hostage in the state of Chao (趙). His mother was a former concubine of the rich merchant Lu Puwei (呂不韋). By 221 B.C., with the help of espionage, extensive bribery, and the ruthlessly effective leadership of gifted generals, he had marked his final triumph: For the first time, China was united, under the supreme rule of the Chin. With unbounded confidence, he claimed that his dynasty would last "10,000 generations." However, it collapsed only four years after his death. It seems certain that Shih Huangdi had an imposing personality and showed an unbending will in pursuing his aim of uniting and strengthening the empire. His despotic rule and the draconian punishments he meted out were dictated largely by his legalistic (法家) ideas. With few exceptions, the traditional historiography of Imperial China has regarded Shih Huangdi as the villain par excellence, in human, uncultivated, and superstitious.

10) 『*Shijing*』(詩經)

"Classics of Poetry", the first anthology of Chinese poetry. It was compiled by the ancient sage Confucius (551~479 B.C.) and cited by him as a model of literary expression; for despite its numerous themes, the subject matter was always "expressive of pleasure without being licentious and of grief without being hurtfully expressive." The book, one of the Five Classics (五經), contains 305 poems (and six poem titles) classified either as popular songs or ballads, courtly songs, or eulogies.

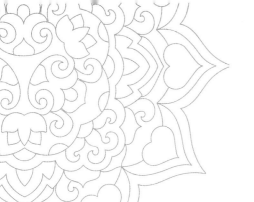

02

Discourse
on the Four Principles

四端論

1   There are four types of human beings based upon the congenital formation of the organs. Those who have a large Lung and a small Liver are greater yang persons. Those who have a large Liver and a small Lung are greater yin persons. Those who have a large Spleen and a small Kidney are lesser yang persons. Those who have a large Kidney and a small Spleen are lesser yin persons.

人禀臟理有四不同肺大而肝小者名曰太陽人肝大而肺小者名曰太陰人脾大而腎小者名曰少陽人腎大而脾小者名曰少陰人

2   There are four kinds of inclinations in the human mind. Those who neglect propriety and who are self-indulgent are called the mean. Those who neglect righteousness and who are idle are called the weak. Those who neglect wisdom and who use flattery are called the sycophantic. Those who neglect benevolence and who are very greedy are called the avaricious.

人趨心慾有四不同棄禮而放縱者名曰鄙人棄義而偸逸者名曰懦人棄智而飾私者名曰薄人棄仁而極慾者名曰貪人

3   Among the five organs, the Heart is the Taichi, the Great Absolute, located in the center. Among the five organs, the Lung, the Spleen, the Liver and the Kidney are the four symbols related to the four corners. The Great Absolute in the center, the Heart, of the sage is higher than that of the ordinary people. The four symbols related to the four corners of the sage are similar to those of the ordinary people.

五臟之心中央之太極也五臟之肺脾肝腎四維之四象也中央之太極聖人之太極高出於衆人之太極也四維之四象聖人之四象旁通於衆人之四象也

4 There are four different categories based upon the formation of the organs, but there is one thing that is common to all, the transformation according to the principles of nature. The sage and the ordinary people are the same. There are four different classes of the mind, and in each class, there are 10,000 different levels, because of the varieties of selfish desires. For this reason, the sage and the ordinary people are different in 10,000 ways.

太少陰陽之臟局短長四不同中有一大同天理之變化也聖人與衆人一同也鄙薄貪懦之心地清濁四不同中有萬不同人欲之濶狹也聖人與衆人萬殊也

5 The changes of yin and yang are based on one principle and have four different aspects. This is the reason why the sage admires heaven. The degree of chasteness and generosity, among the four inclinations of the mind - the mean, the weak, the sycophantic and the avaricious - varies in 10,000 ways. Among this variety, there is one thing in common. This is the reason why the ordinary people admires the sage.

太少陰陽之短長變化一同之中有四偏聖人所以希天也鄙薄貪懦之清濁濶狹萬殊之中有一同衆人所以希聖也

6 There are four types of organ formation in the sage, and there are four types of organ formation in ordinary people, too. When one sage dwells among 10,000 ordinary people, the ordinary people are delighted by his presence. The sage is not avaricious, but the ordinary people are avaricious. When one sage dwells among 10,000 ordinary people, the sage is concerned about the ordinary people.

聖人之臟四端也衆人之臟亦四端也以聖人之一四端之臟處於衆人萬四端之中聖人者衆人之所樂也聖人之心無慾也衆人之心有慾也以聖人一無慾之心處於衆人萬有慾之中衆人者聖人之所憂也

7 The organs of the ordinary people are the same as those of the sage. Their abilities are the same as that of the sage. Since ordinary people have the same Lung, Spleen, Liver and Kidney ability as that of the sage, claiming that they have no ability is the fault not of the ability, but of the Heart.

然則天下衆人之臟理亦皆聖人之臟理而才能亦皆聖人之才能也以肺脾肝腎聖人之才能而自言曰我無才能云者豈才能之罪哉心之罪也

8 The vast flowing qi issues forth from the Lung, the Spleen, the Liver and the Kidney. The vast flowing principle issues forth from the Heart. When the qi of the four organs, which are benevolence, righteousness, propriety and wisdom, is amplified, the vast flowing qi issues forth from those four organs. When the desires of the four types of people, which are the mean, the weak, the sycophantic and the avaricious, are identified, the vast flowing principle issues forth from the Heart.

浩然之氣出於肺脾肝腎也浩然之理出於心也仁義禮智四臟之氣擴而充之則浩然之氣出於此也鄙薄貪懦一心之慾明而辨之則浩然之理出於此也

9　They say that the sage has no desire, but having no desire is not the same as the nothingness of Taoism or the nirvana of Buddhism. This means that the sage is so deeply concerned that the world is not well ordered, that he has no desire about himself, and that, moreover, he has no time to think about it. That the sage is deeply concerned that the world is not ordered, and thus has no time to think about his own desires, certainly means that he learns without satiety, and teaches without being tired. Learning without satiety and teaching without being tired is nothing less than the unselfishness of the sage. If there was even a little desire, it is not the mind of Yao and Shun. If there was no concern even momentarily for the world, it is not the mind of Confucius and Mencius[1).

聖人之心無慾云者非淸淨寂滅如老佛之無慾也聖人之心深憂天下之不治故非但無慾也亦未暇及於一己之慾也深憂天下之不治而未暇及於一己之慾者必學不厭而敎不倦也學不厭而敎不倦者卽聖人之無慾也毫有一己之慾則非堯舜之心也暫無天下之憂則非孔孟之心也

10　For the greater yang person, the nature of his sorrow is distantly dispersed, and the emotion of his anger is quick. Since his sorrow is distantly dispersed, the qi flows into the Lung, and the Lung qi becomes excessive. Since his anger is quick, the qi stimulates the Liver, and the Liver qi becomes depleted. This is why the greater yang's organ formation is "a large Lung and a small Liver." For the lesser yang person, the nature of his anger is widely encompassing, and the emotion of his sorrow is quick. Since his anger is widely encompassing, the qi flows into the Spleen, and the Spleen qi becomes excessive. Since his sorrow is quick, the qi stimulates the Kidney, and the Kidney qi becomes depleted. This is why the lesser yang's organ formation is "a large Spleen and a small Kidney." For the greater yin person, the nature of his joy is broadly extended, and the emotion of his pleasure is quick. Since his joy is broadly extended, the qi flows into the Liver, and the Liver qi becomes excessive. Since his pleasure is quick, the qi stimulates the Lung, and the Lung qi becomes depleted. This is why the greater yin's organ formation is "a large Liver and a small Lung." For the lesser yin person, the nature of his pleasure is firm in depth, and the emotion of his joy is quick. Since his pleasure is firm in depth, the qi flows into the Kidney, and the Kidney qi becomes excessive. Since his joy is quick, the qi stimulates the Spleen, and the Spleen qi becomes depleted. This is why the lesser yin's organ formation is "a large Kidney and a small Spleen."

太陽人哀性遠散而怒情促急哀性遠散則氣注肺而肺益盛怒情促急則氣激肝而肝益削太陽之臟局所以成形於肺大肝小也少陽人怒性宏抱而哀情促急怒性宏抱則氣注脾而脾益盛哀情促急則氣激腎而腎益削少陽之臟局所以成形於脾大腎小也太陰人喜性廣張而樂情促急喜性廣張則氣注肝而肝益盛樂情促急則氣激肺而肺益削太陰之臟局所以成形於肝大肺小也少陰人樂性深確而喜情促急樂性深確則氣注腎而腎益盛喜情促急則氣激脾而脾益削少陰之臟局所以成形於腎大脾小也

Type	Greater Yang (Tai-yang)	Lesser Yang (So-yang)	Greater Yin (Tai-eum)	Lesser Yin (So-eum)
Congenital formation of their organs	a large Lung a small Liver	a large Spleen a small Kidney	a large Liver a small Lung	a large Kidney a small Spleen
Nature	Sorrow	Anger	Joy	Pleasure
Emotion	Anger	Sorrow	Pleasure	Joy

11 The Lung qi extends straight up. The Spleen qi embraces like the shell of the Castaneae Semen. The Liver qi is generous and relaxed. The Kidney qi slowly accumulates.
肺氣直而伸脾氣栗而包肝氣寬而緩腎氣溫而畜

12 Because the Lung exhales and the Liver inhales, the Liver and the Lung are the gates of respiration for air and fluids. Because the Spleen draws in and the Kidney sends out, the Kidney and the Spleen are the storerooms that control the drawing in and sending out of foodstuffs.
肺以呼肝以吸肝肺者呼吸氣液之門戶也脾以納腎以出腎脾者出納水穀之府庫也

13 Sorrow qi ascends straight up. Anger qi ascends obliquely. Joy qi descends obliquely. Pleasure qi drops straight down.
哀氣直升怒氣橫升喜氣放降樂氣陷降

		Lung	Spleen	Liver	Kidney
Qi		Extend straight up	Embrace like the shell of the chestnut	Generous and relaxed	Softly accumulated
		Ascend straight up	Ascend obliquely	Descend obliquely	Drop down
Nature		Distantly disperse	Widely encompassing	Broadly extend	Firm in depth
		Sorrow	Anger	Joy	Pleasure

14 Sorrow qi and anger qi ascend, and joy qi and pleasure qi descend. If ascending qi is excessive, the lower part of the body will be damaged. If descending qi is excessive, the upper part of the body will be damaged.
哀怒之氣上升喜樂之氣下降上升之氣過多則下焦傷下降之氣過多則上焦傷

15 If sorrow qi and anger qi move in an orderly way, they will ascend gently. If joy qi and pleasure qi move in an orderly way, they will descend in a relaxed way. Sorrow qi and anger qi are yang, and this is the reason why if they move smoothly, they will ascend gently. Joy qi and pleasure qi are yin, and this is the reason why if they move smoothly, they will descend gently.
哀怒之氣順動則發越而上騰喜樂之氣順動則緩安而下墜哀怒之氣陽也順動則順而上升喜樂之氣陰也順動則順而下降

16 If sorrow qi and anger qi move in a disorderly manner, they will ascend explosively and amass in the upper part of the body. If joy qi and pleasure qi move in a disorderly manner, they will descend violently and accumulate in the lower part of the body. When the ascending qi moves in a disorderly manner, accumulating in the upper part of the body, the Liver and Kidney will be damaged. When the descending qi moves in a disorderly manner, accumulating in the lower part of the body, the Spleen and Lung will be damaged.

哀怒之氣逆動則暴發而並於上也喜樂之氣逆動則浪發而並於下也上升之氣逆動而並於上則肝腎傷下降之氣逆動而並於下則脾肺傷

17 Due to frequent anger, the waist constricts frequently. The waist is the dwelling place of the Liver, therefore, if the waist becomes constricted irregularly, the Liver will be damaged. Due to sudden fluctuations of joy, the chest will expand and contract. The chest is the dwelling place of the Spleen, so that if the chest expands and contracts irregularly, the Spleen will be damaged. Due to sudden fluctuations of sorrow, the lumbar vertebrae will flex and straighten suddenly. The lumbar vertebrae are the dwelling place of the Kidney, so that if the lumbar vertebrae flex and straighten suddenly, the Kidney will be damaged. Due to repeated fluctuations of pleasure, the upper back will be pushed up and thrust down. The upper back is the dwelling place of the Lung, so that if the upper back is pushed up and thrust down irregularly, the Lung will be damaged.

頻起怒而頻伏怒則腰脇頻迫而頻蕩也腰脇者肝之所住着處也腰脇迫蕩不定則肝其不傷乎乍發喜而乍收喜則胸腋乍濶而乍狹也胸腋者脾之所住着處也胸腋濶狹不定則脾其不傷乎忽動哀而忽止哀則脊曲忽屈而忽伸也脊曲者腎之所住着處也脊曲屈伸不定則腎其不傷乎屢得樂而屢失樂則背䯒暴揚而暴抑也背䯒者肺之所住着處也背䯒抑揚不定則肺其不傷乎

18 The greater yang person is prone to explosive anger and deep sorrow, so he must be cautious about this. The lesser yang person is prone to sudden sorrow and deep anger, so he must be cautious about this. The greater yin person is prone to fluctuating pleasure and deep joy, so he must be cautious about this. The lesser yin person is prone to fluctuating joy and deep pleasure, so he must be cautious about this.

太陽人有暴怒深哀不可不戒少陽人有暴哀深怒不可不戒太陰人有浪樂深喜不可不戒少陰人有浪喜深樂不可不戒

19 Kao Yao said, "Everything lies in knowing others and allowing them to live peacefully." Yu[2] said, "This is so. Yet even King Yao felt this to be difficult. To know others is wisdom. One who knows others can properly award a government post to the right person. To allow people to live peacefully is merciful. People will follow and respect such a merciful leader. If the king is wise and merciful, why should he worry about Huan Dou, and the exile You Miao, or be afraid of the flattery of Kong Ren?"

皐陶曰都在知人在安民禹曰吁咸若時惟帝其難之知人則哲能官人安民則惠黎民懷之能哲而惠何憂乎驩兜何遷乎有苗何畏乎巧言令色孔壬

20 Repeating the above story of King Yu three times and saying admiringly, "Since knowing others is very difficult, King Yao controlled pleasure, anger, sorrow and joy, so that they acted in their due degree. Since he dared not disregard knowing others, King Yu controlled pleasure, anger, sorrow and joy, so that they acted in this due degree. The sudden fluctuation of pleasure, anger, sorrow, and joy in the world comes from insincere deeds and not knowing others well enough. Knowing others was difficult even for King Yao and King Yu lamented over this matter; so what person can easily be satisfied that he know others? One should reflect more on one's own sincerity and never make light of the selection of the right people."

三復大禹之訓而欽仰之曰帝堯之喜怒哀樂每每中節者以其難於知人也大禹之喜怒哀樂每每中節者以其不敢輕易於知人也天下喜怒哀樂之暴動浪動者都出於行身不誠而知人不明也知人帝堯之所難而大禹之所吁也則其誰沾沾自喜乎蓋亦益反其誠而必不可輕易取舍人也

21 Though one has a good and loving mind, if he expresses it in a disorderly way, his virtuous mind will not be clear. Though one has a hatred of the bad mind, if he does so in a disorderly way, his hatred of the bad will not be widely recognized. It is advisable that public affairs be engaged in by good men. If not, joy and pleasure will certainly be disturbed. It is not advisable that public affairs be engaged in by bad men. If so, sorrow and anger will increase.

雖好善之心偏急而好善則好善必不明也雖惡惡之心偏急而惡惡則惡惡必不周也天下事宜與好人做也不與好人做則喜樂必煩也天下事不宜與不好人做也與不好人做則哀怒益煩也

22 Sorrow and anger feed off each other, and joy and pleasure complement each other. If sorrow becomes extreme, anger will be generated. If anger becomes extreme, sorrow will be generated. If pleasure becomes extreme, joy will be generated. If joy becomes extreme, pleasure will be generated. If the greater yang person's sorrow cannot be controlled, in the end, anger will spring forth. If the lesser yang person's anger cannot be controlled, in the end, sorrow will stir deeply within. If the lesser yin person's pleasure cannot be controlled, in the end, joy becomes unstable. If the greater yin person's joy cannot be controlled, in the end, pleasure becomes unrestrained. Such stirring of the emotions is comparable to cutting one's intestines with a sharp knife. Once the emotions are seriously stirred, it may take more than 10 years to recover. This is the key to longevity, so we must be aware of this.

哀怒相成喜樂相資哀性極則怒情動怒性極則哀情動樂性極則喜情動喜性極則樂情動太陽人哀極不濟則忿怒激外少陽人怒極不勝則悲哀動中少陰人樂極不成則喜好不定太陰人喜極不服則侈樂無厭如此而動者無異於以刀割臟一次大動十年難復此死生壽夭之機關也不可不知也

23 The various formations of the four types are due to the changes of yin and yang. We need not mention those congenital formations. In addition, there are incomplete manifestations of the above formations. Such people's destiny is dependent upon their cultivation of human affairs, so we must be cautious.

太少陰陽之臟局短長陰陽之變化也天稟之已定固無可論天稟已定之外又有短長而不全其天稟者

則人事之修不修而命之傾也不可不慎也

24 Just one greater yang person's anger can trigger the anger of a thousand, or tens of thousands of other people; but if his anger cannot handle those people, he will certainly not be equal to the task of dealing with them. Just one lesser yin person's joy can trigger the joy of a thousand, or tens of thousands of other people; but if his joy cannot handle those people, he will certainly not be equal to the task of dealing with them. Just one lesser yang person's sorrow can trigger the sorrow of a thousand, or tens of thousands of other people; but if his sorrow cannot handle those people, he will certainly not be equal to the task of dealing with them. Just one greater yin person's pleasure can trigger the pleasure of a thousand, or tens of thousands of other people; but if his pleasure cannot handle those people, he will certainly not be equal to the task of dealing with them.

太陽人怒以一人之怒而怒千萬人其怒無術於千萬人則必難堪千萬人也少陰人喜以一人之喜而喜千萬人其喜無術於千萬人則必難堪千萬人也少陽人哀以一人之哀而哀千萬人其哀無術於千萬人則必難堪千萬人也太陰人樂以一人之樂而樂千萬人其樂無術於千萬人則必難堪千萬人也

25 The greater yang and lesser yang persons should always be cautious about having too much sorrow and anger; pretending to have joy and pleasure would be useless. If they try to pretend, their joy and pleasure will not be from the bottom of their hearts, and their sorrow and anger will become distorted. The greater yin and lesser yin persons should always be cautious about having too much joy and pleasure; pretending to have sorrow and anger would be useless. If they try to pretend, their sorrow and anger will not be from the bottom of their hearts, and their joy and pleasure will become distorted.

太陽少陽人但恒戒哀怒之過度而不可强做喜樂虛動不及也若强做喜樂而煩數之則喜樂不出於眞情而哀怒益偏也太陰少陰人但恒戒喜樂之過度而不可强做哀怒虛動不及也若强做哀怒而煩數之則哀怒不出於眞情而喜樂益偏也

26 When there are no stirrings of pleasure, anger, sorrow or joy, the mind may be said to be in a state of equilibrium. When those feelings have been stirred, and they act in their due degree, what ensues may be called the state of harmony. When there are no stirrings of pleasure, anger, sorrow or joy, and the mind is always cautious, isn't such a person gradually becoming closer to the state of equilibrium? When pleasure, anger, sorrow, or joy has already been stirred, and one reflects upon them, isn't such a person gradually becoming closer to the state of harmony?

喜怒哀樂之未發謂之中發而皆中節謂之和喜怒哀樂未發而恒戒者此非漸近於中者乎喜怒哀樂已發而自反者此非漸近於節者乎

Notes

1) Mencius (孟子)

(371~239 B.C., ancient state of Tsou (趨), China), early Chinese philosopher whose development of orthodox Confucianism earned him the title "The Second Sage (亞聖)." Chief among his basic tenets was an emphasis on the obligation of rulers to provide for the common people. Mencius' book, 『*Mengzi*』 (孟子) records his doings and sayings and contains statements on the innate goodness of human nature, a topic heatedly debated by Confucianists up to modern times. The philosophical ideas of Mencius might be regarded as an amplification of the teachings of Confucius. Confucius taught the concept of *Ren* (仁), love or humanity, as the basic virtue of mankind. Mencius made the original goodness of human nature the keynote to his system. While Mencius has always been regarded as a major philosopher, special importance was attributed to him and his work by the Neo-Confucianists of the Song dynasty (AD 960~1279). For the last 1,000 years, Mencius has been revered among the Chinese people as the co-founder of Confucianism, second only to Confucius himself.

2) King Yu (禹)

Yu the Great, in Chinese mythology, the Tamer of the Flood, one of China's savior-heroes and reputed founder of China's oldest dynasty, the Xia. King Yu, after years of strenuous labors, dredged outlets to the sea with the aid of dragons, thus making the world suitable for human habitation.

Discourse
on the Establishment and Supplement

擴充論

1 The greater yang person's sorrow is distantly dispersed, and his anger is quick. "Sorrow is distantly dispersed" means that the ears of the greater yang person perceive the times of heaven, and he feels sorrow that people deceive each other. Sorrow is nothing other than "listening." "Anger is quick" means that the Spleen of the greater yang person enters into social acquaintances, and he becomes angry when others disregard him. This anger is nothing other than becoming angry. The lesser yang person's anger is widely encompassing, and his sorrow is quick. "Anger is widely encompassing" means that the eyes of the lesser yang person can see social relationships, and he feels angry that people mutually disregard each other. Anger is nothing other than "observing." "Sorrow is quick" means that the Lung of the lesser yang person engages in appointed roles, and he becomes sorrowful when others deceive him. This sorrow is nothing other than becoming sorrowful. The greater yin person's joy is broadly extended, and his pleasure is quick. "Joy is broadly extended" means that the nose of the greater yin person perceives human relationships, and he feels joy that people help each other. Joy is nothing other than "smelling." "Pleasure is quick" means that the Kidney of the greater yin person engages in living quarters, and he feels pleasure when others protect him. This pleasure is nothing other than becoming pleased. The lesser yin person's pleasure is firm in depth, and his joy is quick. "Pleasure is firm in depth" means that the mouth of the lesser yin person perceives localities, and he feels pleasure when people protect each other. Pleasure is nothing other than "tasting." "Joy is quick" means that the Liver of the lesser yin person engages in clanships, and he becomes joyful when others help him. This joy is nothing other than becoming joyful.

太陽人哀性遠散而怒情促急哀性遠散者太陽之耳察於天時而哀衆人之相欺也哀性非他聽也怒情

促急者太陽之脾行於交遇而怒別人之侮己也怒情非他怒也少陽人怒性宏抱而哀情促急怒性宏抱者少陽之目察於世會而怒衆人之相侮也怒性非他視也哀情促急者少陽之肺行於事務而哀別人之欺己也哀情非他哀也太陰人喜性廣張而樂情促急喜性廣張者太陰之鼻察於人倫而喜衆人之相助也喜性非他嗅也樂情促急者太陰之腎行於居處而樂別人之保己也樂情非他樂也少陰人樂性深確而喜情促急樂性深確者少陰之口察於地方而樂衆人之相保也樂性非他味也喜情促急者少陰之肝行於黨與而喜別人之助己也喜情非他喜也

2　The ears of the greater yang person are able to extensively comprehend the times of heaven, but his nose is unable to extensively comprehend human relationships. The nose of the greater yin person is able to extensively comprehend human relationships, but his ears are unable to extensively comprehend the times of heaven. The eyes of the lesser yang person are able to extensively comprehend social relationships, but his mouth is unable to extensively comprehend localities. The mouth of the lesser yin person is able to extensively comprehend localities, but his eyes are unable to extensively comprehend social relationships.

太陽之耳能廣博於天時而太陽之鼻不能廣博於人倫太陰之鼻能廣博於人倫而太陰之耳不能廣博於天時少陽之目能廣博於世會而少陽之口不能廣博於地方少陰之口能廣博於地方而少陰之目不能廣博於世會

3　The Spleen of the greater yang person is well integrated with social acquaintance, but his Liver cannot get along with clanships. The Liver of the lesser yin person can get along with clanships, but his Spleen cannot be well integrated with social acquaintances. The Lung of the lesser yang person smartly handles appointed roles, but his Kidney cannot maintain constant stability within living quarters. The Kidney of the greater yin person can maintain constant stability within living quarters, but his Lung cannot smartly handle appointed roles.

太陽之脾能勇統於交遇而太陽之肝不能雅立於黨與少陰之肝能雅立於黨與而少陰之脾不能勇統於交遇少陽之肺能敏達於事務而少陽之腎不能恒定於居處太陰之腎能恒定於居處而太陰之肺不能敏達於事務

4　Since the listening of the greater yang person is able to extensively comprehend the times of heaven, his *shen* (mental vitality) is sufficient to fill the brain, and a large amount of it gathers in the Lung. Since the smelling of the greater yang person is unable to extensively comprehend human relationships, his blood is insufficient to fill the lumbar vertebrae, and a small amount of it gathers in the Liver. Since the smelling of the greater yin person is able to extensively comprehend human relationships, his blood is sufficient to fill the lumbar vertebrae, and a large amount of it gathers in the Liver. Since the listening of the greater yin person is unable to extensively comprehend the times of heaven, his mental vitality is insufficient to fill the brain, and a small amount of it gathers in the Lung. Since the sight of the lesser yang person is able to extensively comprehend social relationships, his qi is sufficient to fill the mid-back area, and a large amount of it gathers in the Spleen. Since the tasting of the lesser yang person is unable to extensively comprehend localities, his essence is insufficient to fill the bladders, and a small amount of it gathers in the Kidney. Since the tasting of the lesser yin person is able to extensively comprehend localities, his essence is sufficient to fill the bladders, and a large amount of it gathers in the Kidney. Since the sight of the lesser yin person is unable to extensively comprehend social relationships, his qi is insufficient to fill the midback area, and a small amount of it gathers in the Spleen.

太陽之聽能廣博於天時故太陽之神充足於頭腦而歸肺者大也太陽之嗅不能廣博於人倫故太陽之血不充足於腰脊而歸肝者小也太陰之嗅能廣博於人倫故太陰之血充足於腰脊而歸肝者大也太陰之聽不能廣博於天時故太陰之神不充足於頭腦而歸肺者小也少陽之視能廣博於世會故少陽之氣充足於背膂而歸脾者大也少陽之味不能廣博於地方故少陽之精不充足於膀胱而歸腎者小也少陰之味能廣博於地方故少陰之精充足於膀胱而歸腎者大也少陰之視不能廣博於世會故少陰之氣不充足於背膂而歸脾者小也

5   Since the anger of the greater yang person is well integrated with social acquaintances, he is not disregarded within these acquaintances. Since the joy of the greater yang person cannot keep its standing within clanships, he is disregarded by clanships. The explosive anger of the greater yang person is not caused by social acquaintances, but certainly caused by clanships. Since the joy of the lesser yin person can keep its standing with clanships, he is helped by these clanships. Since the anger of the lesser yin person cannot be well integrated within social acquaintances, he cannot be helped by these acquaintances. The joy experienced by a lesser yin person is not caused by clanships, but certainly caused by social acquaintances. Since the sorrow of the lesser yang person can smartly handle appointed roles, he is not deceived by these appointed roles. Since the pleasure of the lesser yang person is not able to maintain stability within living quarters, he is deceived by living quarters. His overflowing sorrow is not caused by appointed roles, but to these living quarters. Since the pleasure of the greater yin person always maintains stability within living quarters, he is protected by living quarters. Since the sorrow of the greater yin person is not able to smartly handle appointed roles, he cannot be protected by appointed roles. The outpour of pleasure from the greater yin person is not caused by living quarters, but caused by appointed roles.

太陽之怒能勇統於交遇故交遇不侮也太陽之喜不能雅立於黨與故黨與侮也是故太陽之暴怒不在於交遇而必在於黨與也少陰之喜能雅立於黨與故黨與助也少陰之怒不能勇統於交遇故交遇不助也是故少陰之浪喜不在於黨與而必在於交遇也少陽之哀能敏達於事務故事務不欺也少陽之樂不能恒定於居處故居處欺也是故少陽之暴哀不在於事務而必在於居處也太陰之樂能恒定於居處故居處保也太陰之哀不能敏達於事務故事務不保也是故太陰之浪樂不在於居處而必在於事務也

6   The social acquaintances of the greater yang person are governed by anger, but his involvement in clanships should not be constrained by anger. If his anger is directed against clanships, nothing beneficial for these groups can come out of it, and it may even damage his Liver. The involvement in clanships of the lesser yin person is governed by joy, but his social

acquaintances should not be constrained by joy. If his joy is directed towards social acquaintances, nothing beneficial for these acquaintances can come out of it, and it may even damage his Spleen. The appointed roles of the lesser yang person are governed by sorrow, but his living quarters should not be constrained by sorrow. If his sorrow is directed towards living quarters, nothing beneficial for living quarters can come out of it, and it may even damage his Kidney. The living quarters of the greater yin person are governed by pleasure, but his appointed role should not be constrained by pleasure. If his pleasure is directed towards appointed roles, nothing beneficial for appointed roles can come out of it, and it may even damage his Lung.

太陽之交遇可以怒治之而黨與不可以怒治之也若遷怒於黨與則無益於黨與而肝傷也少陰之黨與可以喜治之而交遇不可以喜治之也若遷喜於交遇則無益於交遇而脾傷也少陽之事務可以哀治之而居處不可以哀治之也若遷哀於居處則無益於居處而腎傷也太陰之居處可以樂治之而事務不可以樂治之也若遷樂於事務則無益於事務而肺傷也

7　Due to his temperament, the greater yang person always tends to move forward, not backward. Due to his temperament, the lesser yang person always tends to be active, without finishing what he begins. Due to his temperament, the greater yin person always tends towards stillness, and does not move. Due to his temperament, the lesser yin person always tends to remain in one place, and does not go out.

太陽之性氣恒欲進而不欲退少陽之性氣恒欲舉而不欲措太陰之性氣恒欲靜而不欲動少陰之性氣恒欲處而不欲出

8　The greater yang person always tends to move forward according to his capacity. However, he realizes that his capacities are meager, and when he reflects upon it, he will not be able to move forward. The lesser yang person always tends to be active according to his ability. However, he realizes that his power is not so firm, and when he reflects upon it, he will not be able to be so active. The greater yin person always tends towards stillness according to his comprehension. However, he realizes that his knowledge is not so thorough, and when he reflects upon it, he will not be able to be still. The lesser yin person always tends to remain in one place according to his plans. However, he realizes that his plans are not so far-reaching, and when he reflects upon it, he will not be able to remain in one place.

太陽之進量可而進也自反其材而不莊不能進也少陽之舉量可而舉也自反其力而不固不能舉也太陰之靜量可而靜也自反其知而不周不能靜也少陰之處量可而處也自反其謀而不弘不能處也

9　The emotional character of the greater yang person tends to be masculine, not feminine. The emotional character of the lesser yin person tends to be feminine, not masculine. The emotional character of the lesser yang person tends towards achievements in the outside world and not towards attending to his domestic affairs. The emotional character of the greater yin person tends towards attending to his domestic affairs, but not towards achievement in the outside world.

太陽之情氣恒欲爲雄而不欲爲雌少陰之情氣恒欲爲雌而不欲爲雄少陽之情氣恒欲外勝而不欲內守太陰之情氣恒欲內守而不欲外勝

10 Though the greater yang person tends to be masculine, it is advisable for him to be feminine to some extent. If he tries to be totally masculine, he will become overly self-indulgent. Though the lesser yin person tends to be feminine, it is advisable for him to be masculine to some extent. If he tries to be totally feminine, he will become idle. Though the lesser yang person tends towards achievements in the outside world, it is advisable for him to attend to his domestic affairs to some extent. If he pursues achievements in the outside world totally, he will become overly attached to his own urgencies. Though the greater yin person tends towards attending to his domestic affairs, it is advisable for him to pursue achievements in the outside world to some extent. If he attends but to his domestic affairs, he will become overly avaricious.

太陽之人雖好爲雄亦或宜雌若全好爲雄則放縱之心必過也少陰之人雖好爲雌亦或宜雄若全好爲雌則偸逸之心必過也少陽之人雖好外勝亦宜內守若全好外勝則偏私之心必過也太陰之人雖好內守亦宜外勝若全好內守則物欲之心必過也

11 No matter how stupid the greater yang person is, he can easily comprehend others. Even though he may be very unworthy, he can distinguish between the good and evil in others. No matter how stupid the lesser yang person is, he is highly respectful to others. Even though he may be very unworthy, he can distinguish between cleverness and foolishness in others. No matter how stupid the greater yin person is, he can guide others confidently. Even though he may be very unworthy, he can distinguish between diligence and idleness in others. No matter how stupid the lesser yin person is, he can easily pacify others. Even though he may be very unworthy, he can distinguish between ability and inability in others.

太陽人雖至愚其性便便然猶延納也雖至不肖人之善惡亦知之也少陽人雖至愚其性恢恢然猶式度也雖至不肖人之知愚亦知之也太陰人雖至愚其性卓卓然猶教誘也雖至不肖人之勤惰亦知之也少陰人雖至愚其性坦坦然猶撫循也雖至不肖人之能否亦知之也

12 Since the greater yang person is good at social acquaintances, he always has anger generated by his anxiety when encountering strangers. This anger comes from a fair and respectful mind, so it is very virtuous. Since he neglects clanships, his acquaintances in clanships always create pitfalls for him. Thus, he gets angry, and this damages his organs. The reason is that he is not very sociable.

太陽人謹於交遇故恒有交遇生疎人慮患之怒心此心出於秉彝之敬心也莫非至善而輕於黨與故每爲親熟黨與人所陷而偏怒傷臟以其擇交之心不廣故也

13 Since the lesser yin person is good at clanships, he always has joy coming from acquaintances

with familiar company. This joy comes from a fair and respectful mind, so it is very virtuous. Since he neglects social acquaintances, unfamiliar people could always deceive him. Thus, he becomes excessively joyful, and this damages his organs. The reason is that his anxiety is not very comprehensive.

少陰人謹於黨與故恒有黨與親熟人擇交之喜心此心出於秉彝之敬心也莫非至善而輕於交遇故每爲生踈交遇人所誣而偏喜傷臟以其慮患之心不周故也

14 Since the lesser yang person is cautious of appointed roles, he always has sorrow coming from his tendency to engage in outside business. This sorrow comes from a fair and respectful mind, so it is very virtuous. Since he is not cautious of living quarters, those who always tend to maintain stability within living quarters create pitfalls for him. Thus, he becomes sorrowful, and this damages his organs. The reason is that he cherishes the outside world and neglects his domestic affairs.

少陽人重於事務故恒有出外興事務之哀心此心出於秉彝之敬心也莫非至善而不謹於居處故每爲主內做居處人所陷而偏哀傷臟以其重外而輕內故也

15 Since the greater yin person is cautious of living quarters, he always has pleasure coming from his maintaining stability within living quarters. This pleasure comes from a fair and respectful mind, so it is very virtuous. Since he is not good at appointed roles, he can be deceived by those who always tend to be active in outside affairs. Thus, he indulges in pleasure, and this damages his organs. The reason is that he but pays attention to his domestic affairs and neglects outside matters.

太陰人重於居處故恒有主內做居處之樂心此心出於秉彝之敬心也莫非至善而不謹於事務故每爲出外興事務人所誣而偏樂傷臟以其重內而輕外故也

16 The jaw of the greater yin person has to be cautious about being arrogant. If his jaw has no arrogance, he will possess incomparable cleverness. The chest of the lesser yin person has to be cautious about being overconfident. If his chest has no overconfidence, he will become an incomparable administrator. The navel of the greater yang person has to be cautious about being domineering. If his navel shows no dominance, he will show incomparable moderation. The abdomen of the lesser yang person has to be cautious about being boastful. If his abdomen has no boastfulness, he will display incomparable generosity.

太陰之頷宜戒驕心太陰之頷若無驕心絕世之籌策必在此也少陰之臆宜戒矜心少陰之臆若無矜心絕世之經綸必在此也太陽之臍宜戒伐心太陽之臍若無伐心絕世之行檢必在此也少陽之腹宜戒夸心少陽之腹若無夸心絕世之度量必在此也

17 The head of the lesser yin person has to be cautious about being covetous. If his head has no covetousness, he will certainly possess the magnificent discernment of a great man. The shoulders of the greater yin person have to be cautious about being extravagant. If his shoul-

ders have no extravagance, he will certainly display the magnificent nobility of a great man. The waist of the lesser yang person has to be cautious about being idle. If his waist has no idleness, he will certainly have the magnificent resourcefulness of a great man. The hips of the greater yang person have to be cautious about being greedy. If his hips do not have a greedy nature, he will certainly possess the magnificent method of a great man.

少陰之頭宜戒奪心少陰之頭若無奪心大人之識見必在此也太陰之肩宜戒侈心太陰之肩若無侈心大人之威儀必在此也少陽之腰宜戒懶心少陽之腰若無懶心大人之材幹必在此也太陽之臀宜戒竊心太陽之臀若無竊心大人之方畧必在此也

04

Discourse
on Viscera and Bowels

臟腑論

1 The area of the Lung corresponds to the neck and upper back region. The area of the epigastrium corresponds to the region between the jaw and the upper chest. Between the back and chest is the upper-*jiao*. The area of the Spleen corresponds to the mid-back area. The stomach corresponds to the region of the diaphragm. Between the mid-back area and the diaphragm is the upper-middle-*jiao*. The area of the Liver corresponds to the waist. The area of the small intestine corresponds to the navel level. Between the waist and the navel is the lower-middle-*jiao*. The area of the Kidney corresponds to the area below the lumbar. The area of the large intestine corresponds to the area of lower abdomen. Below the lumbar-navel region is the lower-*jiao*.

肺部位在佳頁下背上胃脘部位在頷下胸上故背上胸上以上謂之上焦脾部位在膋胃部位在膈故膋膈之間謂之中上焦肝部位在腰小腸部位在臍故腰臍之間謂之中下焦腎部位在腰脊下大腸部位在臍腹下故脊下臍下以下謂之下焦

	Four *jiao*	Four region	Four viscera	Four bowels
Heart	upper-*jiao*	between the back and chest	Lung	Epigastrium
	upper-middle-*jiao*	between the mid-back region and the diaphragm	Spleen	Stomach
	lower-middle-*jiao*	between the waist and the navel	Liver	Small Intestine
	lower-*jiao*	between the lumbar-navel region	Kidney	Large Intestine

2 Ingested food moves from the epigastrium into the stomach, then to the small intestine, into the large intestine, and out from the anus. Most ingested food accumulates in the stomach and evaporates into hot qi or is digested in the small intestine and changes into cool qi. The

lighter component of the hot qi rises to the epigastric region and becomes warm qi. The heavier component of cool qi descends into the large intestine and becomes cold qi.

水穀自胃脘而入于胃自胃而入于小腸自小腸而入于大腸自大腸而出于肛門者水穀之都數停畜於胃而薰蒸爲熱氣消導於小腸而平淡爲凉氣熱氣之輕清者上升於胃脘而爲溫氣凉氣之質重者下降於大腸而爲寒氣

3 The epigastric region is connected to the mouth and nose, so the qi of ingested food rises. The large intestine is connected to the anus, so the qi of ingested food descends. The stomach is very large and can contain a large amount of food, so that the qi of ingested food may accumulate there. The small intestine is narrow and convoluted, so that the qi of the ingested food can be digested there.

胃脘通於口鼻故水穀之氣上升也大腸通於肛門故水穀之氣下降也胃之體廣大而包容故水穀之氣停畜也小腸之體狹窄而屈曲故水穀之氣消導也

4 The warm qi of ingested food is transformed into *jin* (thin and clear body fluid) in the epigastric region, and then it rises up to the sublingual area to become the sea of thin and clear body fluid. The sea of thin and clear body fluid is the dwelling place of thin and clear body fluid. The clear qi of the sea of thin and clear body fluid flows out through the ear and becomes mental vitality, which then enters the brain and forms the sea of *ni* (greasy body fluid), which is the dwelling place of mental vitality. The clear fluid of the sea of greasy body fluid ultimately returns to the Lung internally, whereas the turbid substance exits through the skin. Therefore, the epigastric region, tongue, ears, brain and skin all are part of the Lung system.

水穀溫氣自胃脘而化津入于舌下爲津海津海者津之所舍也津海之清氣出于耳而爲神入于頭腦而爲膩海膩海者神之所舍也膩海之膩汁清者內歸于肺濁滓外歸于皮毛故胃脘與舌耳頭腦皮毛皆肺之黨也

5 The hot qi of ingested food transforms into *gao* (paste) in the stomach, and paste enters the area between the breasts to become the sea of paste. The sea of paste is the dwelling place of paste. The clear qi of the sea of paste goes out through the eyes and turns into qi, which then enters the mid-back area and forms the sea of *mo* (membrane), where the qi dwells. The clear fluid of the sea of membrane ultimately goes to the Spleen internally, whereas the turbid substance goes to the tendons externally. Therefore, the stomach, breasts, eyes, mid-back area and tendons all are part of the Spleen system.

水穀熱氣自胃而化膏入于膻間兩乳爲膏海膏海者膏之所舍也膏海之清氣出于目而爲氣入于背膂而爲膜海膜海者氣之所舍也膜海之膜汁清者內歸于脾濁滓外歸于筋故胃與兩乳目背膂筋皆脾之黨也

6   The cool qi of ingested food transforms into *you* (oil) in the small intestine, and then proceeds to the navel area to form the sea of oil, where oil dwells. The clear qi of the sea of oil goes out through the nose, and turns into blood, and finally goes to the lumbar region to form the sea of blood, where blood dwells. The clear fluid of the sea of blood ultimately advances to the Liver internally, whereas the turbid substance enters the muscles externally. Therefore, the small intestine, navel, nose, lumbar region and muscles all are part of the Liver system.

水穀凉氣自小腸而化油入于臍爲油海油海者油之所舍也油海之淸氣出于鼻而爲血入于腰脊而爲血海血海者血之所舍也血海之血汁淸者內歸于肝濁滓外歸于肉故小腸與臍鼻腰脊肉皆肝之黨也

7   The cold qi of ingested food transforms into *ye* (liquid) in the large intestine, and liquid goes to the upper margin of the pubic hair and becomes the sea of liquid, where liquid dwells. The clear qi of the sea of *zhi* (juice) leaves through the mouth and becomes *jing* (essence), and then it advances to the bladder to form the sea of essence, where essence dwells. The clear fluid of the sea of essence ultimately goes to the Kidney internally, whereas the turbid substance goes to the bones externally. Therefore, the large intestine, orifice of the urethra, mouth, bladder and bones all are part of the Kidney system.

水穀寒氣自大腸而化液入于前陰毛際之內爲液海液海者液之所舍也液海之淸氣出于口而爲精入于膀胱而爲精海精海者精之所舍也精海之精汁淸者內歸于腎濁滓外歸于骨故大腸與前陰口膀胱骨皆腎之黨也

8   The ears' capacity to listen to the times of heaven makes it possible to draw out the clear qi from the sea of thin and clear body fluid, which fills the upper-*jiao*. There, the clean qi turns into mental vitality, which then pours into the brain and becomes greasy body fluid. The greasy body fluid accumulates to form the sea of greasy body fluid. The eyes' capacity to see social relationships makes it possible to draw out the clear qi from the sea of paste, which fills the upper-middle-*jiao*. There, the clear qi pours into the mid-back area and becomes membrane. The membrane accumulates to form the sea of membrane. The nose's capacity to smell human relationships makes it possible to draw out the clear qi from the sea of oil, which fills the lower-middle-*jiao*. There, the clear qi turns into blood, which then pours into the lumbar region and becomes concentrated blood. The blood accumulates to form the sea of blood. The mouth's capacity to taste localities makes it possible to draw out the clear qi from the sea of liquid, which fills the lower-*jiao*. There, the clear qi turns into essence, which then pours into the bladder and becomes concentrated essence. The essence accumulates to form the sea of essence.

耳以廣博天時之聽力提出津海之淸氣充滿於上焦爲神而注之頭腦爲膩積累爲膩海目以廣博世會之視力提出膏海之淸氣充滿於中上焦爲氣而注之背脊爲膜積累爲膜海鼻以廣博人倫之嗅力提出油海之淸氣充滿於中下焦爲血而注之腰脊爲凝血積累爲血海口以廣博地方之味力提出液海之淸氣充滿於下焦爲精而注之膀胱爲凝精積累爲精海

9 The Lung's sorrowful power to master appointed roles makes it possible to suck out the clear juice from the sea of greasy body fluid, which enters the Lung. The clear juice nourishes the source of the Lung, supports the sea of thin and clear body fluid internally, stimulates the qi, and concentrates thin and clear body fluid. The Spleen's anger power to master social acquaintances makes it possible to suck out the clear juice from the sea of membrane, which enters the Spleen. The clear juice nourishes the source of the Spleen, supports the sea of paste internally, stimulates the qi, and concentrates paste. The Liver's joy power to master clanships makes it possible to suck out the clear juice from the sea of blood, which enters the Liver. The clear juice nourishes the source of the Liver, supports the sea of oil internally, stimulates the qi, and concentrates oil. The Kidney's pleasure power to master living quarters makes it possible to suck out the clear juice from the sea of essence, which enters the Kidney. The clear juice nourishes the source of the Kidney, supports the sea of liquid internally, stimulates the qi, and concentrates liquid.

肺以鍊達事務之哀力吸得膩海之清汁入于肺以滋肺元而內以擁護津海鼓動其氣凝聚其津脾以鍊達交遇之怒力吸得膜海之清汁入于脾以滋脾元而內以擁護膏海鼓動其氣凝聚其膏肝以鍊達黨與之喜力吸得血海之清汁入于肝以滋肝元而內以擁護油海鼓動其氣凝聚其油腎以鍊達居處之樂力吸得精海之清汁入于腎以滋腎元而內以擁護液海鼓動其氣凝聚其液

10 The ascending power of the epigastrium to collect the turbid substance of the sea of thin and clear body fluid strengthens the epigastrium. The retaining power of the stomach to collect the turbid substance of the sea of paste strengthens the stomach. The removing and digesting power of the small intestine to collect the turbid substance of the sea of oil strengthens the small intestine. The descending power of the large intestine to collect the turbid substance of the sea of liquid strengthens the large intestine.

津海之濁滓則胃脘以上升之力取其濁滓而以補益胃脘膏海之濁滓則胃以停畜之力取其濁滓而以補益胃油海之濁滓則小腸以消導之力取其濁滓而以補益小腸液海之濁滓則大腸以下降之力取其濁滓而以補益大腸

Four bowels	Four Qi	Four front seas	Power	Four back seas
Epigastrium	Warm Qi	Sea of *Jin*	The ascending power	Sea of *Ni*
Stomach	Hot Qi	Sea of *Gao*	The retaining power	Sea of *Mo*
Small Intestine	Cool Qi	Sea of *You*	The removing and digesting power	Sea of Blood
Large Intestine	Cold Qi	Sea of *Ye*	The descending power	Sea of *Jing*

11 The stretching capacity of the head refines and shapes the turbid substance of the sea of greasy body fluid into skin and hair. The grasping capacity of the hands refines and shapes the turbid substance of the sea of membrane into tendons. The dispersing capacity of the waist refines and shapes the turbid substance of the sea of blood into muscle. The flexing capacity of the feet refines and shapes the turbid substance of the sea of essence into bone.

膩海之濁滓則頭以直伸之力鍛鍊之而成皮毛膜海之濁滓則手以能收之力鍛鍊之而成筋血海之濁滓則腰以寬放之力鍛鍊之而成肉精海之濁滓則足以屈强之力鍛鍊之而成骨

12 Therefore, the ears must listen extensively, the eyes must see widely, the nose must smell broadly, and the mouth must taste deeply. The ears, eyes, nose and mouth should use their full capacities so that essence, mental vitality, qi and blood are well developed. If not, essence, mental vitality, qi and blood will be exhausted. The Lung must be good at learning. The Spleen must be good at inquiring. The Liver must be good at thinking. The Kidney must be good at differentiating. The Lung, Spleen, Liver and Kidney should use their capacities so that thin and clear body fluid, liquid, paste and oil are sufficient. If not, thin and clear body fluid, liquid, paste and oil will be consumed.

是故耳必遠聽目必大視鼻必廣嗅口必深味耳目鼻口之用深遠廣大則精神氣血生也淺近狹小則精神氣血耗也肺必善學脾必善問肝必善思腎必善辨肺脾肝腎之用正直中和則津液膏油充也偏倚過不及則津液膏油燥也

13 The sea of greasy body fluid stores mental vitality. The sea of membrane stores *ling* (soul). The sea of blood stores *hun* (ethereal soul). The sea of essence stores *po* (corporeal soul).

膩海藏神膜海藏靈血海藏魂精海藏魄

14 The sea of thin and clear body fluid stores intention. The sea of paste stores consideration. The sea of oil stores integrity. The sea of liquid stores will.

津海藏意膏海藏慮油海藏操液海藏志

15 The sea of greasy body fluid in the head is the source of the Lung. The sea of membrane in the mid-back area is the source of the Spleen. The sea of blood in the lumbar region is the source of the Liver. The sea of essence in the bladders is the source of the Kidney.

頭腦之膩海肺之根本也背膂之膜海脾之根本也腰脊之血海肝之根本也膀胱之精海腎之根本也

16 The sea of thin and clear body fluid in the sublingual area is the source of the ears. The sea of paste in the breasts is the source of the eyes. The sea of oil in the navel is the source of the nose. The sea of liquid in the bladder is the source of the mouth.

舌之津海耳之根本也乳之膏海目之根本也臍之油海鼻之根本也前陰之液海口之根本也

17 The Heart is the supreme ruler of the whole body, located in the center of the chest, and is very bright and shiny. The ears, eyes, nose, and mouth observe all things. The Lung, Spleen, Liver and Kidney consider all things. The jaw, chest, navel and abdomen are sincere in all things. The head, hands, waist and feet respect all things.

心爲一身之主宰負隅背心正向膻中光明瑩徹耳目鼻口無所不察肺脾肝腎無所不忖頜臆臍腹無所不誠頭手腰足無所不敬

05

Discourse
on the Origin of Eastern Medicine

醫源論

1 In the 『*Shujing*』[1] ("Classic of Document"), we read, "If the medicine does not cause a kind of dizziness, the illness cannot be cured." During the reign of Gaozong in the Shang dynasty, Gaozong experienced such dizziness after taking some medicine, and he greatly appreciated its effect. This tradition in medicine is very old, dating to before the era of Shennong[2] and Huangdi[3]. This is plausible, but most people believe that the 『*Bencao*』[4] ("Materia Medica") and 『*Suwen*』[5] ("Plain Questions") were written by Shennong and Huangdi themselves. This is not possible. The reason is as follows. During the eras of Shennong and Huangdi, there were no written characters. Likewise, in the following era, the usage of written language was very approximate, so they could not have written those books. After the Zhou and during the Chin-Han dynasties, Bianque was the preeminent physician. Followed by him, Zhang Zhongjing[6] compiled the medical knowledge of that time. Soon afterwards, the practice of medicine began to flourish. After Zhang Zhongjing, following the Southern and Northern, Sui and Tang dynasties, and during the Song dynasty, Zhu Gong[7] also compiled the existing medical knowledge into the 『*Huorenshu*』[8] ("Book for Saving Life"). After Zhu Gong, the Yuan dynasty's Li Gao[9], Wang Haogu[10], Zhu Zhenheng[11] and Wei Yilin[12] continued this tradition. Li Chan[13] and Gong Xin[14] inherited these medical teachings during the Ming dynasty, and later Heo Jun[15] propagated them in the form of the 『*Dongui Bogam*』[16] ("Treasure Mirror of Eastern Medicine"). This led to a renaissance in traditional medicine. Zhang Zhongjing propagated the medical and pharmacological theories dating back from the era of Shennong and Huangdi to the Chin-Han dynasties. Following this, Zhu Gong promoted similar medical and pharmacological theories from the era of the Wei and the Jin dynasties to the times of Sui and the Tang dynasties. Likewise, Li Chan and Gong Xin and Heo Jun

spread the medical theories of the Song, Yuan and Ming dynasties. If we evaluate their contributions, Zhang Zhongjing, Zhu Gong and Heo Jun deserve the highest recognition, and Li Chan and Gong Xin follow just behind them.

書曰若藥不瞑眩厥疾不瘳商高宗時已有瞑眩藥驗而高宗至於稱歎則醫藥經驗其來已久於神農黃帝之時其說可信於眞也而本草素問出於神農黃帝之手其說不可信於眞也何以言之神農黃帝時文字應無後世文字澆漓例法故也哀周秦漢以來扁鵲有名而張仲景具備得之始爲成家著書醫道始興張仲景以後南北朝隋唐醫繼之而至于宋朱肱具備得之著活人書醫道中興朱肱以後元醫李杲王好古朱震亨危亦林繼之而至于明李梃龔信具備得之許浚具備傳之著東醫寶鑑醫道復興盖自神農黃帝以後秦漢以前病證藥理張仲景傳之魏晉以後隋唐以前病證藥理朱肱傳之宋元以後明以前病證藥理李梃龔信許浚傳之若以醫家勤勞功業論之則當以張仲景朱肱許浚爲首而李梃龔信次之

2   As for the 『*Bencao*』 ("Materia Medica"), beginning with the days of Shennong and Huangdi, the knowledge of herbal medicine was used for several thousand years. In the era of Shennong, the 『*Bencao*』 already existed. The 『*Tangye Bencao*』[17] ("Materia Medica of Decoction") came into being during the Yuan dynasty. During the Tang dynasty, the 『*Shiliao Bencao*』[18] ("Dietetic Materia Medica") was written by Meng Xian[19], and Chen Zangqi[20] wrote the 『*Bencao Shiyi*』[21] ("Supplement to Materia Medica"). During the Song dynasty, the 『*Bencao Buyi*』 ("Reinforcing the Materia Medica") was written by Fang Anshang[22], and the 『*Rihuazi Bencao*』[23] ("Rihuazi Materia Medica") was published. During the Yuan dynasty, the 『*Tangye Bencao*』 was written by Wang Haogu.

本草自神農黃帝以來數千年世間流來經驗而神農時有本草殷時有湯液本草唐時有孟詵食療本草陳藏器本草拾遺宋時有龐安常本草補遺日華子本草元時有王好古湯液本草

3   The medical and pharmacological theories related to the lesser yin type were explained in detail by Zhang Zhongjing. However, it took the doctors of the Song, Yuan and Ming dynasties to develop these ideas to near completion. The medical and pharmacological theories related to the lesser yang type were partially explained by Zhang Zhongjing. Later, the doctors of the Song, Yuan and Ming dynasties also developed these ideas in detail. As for the medical and pharmacological ideas related to the greater yin type, Zhang Zhongjing only roughly sketched them out. The doctors of the Song, Yuan and Ming dynasties imparted more details to those ideas. For the greater yang type, the medical and pharmacological theories were also only roughly sketched out by Zhu Zhenheng, and in the 『*Bencao*』, pharmacological theories were briefly mentioned, too.

少陰人病證藥理張仲景庶幾乎昭詳發明而宋元明諸醫盡乎昭詳發明少陽人病證藥理張仲景半乎昭詳發明而宋元明諸醫庶幾乎昭詳發明太陰人病證藥理張仲景略得影子而宋元明諸醫太半乎昭詳發明太陽人病證藥理朱震亨畧得影子而本草畧有藥理

4   Five to six thousand years after the development of this medical tradition, I perceived the principles of the four constitutional types by chance, and wrote a book titled the 『*Suse Bo-*

won」[24] ("Longevity and Life Preservation"). The designations of greater yang disease, lesser yang disease, yang brightness disease, greater yin disease, lesser yin disease and reverting yin disease, mentioned by Zhang Zhongjing, were based on the terminology of symptoms. In my system, however, the designations of greater yang, lesser yang, greater yin and lesser yin types are based on the person's constitutions. We must not confuse these two viewpoints. First, we must perceive the roots and trunk, and afterward the branches and leaves. Taking the pulse is one of the methods for diagnosing symptoms and signs. When taking a pulse, we must remember that, fundamentally, there are but four main types of pulse, i. e. floating (superficial), deep, slow and fast. Aside from these, there is not much else of importance for diagnosis. The three yins and three yangs are differentiated according to their symptoms and the signs. Those principles originated from the symptoms and signs of the abdomen and back, and the outside and inside of the body, so there is no need to try to detect changes in the meridians.

余生於醫藥經驗五六千載後因前人之述偶得四象人臟腑性理著得一書名曰壽世保元原書中張仲景所論太陽病少陽病陽明病太陰病少陰病厥陰病以病證名目而論之也余所論太陽人少陽人太陰人少陰人以人物名目而論之也二者不可混看又不可厭煩然後可以探其根株而採其枝葉也若夫脈法者執證之一端也其理在於浮沈遲數而不必究其奇妙之致也三陰三陽者辨證之同異也其理在於腹背表裏而不必求其經絡之變也

5   In ancient times, doctors explained disease according to the theories of six meridians related to yin and yang, so when Zhang Zhongjing wrote his 『*Shanghanlun*』[25], he also classified symptoms according to those assumptions. If the patient had a headache, aching of the body, fever, chills and a floating pulse, we can say that he has a greater yang disease. Bitterness in the mouth, parched throat, vertigo, deafness, fullness in the chest, chills and fever that come and go, headache, fever, and a tight and slender pulse indicate the lesser yang disease. Spontaneous perspiration, with an aversion to heat during fever, but no aversion to cold, and constipation indicate the yang brightness disease. Abdominal distention with occasional pain, without a thirst for water, or heartburn and diarrheas indicate the greater yin disease. A feeble and weak pulse, constant drowsiness, thirst, heartburn, and diarrheas indicate the lesser yin disease. No abdominal pain and diarrheas at the onset, but appearing after the sixth or seventh day, feeble and loose pulse, cold limbs, curled tongue, and shrinkage of the scrotum indicate the reverting yin disease. Among the above six diseases, the three yin diseases are closely related to the lesser yin type. The lesser yang disease is closely related to the lesser yang type. The greater yang and yang brightness diseases may affect the lesser yang, lesser yin and greater yin types, but mostly they affect the lesser yin type. From ancient times, medical ideas and principles were widespread. Zhang Zhongjing compiled the prevalent ideas, as well as clinical experiences from ancient times, and wrote his 『*Shanghanlun*』. However, most ancient doctors did not understand that the propensities for love, hate, avarice, joy, anger, sorrow and pleasure in the mind were the causes of disease. Rather, they thought that an improper diet, wind, cold, summer heat and dampness were the causes of disease. If we analyze their ideas re-

garding disease and medicine, we can see that most of them were focused on the improper diet of the lesser yin type. Stomach-heat pattern of the lesser yang type was described only a little, and disease situation of the greater yin and the greater yang persons were not described at all.

古人以六經陰陽論病故張仲景著傷寒論亦以六經陰陽該病證而以頭痛身疼發熱惡寒脈浮者謂之太陽病證以口苦咽乾目眩耳聾胸脇滿寒熱往來頭痛發熱脈弦細者謂之少陽病證以不惡寒反惡熱汗自出大便秘者謂之陽明病證以腹滿時痛口不燥心不煩而自利者謂之太陰病證以脈微細但欲寐口燥心煩而自利者謂之少陰病證以初無腹痛自利等證而傷寒六七日脈微緩手足厥冷舌卷囊縮者謂之厥陰病證六條病證中三陰病證皆少陰人病證也少陽病證即少陽人病證也太陽病證陽明病證則少陽人少陰人太陰人病證均有之而少陰人病證居多也古昔以來醫藥法方流行世間經歷累驗者仲景採摭而著述之盖古之醫師不知心之愛惡所欲喜怒哀樂偏着者爲病而但知脾胃水穀風寒暑濕觸犯者爲病故其論病論藥全局都自少陰人脾胃水穀中出來而少陽人胃熱證藥間或有焉至於太陰人太陽人病情則全昧也

6 Qibo[26] answered, "On the first day, the febrile disease caused by cold is received by the greater yang meridian. Therefore, the head and the neck are in pain, and the waist and the back become rigid. On the second day, the yang brightness meridian contracts the disease. The yang brightness controls the flesh, its meridian supports the nose, and it is connected to the eyes. Thus the body is feverish, there is eyeball pain, the nose is dry and parched, and the patient finds it impossible to rest. On the third day, the lesser yang meridian contracts the disease. The region of the lesser yang controls the gall bladder. Its meridian follows the flanks and is connected to the ears. Thus, the ribs and chest are in pain, and the ears grow deaf. Now, the meridian of the three yangs have contracted the disease, but it has not yet entered the viscera; therefore, if one can produce perspiration, one can cure the disease. On the fourth day, the greater yin meridian contracts the disease. The meridian of greater yin leads into the interior of the stomach and is connected to the throat. Thus, the stomach becomes replete (full), and the throat becomes dry and parched. On the fifth day, the lesser yin meridian contracts the disease. The meridian of lesser yin penetrates into the Kidney and is connected to the Lung; it is also connected to the root of the tongue. Thus, the mouth is dry, and the tongue is parched and dry. On the sixth day, the reverting yin meridian contracts the disease. The meridian of reverting yin passes through the sex organs and is connected to the Liver. The results are an affliction of fullness and shrinkage of the scrotum. Now, if the three yins, the three yangs, the five viscera and the six bowels have all contracted the disease, there is stagnation of the *ying* (nutrient) and the *wei* (defense), and no circulation of the five viscera. Death follows."

岐伯曰傷寒一日巨陽受之故頭項痛腰脊强二日陽明受之陽明主肉其脈挾鼻絡於目故身熱目疼而鼻乾不得臥也三日少陽受之少陽主膽其脈循脇絡於耳故胸脇痛而耳聾三陽經絡皆受其病而未入於藏故可汗而已四日太陰受之太陰脈布胃中絡於嗌故腹滿而嗌乾五日少陰受之少陰脈貫腎絡於肺繫舌本故口燥舌乾而渴六日厥陰受之厥陰脈循陰器而絡於肝故煩滿而囊縮三陰三陽五臟六腑皆受病榮衛不行五藏不通則死矣

7 "If there is a patient in the simultaneous occurrence of patterns of both the yang and yin meridians caused by cold, he will die. When the patterns of both the yang and yin meridians caused by cold simultaneously occur, both the greater yang and lesser yin meridians are affected on the first day of illness. There will be a headache, a parched mouth, and discomfort in the chest. On the second day of illness, the yang brightness and greater yin meridians are both affected. The patient's abdomen feels full, and his body feverish. He does not want food and speaks deliriously. On the third day of illness, the lesser yang and reverting yin meridians are both affected. The ears grow deaf, and the scrotum shrinks and becomes cold. Water and broth cannot be ingested, the patient cannot recognize other people, and on the sixth day, he will die. Their death always takes a period of six or seven days, their improvement ten days."

兩感於寒者必不免於死兩感於寒者一日巨陽少陰俱病則頭痛口乾而煩滿二日陽明太陰俱病腹滿身熱不飲食譫語三日少陽厥陰俱病耳聾囊縮而厥水漿不入口不知人六日死其死皆以六七日之間其愈皆以十日已上

8 I have said, "The idea that the 『*Lingshu*』[27] and 『*Suwen*』 were attributed to Huangdi is nonsense and confuses the people. However, in those days, it was a common belief, so we need not criticize it. Since those books contain the medical experiences of ancient times concerning the theories of the five viscera, the six bowels, the meridians, acupuncture, disease and the cultivation of health, as well as many enlightening ideas, they are sovereign in providing doctors with insightful knowledge of medical laws. Despite the fact that these books are not perfect, we must not criticize them or detract from their contributions. They recorded the wisdom and widespread knowledge of ancient times, including original ideas concerning the cultivation of health. We must take them into consideration, but should not accept them at face value."

論曰靈樞素問假托黃帝異怪幻惑無足稱道方術好事者之言容或如是不必深責也然此書亦是古人之經驗而五臟六腑經絡鍼法病證修養之辨多有所啓發則實是醫家格致之宗主而苗脈之所自出也不可全數其虛誕之罪而廢其啓發之功也盖此書亦古之聰慧博物之言方士淵源修養之述也其理有可考而其說不可盡信

9 "The greater yang, lesser yang and lesser yin meridian diseases mentioned by Qibo are actually diseases of the lesser yang person. The yang brightness and greater yin meridian diseases spoken of by Qibo are actually diseases of the greater yin person. The reverting yin meridian disease referred to by Qibo is actually a disease of the lesser yin person."

岐伯所論巨陽少陽少陰經病皆少陽人病也陽明太陰經病皆太陰人病也厥陰經病少陰人病也

Notes

1) 『*Shujing*』 (書經)

The "Classic of Document", also called the 『*Shangshu*』 (商書: "Official History"), one of the Five Classics of Chinese antiquity. The 『*Shujing*』 consists of fifty eight chapters. The first five chapters purport to preserve the sayings and to recall the deeds of such illustrious emperors as Yao and Shun. Chapters six to nine are devoted to the Xia dynasty (c. 2205~1766 B.C.), the historicity of which has not been definitively established. The next 17 chapters deal with the Shang dynasty and its collapse in 1122 B.C.. The final 32 chapters cover the Western Zhou dynasty that ruled China until 771 B.C..

2) Shennong (神農)

The second of ancient China's mythical emperors, said to have been born in the 28th century B.C., with the head of a bull and the body of a man. By inventing the cart and plow, taming the ox, yoking the horse, and teaching his people to clear the land with fire, Shennong is said to have established a stable agricultural society in China. His catalog of 365 species of medicinal plants became the basis of later herbological studies. Marvelous tales of his youth relate that he spoke after three days, walked within a week, and could plow a field at the age of three.

3) Huangdi (黃帝)

The third of ancient China's mythological emperors, a cultural hero and patron saint of Taoism. Huangdi is reputed to have been born in 2,704 B.C., and begun his rule as emperor in 2,697 B.C.. His legendary reign is credited with the introduction of wooden houses, carts, boats, the bow and arrow, and writing. Huangdi himself is credited with defeating "barbarians" in a great battle somewhere in what is now Shansi. The victory won him the leadership of tribes throughout the Huang He (黃河: Yellow River) plain. Some traditions also credit him with the introduction of governmental institutions and the use of coined money. His wife was reputed to have discovered sericulture (silk production) and to have taught women how to breed silkworms and weave fabrics of silk. Huangdi is held up in some ancient sources as a paragon of wisdom whose reign was a golden age. He is said to have dreamed of an ideal kingdom whose tranquil inhabitants lived in harmonious accord with natural law and possessed virtues remarkably like those espoused by early Taoism. Upon waking from his dream, Huangdi sought to inculcate these virtues in his own kingdom and to ensure order and prosperity among the inhabitants. Upon his death, he was said to have become an immortal.

4) 『Bencao』(本草)

The "Materia Medica", 『Shennong Bencaojing』(神農本草經), the earliest book on Materia Medica, and believed to have been a product of the first century B.C., with its authorship attributed to the ancient emperor "the Divine Peasant" Shennong. There are 365 kinds of drugs listed. The drugs are divided into three classes: superior, common and inferior.

5) 『Suwen』(素問)

The "Plain Questions", also called the 『Huangdi Neijing Suwen』(黃帝內經 素問), originally consisting of nine volumes, with 81 articles. After the Wei and Jin dynasties, there were only eight volumes extant. In the Tang dynasty, while making notes and commentaries on the book, Wang Bing (王氷) divided it into 24 volumes and supplemented some of the lost articles. In the Northern Song dynasty, Lin Yi (林億) and other scholars, read proofs and made notes on it again. All later extant editions were based on the Northern Song version. The book includes a variety of subjects, such as human anatomy, physiology, etiology, pathology, diagnosis, pattern identification, treatment, disease prevention, health preservation, relations between man and nature, the application of yin-yang and five phases in medicine, the theory of promoting the flow of qi, etc. The book has been prized by physicians of all generations.

6) Zhang Zhongjing (張仲景)

(150~219 A.D.) Also called Zhang Ji (張機), and is considered one of the most influential figures in the history of Chinese medicine. He was the first to advocate the methods of analyzing and differentiating pathological conditions in accordance with the six stages and the eight principal patterns. He stressed the principle of treating diseases according to the method of differentiating symptoms and signs. He is also ascribed the authorship of several medical books on various topics, the most important of which, now extant, are the 『Shanghan Zabinglun』(傷寒雜病論: "Treatise on Cold-induced and Miscellaneous Diseases") and 『Jinkui Yaolue Fanglun』(金匱要略方論: "Synopsis of Prescriptions of the Golden Chamber").

7) Zhu Gong (朱肱)

A famous physician in the Song dynasty. He studied Zhang Zhongjing's theory for many years, and wrote the 『Shanghan Baiwen』(傷寒百問, 1108), which is in the form of 100 questions and answers. In 1114 (A.D.), he wrote the 『Huorenshu』(活人書), which is a 22 volume rewrite of the 『Shanghan Baiwen』. In this book, he analyzed Zhang Zhongjing's liujing (六經) through the theory of the six meridians.

8) 『Huorenshu』(活人書)

The "Book for Saving Life", also called the 『Nanyang Huorenshu』(南陽活人書), 『Leizheng Huorenshu』(類證活人書), written in 22 volumes by Zhu Gong (朱肱) in 1108 A.D.. He divided the volumes into four parts and introduced the febrile diseases and miscellaneous diseases separately. The 『*Huorenshu*』 was influential to the early commentaries pertaining to Zhang Zhongjing's theory.

9) Li Gao (李杲)

(1180~1251 A.D.) Also called Li Mingzhi (李明之) or Li Dongyuan (李東垣), a disciple of Zhang Yuansu (張元素), who held that diseases, apart from external changes, were mainly caused by the "internal injury"of the Spleen and stomach (i.e., intemperance in drinking and eating or overwork), and advocated the regulation of the Spleen and stomach and nourishing the original qi. He is considered the founder of the school of strengthening the Spleen and stomach. His masterpiece was the 『*Piweilun*』(脾胃論: "Treatise on the Spleen and Stomach").

10) Wang Haogu (王好古)

Also called Wang Jinzhi (王進之), or Wang Haizang (王海藏). A distinguished physician in the 13th century, whose chief contribution was his plea in support of using tonics and stimulants for infectious diseases in the later stage when the metabolic function is weakened, and the avoidance of purgatives. Five of his publications are still in existence, including the 『*Tangye Bencao*』(湯液本草: "Materia Medica of Decoction",1289 A.D.).

11) Zhu Zhenheng (朱震亨)

(1282~1358 A.D.) A native of Danxi (丹溪), Jinhua County, Zhejiang Province, also known as the Master of Danxi, who took indulgence as the root of all troubles and exhorted the value of tonics for the purpose of supplementing the yin deficiency. He advocated the theory that yang was always in excess while yin was often deficient, and thus belonged to the school of nourishing yin. He was the author of 『*Gezhi Yulun*』(格致餘論: "Inquiry into the Properties of Things", 1347 A.D.) and 『*Jufang Fahui*』(局方發揮: "Expounding on the Formularies of the Bureau of People's Welfare Pharmacies").

12) Wei Yilin (危亦林)

(1277~1347 A.D.) Also called Wei Dazhai (危達齋) was thought to have been a bone physician famous for setting bones. Based on the experience and findings of his ancestors, not a few of whom were noted physicians, he compiled a large number of prescriptions in a book entitled 『*Shiyi Dexiaofang*』(世醫得效方: "Effective Formulas Tested by Physicians for Generations").

13) Li Chan (李梴)

Also called Li Jianzhai (李健齋). A physician in the 16th century who summarized the prescriptions used at that period in medical practice and divided them into 18 different categories. Li was the author of the 『*Yixue Rumen*』(醫學入門: "Introduction to Medicine", 1575 A.D.), and 『*Xiyi Guige*』(習醫規格: "Rules for the Study of Medicine", 1575 A.D.).

14) Gong Xin (龔信)

A famous physician of the Ming dynasty and the author of the 『*Yijianshu*』(醫鑑書), which was completed by his son, Gong Tingxian.

15) Heo Jun (許浚)

Heo Jun was born in 1546, and became the head physician during the reign of King Seonjo (宣祖) and Gwanghaegun (光海君) in the Joseon dynasty. Additionally, Heo Jun contributed several works to the literature of traditional Korean medicine. The most brilliant of them is the 『*Dongui Bogam*』, which he finished compiling in 1610. His medical philosophy drew heavily from the 『*Suwen*』, 『*Lingshu*』 and 『*Nanjing*』. The theories of Zhang Zhongjing and the "Four Masters" of the Jin-Yuan dynasties were influential as well.

16) 『*Dongui Bogam*』(東醫寶鑑)

The "Treasure Mirror of Eastern Medicine" was compiled by Heo Jun and was published in 1611 A.D. (Joseon dynasty) in 25 volumes. Heo Jun gathered and organized the traditional Chinese medical books, which had been published until the Ming dynasty. The 『*Dongui Bogam*』 consisted of five parts: Internal Medicine (內景篇), External Diseases (外形篇), Miscellaneous Diseases (雜病篇), Drugs and Decoctions (湯液篇), and Acupuncture and Moxibustion (鍼灸篇). The scope of this work is very broad and well organized. Eventually, it became one of the most important books in east Asian traditional medicine.

17) 『*Tangye Bencao*』(湯液本草)

The "Materia Medica of Decoction", written by Wang Haogu (王好古) and published in 1298 A.D., lists 238 kinds of drugs, in which the flavor, taste, therapeutic properties as well as the mutual influence of mixing medicines are all described. This text is used in combination with the study of the Materia Medica.

18) 『*Shiliao Bencao*』(食療本草)

The "Dietetic Materia Medica" is a monograph by the Tang dynasty's Meng Xian (孟詵), recording herbs, which can be used as both food and drugs. The original has been lost, but its text can be found in the 『*Leizheng Bencao*』(類證本草: "Classified Materia Medica").

19) Meng Xian (孟詵)

(621~713 A.D.) A herbalist in the Tang dynasty and author of the 『*Shiliao Bencao*』. The original has been lost, but the text can be found in the 『*Leizheng Bencao*』.

20) Chen Zangqi (陳藏器)

An herbalist in the Tang dynasty, and author of the 『*Bencao Shiyi*』(本草拾遺).

21) 『*Bencao Shiyi*』 (本草拾遺)

The "Supplement to Materia Medica" was written in ten volumes by Chen Zangqi (陳藏器) in the Tang dynasty, and added medical substances not included in the 『*Xinxiu Bencao*』 (新修本草: "Newly Compiled Materia Medica").

22) Fang Anshang (龐安常)

Also called Fang Anshi, a noted physician known for having written several medical works, among which the most widely read was a detailed and comprehensive treatise on various kinds of fevers under the title of 『*Shanghan Zhongbinglun*』 (傷寒總病論: "General Treatise on Cold-induced Disease", 1100 A.D.).

23) 『*Rihuazi Bencao*』 (日華子本草)

Written in 20 volumes by Rihuazi (日華子). The original copy is lost, but parts of its contents are found in the 『*Zhenglei Bencao*』 (證類本草).

24) 『*Suse Bowon*』 (壽世保元)

The "Longevity and Life Preservation", written by Lee Je-ma and published in 1894. Its full name is 『*Dongui Suse Bowon*』 (東醫壽世保元), and is the text upon which Sasang Constitutional Medicine is based.

25) 『*Shanghanlun*』 (傷寒論)

The "Treatise on Cold-induced Diseases", a new edition of Zhang Zhongjing's "Treatise on Cold-induced and Miscellaneous Diseases", rearranged by Wang Shuhe (王叔和) in the Jin dynasty. In this work, acute febrile diseases are analyzed and differentiated in accordance with the theory of the six stages. The book is regarded as one of the most influential works in the traditional practice of Chinese medicine.

26) Qibo (岐伯)

A famous mythical physician in the reign of Huangdi, the Yellow Emperor (2698~2589 B.C.), who was asked by the Emperor to taste various kinds of herbs and to study medicine and pharmacy. The first and greatest medical work in China, the 『*Huangdi Neijing*』, consists of questions and answers between Huangdi and Qibo and other officials on problems of medicine and pharmacy.

27) 『*Lingshu*』 (靈樞)

The "Miraculous Pivot" or "Divine Axis", one of the two parts of the 『*Huangdi Neijing*』, also called 『*Huangdi Neijing Lingshujing*』 (黃帝內經 靈樞經: "Miraculous Pivot of Yellow Emperor's Canon of Internal Medicine"). The subjects of "Miraculous Pivot" are similar to those of 『*Suwen*』 ("Plain Questions") but the former has a more detailed description of meridians and needling, and is less concerned with the basic theories about the functions of the internal organs and the vital substances. In introducing basic theories and clinical practice, the two books supplement each other. This book, like 『*Suwen*』, has been prized by physicians of all generations.

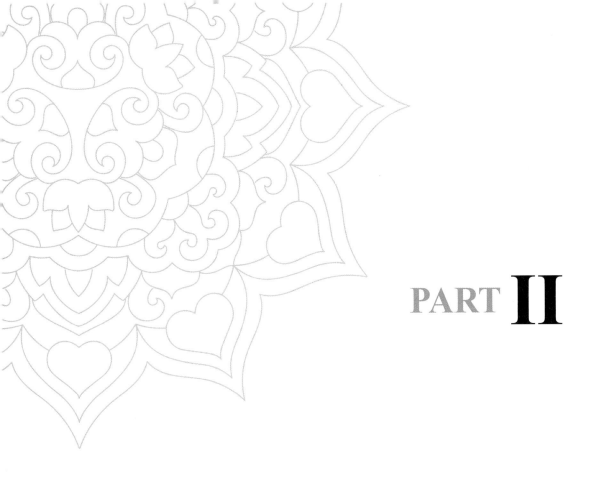

PART II

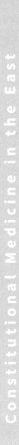

Discourse on the Soeum (Lesser Yin) Person's Exterior Febrile Disease Induced from the Kidney Affected by Heat

少陰人腎受熱表熱病論

1 In the 『*Shanghanlun*』, Zhang Zhongjing said, "Fever, chills and a floating pulse are the general symptoms and signs of the greater yang pattern, which is in the exterior stage."

張仲景傷寒論曰發熱惡寒脈浮者屬表卽太陽證也

2 The pulse of the greater yang febrile disease caused by wind is floating when felt at the surface level and weak at the depth level. A pulse floating at the surface signifies spontaneous fever. A pulse weak in depth signifies spontaneous perspiration. Guizhi Tang (Cinnamon Twig Decoction) should be used when the patient feels chills and an aversion to wind, uneasy because of fever and nauseous with a tendency to snore.

太陽傷風脈陽浮而陰弱陽浮者熱自發陰弱者汗自出嗇嗇惡寒淅淅惡風翕翕發熱鼻鳴乾嘔桂枝湯主之

3 In the 『*Dexiaofang*』[1] ("Effective Formulas"), Wei Yilin said, "The pestilences of the four seasons can be treated with Xiangsu San (Cyperus and Perilla Leaf Powder)."

危亦林得效方曰四時瘟疫當用香蘇散

4 In the 『*Yijian*』[2] ("Mirror of Medicine"), Gong Xin said, "The exogenous febrile disease with the symptoms of headache and aching of the body can be treated with Huoxiang Zhengqi San (Agastache Powder to Rectify the Qi). It is difficult to determine whether this disease belongs to the exterior or interior pattern."

龔信醫鑑曰傷寒頭痛身疼不分表裏證當用藿香正氣散

5　I have said, "The fever with chills in the greater yang febrile disease caused by wind mentioned by Zhang Zhongjing is the same as the lesser yin person's exterior febrile disease induced from the Kidney affected by heat. Fever and chills without perspiration should be treated with Guizhi Tang, Cheongung Gyeji Tang (Chuanxiong Rhizoma and Cinnamomi Ramulus Decoction), Xiangsu San, Gunggwi Hyangso San (Cyperus and Perilla Leaf Powder with Chuanxiong Rhizoma and Angelicae Gigantis Radix) and Huoxiang Zhengqi San. Fever and chills with perspiration is the start of *mangyang* (yang collapse), and should not be ignored. Begin treatment with Hwanggi Gyeji Tang (Astragalus and Cinnamon Twig Decoction), Bojung Ikgi Tang (Tonify the Middle to Augment the Qi Decoction) and Seungyang Ikgi Tang (Decoction for Ascending Yang and Replenishing Qi) for three days. If sweating persists after the treatment, treat with Guizhi Fuzi Tang (Cinnamon Twig and Aconite Decoction), Insam Gyeji Buja Tang (Ginseng, Cinnamon Twig, and Aconiti Accessory Root Decoction) and Seungyang Ikgi Buja Tang (Decoction of Aconiti Lateralis Radix Praeparata for Lifting Yang and Replenishing Qi)."

論曰張仲景所論太陽傷風發熱惡寒者卽少陰人腎受熱表熱病也此證發熱惡寒而無汗者當用桂枝湯川芎桂枝湯香蘇散芎歸香蘇散藿香正氣散發熱惡寒而有汗者此亡陽初證也必不可輕易視之先用黃芪桂枝湯補中益氣湯升陽益氣湯三日連服而汗不止病不愈則當用桂枝付子湯人蔘桂枝付子湯升陽益氣付子湯

6　Zhang Zhongjing said, "If a patient suffering from greater yang disease has a fever, a floating and tense pulse and no perspiration, he will recover spontaneously after epistaxis."

張仲景曰太陽病脈浮緊發熱無汗而衄者自愈也

7　In the case of the greater yang disease, after six to seven days, if the exterior pattern still remains and the pulse is feeble and deep, the patient does not suffer from *jiexiong* (accumulation of pathogen in the chest), but behaves in a manic way. This is because the pathogenic heat has congealed in the lower-*jiao* and has formed a hard distension in the lower abdomen. If the patient's urination was normal, he can recover after discharging blood clots. Didang Tang (Appropriate Decoction) is a curative.

太陽病六七日表證因在脈微而沈反不結胸其人如狂者以熱在下焦小腹當滿小便自利者下血乃愈抵當湯主之

8　In the greater yang pattern, jaundiced skin, manic behavior, a hard distension in the lower abdomen and normal urination are the symptoms and signs of blood stasis. Didang Tang will be the curative. If a patient with an exogenous febrile disease caused by cold has a distension of the lower abdomen, there ought to be dysuria. However, if the patient's urination is normal, he has blood stasis.

太陽證身黃發狂小腹硬滿小便自利者血證宜抵當湯傷寒小腹滿應小便不利今反利者以有血也

9　Before the greater yang disease is gone, pathogenic heat congeals in the urinary bladder, and then the patient turns manic. The disease is gone when blood is passed. If the patient feels tightness and pain in the lower abdomen below the umbilicus, a purgative, Taoren Chengqi Tang (Peach Pit Decoction for Purgation), can be used.

太陽病不解熱結膀胱其人如狂血自下者自愈但小腹急結者宜攻之宜桃仁承氣湯

10　For the greater yang disease, there will be repeated diarrheas if purgatives are used several times before the exterior pattern disperses. This shows that the exterior and interior patterns still remain with hardness and stagnancy at the esophagus. Renshen Guizhi Tang (Ginseng and Cinnamon Twig Decoction) can be adopted as a curative.

太陽病外證未除而數下之遂下利不止心下痞硬表裏不解人蔘桂枝湯主之

11　I have said, "The cause of the mania mentioned above is Kidney yang confronted by the heat. Meanwhile, the hardness and fullness in the lower abdomen indicates that his large intestine is averse to cold. When these two symptoms co-exist, we must treat the most urgent case first. If the former is urgent, the ascending supplement of Cheongung Gyeji Tang, Hwanggi Gyeji Tang and Palmul Gunja Tang (Decoction of Eight Noble Ingredients) should be prescribed; if the latter is urgent, regulating with Gwakhyang Jeonggi San and Hyangsa Yangwi Tang (Nourish the Stomach Decoction with Auklandia and Amomum) should be adopted. If the exterior heat embraces the interior cold, then the poisonous qi gathers inside, becoming stronger as when one raises a tiger to know disaster later. If so, we must use Padu Dan (Crotonis Fructus Pill) to induce a bit of diarrheas, then give Gwakhyang Jeonggi San and Palmul Gunja Tang, which are regulating and strong tonifying drugs."

論曰此證其人如狂者腎陽困熱也小腹硬滿者大腸怕寒也二證俱見當先其急腎陽困熱則當用川芎桂枝湯黃芪桂枝湯八物君子湯升補之大腸怕寒則當用藿香正氣散香砂養胃湯和解之若外熱包裹冷而毒氣重結於內或將有養虎遺患之獘則當用巴豆丹下利一二度因以藿香正氣散八物君子湯和解而峻補之

12　What Zhang Zhongjing referred to, as a blood disease of the lower-*jiao* is the same as the pattern of the lesser yin patient whose Spleen yang qi is covered by cold and whose Kidney yang qi is obstructed by a pathogenic factor. Thus, the yang qi cannot go straight up to connect with the Spleen and is contracted in the bladder. "The manic behavior" means to speak in a confused state. "Having met a ghost" means emotional excitement and delirium. "The exterior pattern of the greater yang disease still remains" means that the patient sometimes has the symptoms of fever with uneasiness and chills. "The exterior pattern of the greater yang disease is dispersed" means that the patient has no symptoms of fever with uneasiness and chills. The best way to treat this disease is to supplement the qi and to help the yang ascend, but to remove the blood stasis and to dispel the fever is not a good idea. Diarrhea caused by treatment with the purgative method described earlier indicates that treating the patients, who display the exterior symptoms of the greater yang disease, with Chengqi Tang (Decoction for Purgation) is not suitable. Rather, one should replace it with Didang Tang or Taoren Tang (Peach Pit Decoction). While the exterior symptoms of the greater yang disease still remain, the yang qi is capable of fighting the pathogenic cold at the exterior level, although it is somewhat weakened. If the exterior symptoms have passed completely, then the yang qi is too weak to fight with the cold anymore. Finally, the yang qi is forced down by the cold. For this situation, how is it possible that purgative drugs are considered the ideal treatment? We do not have to wait until the yang qi reaches this stage to treat at with Renshen Guizhi Tang. By then, it is too late, is it not?

張仲景所論下焦血證卽少陰人脾局陽氣爲寒邪所掩抑而腎局陽氣爲邪所拒不能直升連接於脾局鬱縮膀胱之證也其人如狂者其人亂言也如見鬼狀者怳惚譫語也太陽病表證因在者身熱煩惱而惡寒之證間有之也太陽病外證除者身熱煩惱而惡寒之證都無之也此證益氣而升陽則得其上策也破血而解熱則出於下計也太陽病外證未除而數下之逐下利不止云云者亦可見古人之於此證用承氣湯則下利不止故逐變其方而用抵當桃仁湯耳太陽病外證未除則陽氣其力雖有鬱抑猶能振寒而與寒邪相爭於表也若外證盡除則陽氣其力不能振寒而逐爲窮困縮伏之勢也攻下之藥何甚好藥而必待陽氣窮困縮伏之時而應用耶人蔘桂枝湯不亦晚乎

13 Zhang Zhongjing mentioned the febrile disease for women caused by the cold: At the onset of menstruation, the patient is feverish, delirious and insane at night, but returns to consciousness in the day. These are the symptoms of heat entering the blood chamber. Be careful not to disturb the stomach vital qi and the upper-middle-*jiao*. Self-healing will occur.

張仲景曰婦人傷寒發熱經水適來斷晝日明了夜則譫語如見鬼狀此爲熱入血室無犯胃氣及上二焦必自愈

14 Yang brightness disease: Even though the patient has a parched throat with a thirst for water, if he can only hold the water in his mouth and cannot swallow, then certainly he has epistaxis. Do not use a purgative.

陽明病口燥嗽水不欲嚥此必衄不下

15 Yang brightness disease: If the remedy of heat-elimination is adopted when anorexia is observed, hiccupping will occur. During the febrile disease caused by cold, if the patient has repeated nausea and vomiting, a purgative is prohibited, even though the yang brightness pattern is observed. *Weijiashi* (Excess of the stomach and intestines) with constipation indicates that the exterior symptoms are not gone or the pattern is half-exterior. A purgative will be applicable after regulation is achieved by taking Cinnamomi Ramulus and Bupleuri Radix .

陽明病不能食攻其熱必噦傷寒嘔多雖有陽明不可攻胃家實不大便若表未解及有半表者先以桂枝柴胡和解乃可下也

16 I have said, "The pattern mentioned above should be treated with Gwakhyang Jeonggi San, Hyangsa Yangwi Tang and Palmul Gunja Tang."

論曰右諸證當用藿香正氣散香砂養胃湯八物君子湯

17 Zhang Zhongjing said, "The cause of the yang brightness disease is the excess of the stomach and intestines." One asked, "How does the yang brightness disease come into being?" Zhang Zhongjing answered, "When a diaphoretic, a purgative, or a diuretic is adopted for the greater yang disease, it will cause a loss of body fluid; and if the stomach is suffering from pathogenic dryness, then the disease transforms into the yang brightness. The patient suffering from interior excess will not change clothes (make stools) and experience constipation. What is described above is the so-called yang brightness disease."

張仲景曰陽明之爲病胃家實也問曰緣何得陽明病答曰太陽病發汗若下若利小便者此亡津液胃中乾燥因轉屬陽明不更衣內實大便難者此名陽明病也

18 If the exogenous febrile disease caused by cold changes into yang brightness, then a continuous light perspiration making the body wet will show itself; hence, the body becomes wet.

傷寒轉屬陽明其人濈然微汗出也

19 The exogenous febrile disease caused by cold: The pattern is not gone after the adoption of an emetic or a purgative. There is no stool for five to six days, or even ten days, with tidal fever in the afternoon, but no chills. The patient speaks to himself in an insane manner, as though he were observing ghosts. In a serious case, the patient unconsciously gropes at his clothes and bed in terror. He also has a slight dyspnea and stares out into nothingness. A tight pulse will indicate a curable case, while a hesitant pulse is the sign of a fatal case.

傷寒若吐若下後不解不大便五六日至十餘日日晡所發潮熱不惡寒狂言如見鬼狀若劇者發則不識人循衣摸床惕而不安微喘直視脈弦者生脈濇者死

20 I have said, "When a doctor of the Chin-Han dynasties treated constipation, there was Rhei Radix et Rhizoma treatment, but no Crotonis Fructus treatment. So Zhang Zhongjing also used Da Chengqi Tang (Drastic Purgative Decoction), which contains Rhei Radix et Rhizoma to treat a lesser yin patient who has the yang brightness disease transmitted from the greater yang disease. When a patient has continuous light perspiration, no stool for five to six days, or for even longer than ten days, due to dryness, fidgetiness and excessiveness of the stomach, tidal fever in the afternoon, but no chills, and speaks to himself in an insane manner, as though he were observing ghosts, the decoction will bring about a dramatic recovery. However, if the patient's condition is serious, he loses consciousness and gropes at his clothes and bed in terror, has a slight dyspnea and stares out into nothingness. After taking this decoction, if his pulse is tight, he will survive, while a hesitant pulse is the sign of a fatal case. This decoction can be applied to lesser yin patients who have had no stool for five to six days

with tidal fever in the afternoon as a result of the yang brightness disease transmitted from the greater yang disease. Zhang Zhongjing knew when to use this drug. Hence, he also knew that the symptoms and signs which show the transmission of the yang brightness disease from the greater yang disease in a lesser yin person. Zhang Zhongjing devoted his energy to determining the most suitable time to use Da Chengqi Tang in the treatment of this disease. Hence, he also knew when not to use this decoction. He found out that Guizhi Tang and Renshen Guizhi Tang are the only suitable drugs in the treatment of the greater yang and yang brightness diseases. To use this Da Chengqi Tang is like leaving the patient up to fate on the endless seaside (or the vast barren wasteland), waiting until the decoction can be used. In using Da Chengqi Tang, you must wait until the patient has had no stool for five to six days, with tidal fever in the afternoon, and speaks to himself in an insane manner. How can it be said that this is an ideal treatment? Generally, if a lesser yin person has no spontaneous perspiration, his Spleen is not weak. Difficulties in defecation and dry stool indicate that his stomach is excess. That the lesser yin person with the greater yang and yang brightness diseases has no spontaneous perspiration means his Spleen is in fine condition. In this case, the illness is not so severe, even though the stools are very hard. There are drugs available to treat this condition easily. Rhei Radix et Rhizoma, Aurantii Fructus immaturus, Magnoliae officinalis Cortex, and Natrii Sulfas are suitable for this case. In patients whose conditions are even more serious, there is only a fifty-percent chance of survival. When the condition is serious, we use Palmul Gunja Tang and Seungyang Ikgi Tang with Padu Dan. The result is dependent upon the following principles that in the case his pulse is tight, then he will survive, while a hesitant pulse is the sign of a fatal case. When the exterior symptoms of the greater yang disease remain, why do we not use the tonifying treatments to prevent and treat? For example, Crotonis Fructus, a drug warm in nature and in vital function invigorating. Why should we wait till the occurrence of the yang brightness disease, which is accompanied by the tidal fever in the afternoon, and the patient speaks to himself in an insane manner? If Chengqi Tang is used, there is only a fifty percent chance of survival."

論曰秦漢時醫方治法大便秘燥者有大黃治法無巴豆治法故張仲景亦用大黃大承氣湯治少陰人太陽病轉屬陽明其人濈然微汗出胃中燥煩實不大便五六日至十餘日日晡發潮熱不惡寒狂言如見鬼狀之時而用之則神效若劇者發則不識人循衣摸床惕而不安微喘直視用之於此則脈弦者生脈濇者死盖此方治少陰人太陽病轉屬陽明不大便五六日日晡發潮熱者可用而其他則不可用也仲景知此方有可用不可用之時候故亦能昭詳少陰人太陽陽明病證候也盖仲景一心精力都在於探得大承氣湯可用時候故不可用之時候亦昭詳知之也仲景太陽陽明病藥方中惟桂枝湯人蔘桂枝湯得其彷彿而大承氣湯則置人死生於茫無津涯之中必求大承氣湯可用之時候而待其不大便五六日日晡發潮熱狂言時是豈美法也哉盖少陰人病候自汗不出則脾不弱也大便秘燥則胃實也少陰人太陽陽明病自汗不出脾不弱者輕病也大便雖硬用藥則易愈也故大黃枳實厚朴芒硝之藥亦能成功於此時而劇者猶有半生半死若用八物君子湯升陽益氣湯與巴豆丹則雖劇者亦無脈弦者生脈濇者死之理也又太陽病表證因在時何不早用溫補升陽之藥與巴豆預圖其病而必待陽明病日晡發潮熱狂言時用承氣湯使人半生半死耶

21 In the 『*Benshifang*』3) ("Effective Prescriptions"), Xu Shuwei4) said, "There was a patient suffering from the febrile disease caused by cold who had dyspnea, tachypnea, difficulty in defecation, tidal fever recurring daily in the afternoon, and groping at his clothes, waving his hands in the air, looking straight ahead. Many doctors came to see him, but the patient's condition was very bad. Zhang Zhongjing wrote down these symptoms, but mentioned no effective treatment. He just said, 'The tight pulse indicates life, while the hesitant pulse indicates death.' At that time, I gave one pack of Xiao Chengqi Tang (Mild Purgative Decoction). Afterwards, he had a bowel movement, his symptoms began to disappear gradually, and his pulse also showed slight tautness. In a fortnight, he had completely recovered."

許叔微本事方曰一人病傷寒大便不利日晡發潮熱手循衣縫兩手撮空直視喘急諸醫皆走此誠惡候仲景雖有證而無法但云脈弦者生脈濇者死謾且救之與小承氣湯一服而大便利諸疾漸退脈且微弦半月愈

22 In the 『*Haizangshu*』5) ("Book of Haizang"), Wang Haogu said, "Once there was a patient suffering from the disease caused by cold who became insane enough with emotional excitement to run away, and had a weak, but rapid pulse. His condition worsened after he took Chaihu Tang (Decoction of Bupleuri Radix). Then he was treated with one pack of Ginseng Radix, Astragali Radix, Angelicae Gigantis Radix, Atractylodis Rhizoma Alba, Citri Reticulatae Pericarpium, and Glycyrrhizae Radix et Rhizoma decoction, his condition stabilized, and with one more dose, he slept soundly and was cured."

王好古海藏書曰一人傷寒發狂欲走脈虛數用柴胡湯反劇以蔘芪歸尤陳皮甘草煎湯一服狂定再服安睡而愈

23 In the 『*Yixue Gangmu*』6) ("Compendium of Medicine"), we read, "I have used qi invigorator and blood invigorator to cure some patients displaying symptoms of groping at their clothes and bed; only one of them showed eyelid fasciculation and arrhythmia. I treated him with the same drugs, adding Cinnamomi Ramulus, after which the symptoms subsided."

醫學綱目曰嘗治循衣摸床者數人皆用大補氣血之劑惟一人兼瞤振脈代遂於補劑中畧加桂亦振止脈和而愈

24 In the 『*Minglilun*』7) ("Expounding on the Treatise"), Cheng Wuji said, "The tidal fever is a symptom of yang brightness disease, but only the fever occurring in the afternoon can be called the tidal fever. The yang brightness disease means the excess of the stomach and intestines. If there was the excess of the stomach and intestines, the patient shows symptoms of delirium and sticky perspiration on the hands and feet, accompanied by hard stool. If a patient displays the symptoms of delirious speech and tidal fever, we may give him Chengqi Tang, but if the fever is not recurring tidal in the afternoon, the purgative must not be taken."

成無己明理論曰潮熱屬陽明必於日晡時發者乃爲潮熱也陽明之爲病胃家實也胃實則譫語手足濈

然汗出者此大便已硬也譫語有潮熱承氣湯下之熱不潮者勿服

25 In the 『*Danxi Xinfa*』8) ("Danxi's Experiential Therapy"), Zhu Zhenheng said, "Whenever a deteriorated case of febrile disease caused by cold went into a coma, the nearly dying patient was made to drink 37.5g of Ginseng Radix boiled in water. Sweat then began to run down from the bridge of his nose."

朱震亨丹溪心法曰傷寒壞證昏沈垂死一切危急之證好人蔘一兩水煎一服而盡汗自鼻梁上出涓涓如水

26 I have said, "The discussions above indicate the difficulties in knowing when to use Da Chengqi Tang, so Zhang Zhongjing's Da Chengqi Tang cannot be relied upon. As shown already, there has been much confusion caused by his words. Zhang Zhongjing's Da Chengqi Tang might kill a person instead of curing him, so it should not be emphasized. The excess of the stomach and intestines, including difficulty in defecation and madness, should be treated with either whole Crotonis Fructus or Doksam Palmul Gunja Tang (Decoction of Eight Noble Ingredients with Heavy Dose of Ginseng Radix), or use Crotonis Fructus first, then add Palmul Gunja Tang."

論曰右論皆以張仲景大承氣湯始作俑而可用不可用時候難知故紛紜多惑而始知張仲景之不可信也張仲景大承氣湯元是殺人之藥而非活人之藥則大承氣湯不必舉論此胃家實病不更衣發狂證當用巴豆全粒或用獨蔘八物君子湯或先用巴豆後用八物君子湯以壓之

27 Zhang Zhongjing said, "The exterior symptoms of the yang brightness disease are fever, spontaneous perspiration with an aversion to heat during fever, but no chills."

張仲景曰陽明病外證身熱汗自出不惡寒反惡熱

28 Yang brightness disease caused by cold: If a patient has spontaneous perspiration and frequent urination, then the loss of body fluid will result in constipation and *piyue* (Spleen restriction). Maren Wan (Hemp Seed Pill) will be a curative.

傷寒陽明病自汗出小便數則津液內竭大便必難其脾為約麻仁丸主之

29 Yang brightness disease with spontaneous perspiration and normal urination will induce the exhaustion of the body fluid. Although there is constipation, no purgative should be adopted. Honey can be used as a constipation-dredging medication.

陽明病自汗出小便自利者此為津液內竭大便雖硬不可攻之宜用蜜導法通之

30 Da Chengqi Tang should be adopted immediately against yang brightness disease with fever and profuse sweating.

陽明病發熱汗多者急下之宜大承氣湯

31 In the 『*Yixue Rumen*』9) ("Introduction to Medicine"), Li Chan said, "If the sweating cannot be stopped, it is called yang collapse. If symptoms such as a feeling of stuffiness in the esophageal region, vexation in the chest, pale complexion, and twitching of muscles appear, the disease is difficult to treat. If the skin has a yellowish complexion and the limbs feel warm, the patient can be cured. When the sweating cannot be stopped, and genuine yang is lost, it is called yang collapse, and the body must be made cold. Numbness with coldness and contraction of the four limbs will appear, so Guizhi Fuzi Tang should be used."

李梴醫學入門曰汗多不止謂之亡陽如心痞胸煩面青膚瞤者難治色黃手足溫者可治凡汗漏不止眞陽脫亡故謂之亡陽其身必冷多成痺寒四肢拘急桂枝附子湯主之

32 Once, I treated an 11 year old lesser yin child who had yang collapse from too much sweating. He was always thinking seriously and suffered from diarrheas for a long time, and had heavy facial sweating at every meal. One day, headache, fever, spontaneous perspiration and constipation occurred suddenly. Since I was anxious about his frequent diarrheas, I didn't pay attention to the febrile symptoms such as headache, fever, constipation and perspiration, and just tried to dispel the exterior patterns with Astragali Radix, Cinnamomi Ramulus, and Paeoniae Radix Alba, etc. Four to five days after the treatment, the headache and fever had not disappeared. On the sixth day, I carefully observed his symptoms. The constipation lasted for four to five days. He urinated uncomfortably only two to three spoons of reddish urine two to three times a day. There were no chills with fever, and two to four times a day, he perspired over his face and whole body, and sometimes on the Renzhong (GV 26) point. The symptom was very serious, and I noticed that he got yang collapse from too much sweating. This pattern was very serious, so I prescribed one bean of Crotonis Fructus and Hwanggi Gyeji Buja Tang (Decoction of Astragali Radix, Cinnamomi Ramulus, and Aconiti Lateralis Radix Praeparata), and he took two packs continuously. Later, at two o'clock in the afternoon, he had bowel movements and his urine became clean and slightly increased. The next day was the seventh day after the onset, and since I worried that he had taken too much Aconiti Lateralis Radix Praeparata, I prescribed one pack of Hwanggi Gyeji Buja Tang for two days. Two days later, yang collapse symptoms such as fever with no chills, profuse sweating, reddish and difficult urination, and constipation, a bluish face, and an intermittent tight cough appeared. His symptoms became more serious than before. It was around ten o'clock on the ninth day. Quickly, I gave him one bean of Crotonis Fructus and two packs of Insam Gyeji Buja Tang containing 18.75g of Ginseng Radix and 7.5g of Aconiti Lateralis Radix Praeparata continuously. In the afternoon, bowel movement was possible, urination slightly increased, and the color of the urine was red, the same as before. Another pack of Insam Gyeji Buja Tang containing 18.75g of Ginseng Radix and 7.5g of Aconiti Lateralis Radix Praeparata was taken again. At midnight, the child was lying down laterally and could not raise his head. He vomited one or two spoonfuls of sputum, and consequently the tight coughing stopped. The next day, he took three packs of Insam Gyeji Buja Tang with 18.75g of Ginseng Radix and 7.5g

of Aconiti Lateralis Radix Praeparata, and ate two or three spoonfuls of rice gruel. After each administration, he felt comfortable, stopped sweating, urinated a little more than before, and experienced no more constipation. The next day, he took another two packs, and could eat half a bowl of rice gruel. The next day, he took two more packs, and could eat more than half a bowl of rice gruel, felt comfortable without fever, and could move about in his house. It was the twelfth day after onset. During the last three days, the reason for his body experiencing no fever, no sweating, no constipation, and clean and fluent urine was due to taking 7.5g of Aconiti Lateralis Radix Praeparata two or three times a day. On the thirteenth day, he walked down to the garden, but he could not keep his head upright. Since I worried that he had taken too much Aconiti Lateralis Radix Praeparata, I gave him Hwanggi Gyeji Buja Tang, including 3.75g of Aconiti Lateralis Radix Praeparata only twice a day. After seven to eight days, he could bring his head into a slightly upright position and his facial edema was relieved. Thus, the same drug was used twice per day. After seven to eight days, he could put his head upright and his facial edema became milder than before. Afterwards, two packs of the drug were used every day. From the beginning, he took about 300g of Aconiti Lateralis Radix Praeparata for a month or more.

嘗治少陰人十一歲兒汗多亡陽病此兒勞心焦思素證有時以泄瀉爲憂而每飯時汗流滿面矣忽一日頭痛發熱汗自出大便秘燥以此兒素證泄瀉爲憂故頭痛身熱便秘汗出之熱證以其反於泄瀉寒證而曾不關心尋常治之以黃芪桂枝白芍藥等屬發表矣至于四五日頭痛發熱不愈六日平明察其證候則大便燥結已四五日小便赤澁二三匙而一晝夜間小便度數不過二三次不惡寒而發熱汗出度數則一晝夜間二三四次不均而人中則或有時有汗或有時無汗汗流滿面滿體其證可惡始覺汗多亡陽證候眞是危證也急用巴豆一粒仍煎黃芪桂枝附子湯用附子一錢連服二貼以壓之至于未刻大便通小便稍清而稍多其翌日卽得病七日也以小兒附子太過之慮故以黃芪桂枝附子湯一貼分兩日服矣兩日後其兒亡陽證又作不惡寒發熱汗多而小便赤澁大便秘結如前面色帶靑間有乾咳病勢比前太甚其日卽得病九日也時則巳時末刻也急用巴豆一粒仍煎人蔘桂枝附子湯用人蔘五錢附子二錢連二貼以壓之至于日晡大便始通小便稍多而色赤則一也又用人蔘桂枝附子湯人蔘五錢附子二錢一貼服矣至于二更夜其兒側臥而頭不能舉自吐痰一二匙而乾咳仍止其翌日又用人蔘桂枝附子湯人蔘五錢附子二錢三貼食粥二三匙每用藥後則身清凉無汗小便稍多而大便必通又翌日用此方二貼食粥半碗又翌日用此方二貼食粥半碗有餘身清凉自起坐房室中此日卽得病十二日也此三日內身清凉無汗大便通小便清而多者連用附子二錢日二三貼之故也至于十三日又起步門庭而舉頭不能仰面懲前小兒附子太過之慮用黃芪桂枝附子湯用附子一錢每日二貼服至于七八日頭面稍得仰舉而面部浮腫又每日二貼服至于七八日頭面又得仰舉而面部浮腫亦減其後用此方每日二貼服自得病初至於病解前後一月餘用附子凡八兩矣

33 Zhang Zhongjing said, "There are three types of the yang brightness disease. *Piyue* (Spleen restriction) is called the yang brightness disease of the greater yang. The excess of the stomach and intestines is called the yang brightness disease of the yang brightness. The yang brightness disease of the lesser yang, which is caused by the adoption of a diaphoretic and a diuretic, manifests itself as dryness, fidgetiness and excessiveness of the stomach with constipation."

張仲景曰陽明病有三病太陽陽明者脾約是也正陽陽明者胃家實是也少陽陽明者發汗利小便胃中燥煩實大便難是也

34 I have said, "Among the three types of the yang brightness disease mentioned by Zhang Zhongjing, the first one is the Spleen restriction, which displays symptoms such as spontaneous perspiration and smooth urination. The second one is the excess of the stomach and intestines, which contains symptoms such as the inability to change clothes and difficulty in defecation. The third one has symptoms such as dryness, fidgetiness and excessiveness of the stomach due to the adoption of a diaphoretic and a diuretic. This also belongs to the excess of the stomach and intestines, so there are not three, but only two types. Zhang Zhongjing regarded the Spleen restriction as the gradual decrease of body fluid, and the excess of the stomach and intestines as the dryness and excessiveness of the whole stomach region as the body fluid becomes exhausted. During the ancient middle ages, e.g. Warring States and Chin-Han dynasties, diaphoretic, emetic and purgative treatment began to be widely used after a long period of experiments using simpler drugs. For the exterior patterns of the greater yang disease, one might use Mahuang Tang (Ephedra Decoction) to induce sweating, or Zhuling Tang (Polyporus Decoction) to induce smoother urination, or Chengqi Tang (Purgative Decoction) to induce defecation. Inducing defecation by Chengqi Tang may cause unceasing diarrheas. Taking Mahuang Tang and Zhuling Tang, which induce sweating and urination, will cause dryness, fidgetiness and excessiveness of the stomach with constipation. Zhang Zhongjing thought that the gradual restriction of Spleen fluid induced by the spontaneous perspiration and the smooth urination of the Spleen restriction turned into dryness, fidgetiness and excessiveness of stomach. However, the Spleen restriction comes from the Spleen restriction, and the excess of the stomach and intestines comes from the excess of the stomach and intestines. It is unreasonable to assume that Spleen restriction should induce the excess of the stomach and intestines."

論曰張仲景所論陽明三病一曰脾約者自汗出小便利之證也二曰胃家實者不更衣大便難之證也三曰發汗利小便胃中燥煩實者此亦胃家實也其實非三病也二病而已仲景意脾約云者津液漸竭脾之潤氣漸約之謂也胃家實云者津液已竭胃之全局燥實之謂也中古戰國秦漢之時醫家單方經驗其來已久汗吐下三法始爲盛行太陽病表證因在者或以麻黃湯發汗或以猪苓湯利小便或以承氣湯下之承氣湯下之則下利不止之證作矣麻黃湯猪苓湯發汗利小便則胃中燥煩實大便難之證作矣仲景有見於此故以脾約之自汗出自利小便者脾之潤氣漸約亦將爲胃燥實之張本矣然脾約自脾約也胃家實自胃家實也寧有其病先自脾約而後至於胃家實之理耶

35 The excess of the stomach and intestines and the Spleen restriction are as different from each other as the deficient and excessive symptoms of greater yin and lesser yin disease, which belong to the yin pattern. At the exterior pattern of the greater yang disease, they have already separated into their own paths and cannot be remingled. When the exterior pattern of the greater yang disease still remains and the patient behaves in a manic way, it is the initial stage

symptoms of *yukuang* (oppressive mania). The inability to experience a bowel movement due to yang brightness disease with excess of the stomach and intestines belongs to the midstage symptoms of oppressive mania. Yang brightness disease with tidal fever, manic speech, minor dyspnea, and staring straight are the terminal stage symptoms of oppressive mania. Greater yang disease with fever, chills, and spontaneous perspiration is the initial stage of yang collapse. Yang brightness disease with no chills, but rather an aversion to heat, and spontaneous perspiration are the midstage symptoms of yang collapse. Yang brightness disease with fever and profuse sweating are the terminal stage symptoms of yang collapse. Generally, most oppressive mania symptoms include fever with no sweating, while most yang collapse symptoms include fever with spontaneous sweating.

胃家實脾約二病如陰證之太陰少陰病虛實證狀顯然不同自太陽病表證因在時已爲兩路分岐元不相合太陽病表證因在而其人如狂者鬱狂之初證也陽明病胃家實不更衣者鬱狂之中證也陽明病潮熱狂言微喘直視者鬱狂之末證也太陽病發熱惡寒汗自出者亡陽之初證也陽明病不惡寒反惡熱汗自出者亡陽之中證也陽明病發熱汗多者亡陽之末證也盖鬱狂證都是身熱自汗不出也亡陽證都是身熱自汗出也

36 Among the yin patterns, abdominal pain, diarrheas and the absence of abnormal sensation in the mouth are symptoms of the greater yin disease, while abnormal sensations in the mouth, abdominal pain and diarrheas are symptoms of the lesser yin disease. Among the yang patterns, no spontaneous perspiration with headaches and fever are the oppressive maniac patterns of the yang brightness disease of the greater yang, and spontaneous perspiration, headaches and fever are the yang collapse patterns of the yang brightness disease of the greater yang. Among the greater yin disease of yin pattern and the oppressive maniac disease of yang pattern, there are mild and severe symptoms. Among the lesser yin disease of yin pattern and the yang collapse disease of yang pattern, there are dangerous and critical symptoms, too. From the onset, yang collapse and the lesser yin disease already show a dangerous condition and which will grow increasingly critical.

陰證口中和而有腹痛泄瀉者太陰病也口中不和而有腹痛泄瀉者少陰病也陽證自汗不出而有頭痛身熱者太陽陽明病鬱狂證也自汗出而頭痛身熱者太陽陽明病亡陽證也陰證之太陰病陽證之鬱狂病有輕證重證也陰證之少陰病陽證之亡陽病有險證危證也亡陽少陰病自初痛已爲險證繼而危證也

37 Among the yang collapse symptoms, we should pay attention to the sweating, and, also, to the amount of urine. If there is clear and profuse urine flow and spontaneous perspiration, it belongs to the Spleen restriction. They are dangerous symptoms. If there is yang collapse with reddish and difficult urination and spontaneous perspiration, it belongs to the yang brightness disease with fever and profuse sweating. This too indicates a critical condition. However, there is also profuse sweating with reddish and difficult urination in the interior heat pattern of the lesser yang person and the exterior heat pattern of the greater yin person, so we should

differentiate those diseases and avoid adopting the wrong drugs.

亡陽病證非但觀於汗也必觀於小便多少也若小便清利而自汗出則脾約病也此險證也小便赤澁而自汗出則陽明病發熱汗多也此危證也然少陽人裡熱證太陰人表熱證亦有汗多而小便赤澁者宜察之不可誤藥

38 In the beginning of excess of the stomach and intestines, the symptoms are aversion to heat during fever, but no sweating or chills. When the condition becomes critical, there should be a little sticky sweating and tidal fever. A little sticky sweating and tidal fever indicate that the force dispersing and expelling the exterior cold evil is thoroughly exhausted. This is a sign of *weijie* (Stomach exhaustion). In the beginning of the Spleen restriction, the symptoms are fever, spontaneous sweating, but no chills. When the condition becomes critical, the patient should display symptoms such as fever, profuse sweating and chills. Fever, profuse sweating and chills indicate that the force supporting the interior heat is already exhausted; this is also a sign of *pijue* (Spleen failure).

胃家實病其始焉汗不出不惡寒但惡熱而其病垂危則濈然微汗出潮熱也濈然微汗出潮熱者表寒振發之力永竭故也胃竭之候也脾約病其始焉身熱汗自出不惡寒而若其病垂危則發熱汗多而惡寒也發熱汗多而惡寒者裏熱撑支之勢已窮故也脾絕之候也

39 Zhang Zhongjing mentioned, "The reverting yin pattern: Danggui Sini Tang (Tangkuei Decoction for Frigid Extremities) is the curative for a case of cold limbs, lower abdominal pain, restlessness and fullness in the chest, constriction of the scrotum, and a slender pulse that is hardly detectable."

張仲景曰厥陰證手足厥冷小腹痛煩滿囊縮脈微欲絕宜當歸四逆湯

40 When the yin qi and yang qi cannot connect with each other, *jue* (syncope) will occur. The symptoms of syncope are a feeling of coldness on the hands and feet.

凡厥者陰陽氣不相順接便爲厥厥者手足逆冷是也

41 Six to seven days after the onset of exogenous febrile disease caused by cold, if the *chi* (cubit) and *cun* (inch) pulses are slightly moderate, it is the stage of reverting yin. When the symptoms of reverting yin include fullness in the lower abdomen and constriction of the scrotum, Chengqi Tang may be used.

傷寒六七日尺寸脈微緩者厥陰受病也其證小腹煩滿而囊縮宜用承氣湯下之

42 Six to seven days after the onset of exogenous febrile disease caused by cold, if there is a big pulse, severe restlessness, stiffness of the mouth inducing an inability to speak and discomfort, he will certainly recover.

六七日脈至皆大煩而口噤不能言躁擾者必欲解也

43 In the 『*Huorenshu*』, Zhu Gong said, "When one's limbs are cold, it is called syncope. When the tips of one's fingers and toes are slightly cold, it is called 'cool' and is a mild case. If one gets yin syncope, from the beginning, one will have cold limbs, a deep, weak, slow pulse pattern, and the feet may tremble."

朱肱活人書曰厥者手足逆冷是也手足指頭微寒者謂之清此疾爲輕陰厥者初得病便四肢厥冷脈沈微而不數足多攣

44 Six to seven days after the onset of an exogenous febrile disease caused by cold, if there is restlessness and fullness in the chest, constriction of the scrotum and the inch and cubit pulses are moderate in nature; it means that the Liver meridian has been affected. If his pulse type is weak and floating, it indicates that he will recover; but if his pulse type is not floating, it indicates that his condition is difficult to cure. If his pulse type was floating and moderate, his scrotum is not constricted. If the patient had the exterior symptoms such as fever and chillness, his illness is about to be cured. Guima Geban Tang (Half and Half Combination of Guizhi Tang and Mahuang Tang) may be used. If his pulse type is deep and short on the inch and cubit, the scrotum constricts, and the toxic evil invades his abdomen, Chengqi Tang should be used. Emergency administration of Chengqi Tang could save five in six patients. When a patient's pulse type becomes weak and floating on the sixth and seventh day, it means the condition is one of going up of water and going down of fire, according to the following principle: "If the Pi (☷) goes to extremes, the Tai (☷) will come." He will be fine after some chills and fever with profuse sweating.

傷寒六七日煩滿囊縮尺寸俱微緩者足厥陰經受病也其脈微浮爲欲愈不浮爲難愈脈浮緩者必囊不縮外證必發熱惡寒爲欲愈宜桂麻各半湯若尺寸俱沈短者必囊縮毒氣入腹宜承氣湯下之速用承氣湯可保五生一死六七日脈微浮者否極泰來水升火降寒熱作而大汗解矣

45 A symptom such as cold limbs belongs to reverting yin, and we cannot adopt the diaphoretics and the purgative. However, the diaphoretics and the purgative can be used when the limbs of the patient get warm and the palms of the hands and feet feel warm from time to time. This is not *zhengjueni* (genuine cold limbs), so we must be careful.

諸手足逆冷皆屬厥陰不可汗下然有須汗須下者謂手足雖逆冷時有溫時手足掌心必煖非正厥逆當消息之

46 Li Chan said, "If there are symptoms such as curled tongue, coldness over the elbow and the knee, and colic pain in the lower abdomen, Sanwei Shenyu Tang (Decoction of Three Drugs including Ginseng and Evodia) and Sishun Tang (Decoction of Four Drugs for Favorable Condition) can be used. If there are symptoms such as constriction of the scrotum, alternating hot and cold limbs, and restlessness, Da Chengqi Tang may be used."

李梴曰舌卷厥逆冷過肘膝小腹絞痛三味蔘萸湯四順湯主之囊縮手足乍冷乍溫煩滿者大承氣湯主之

47 I have said, "The reverting yin disease, mentioned by Zhang Zhongjing, in which there is no abdominal pain or diarrhea at the onset, and sudden cold limbs on the sixth and seventh days, is not a case of yin pattern. For a lesser yin person, the greater yang disease caused by wind has symptoms such as chills, fever and spontaneous perspiration. These symptoms indicate a long-term conflict between the healthy qi and the pathogen. Eventually, this conflict brings about this pattern, and this should be called the reverting yin pattern of the greater yang disease. It is not suitable to use Danggui Sini Tang or Guima Geban Tang, but Shenyu Tang, Insam Osuyu Tang or Doksam Palmul Tang could be used. Da Chengqi Tang is not suitable, but Crotonis Fructus must be adopted."

論曰張仲景所論厥陰病初無腹痛下利等證而六七日猝然而厥手足逆冷則此非陰證之類也乃少陰人太陽傷風惡寒發熱汗自出之證正邪相持日久當解不解而變爲此證也此證當謂之太陽病厥陰證也此證不必用當歸四逆湯桂麻各半湯而當用蔘萸湯人蔘吳茱萸湯獨蔘八物湯不當用大承氣湯而當用巴豆

48 A lesser yin person who gets an exogenous disease and cannot sweat for six to seven days will die from the reverting yin disease. After careful observation of his condition for four to five days, if the patient takes three to five packs of Hwanggi Gyeji Tang and Palmul Gunja Tang, death will be prevented.

凡少陰人外感病六七日不得汗解而死者皆死於厥陰也四五日觀其病勢用黃芪桂枝湯八物君子湯三四五貼預防可也

49 Zhu Gong said, "The reverting yin disease displays the following symptoms: great thirst with frequent urination, an uncomfortable feeling of ascending qi rushing up from below the esophagus, a hot and painful feeling in the chest, and hunger without being able to take in food. Once food is taken, ascarides will be regurgitated."

朱肱曰厥陰病消渴氣上衝心心中疼熱飢不欲食食則吐蚘

50 Gong Xin said, "Avoid adopting a purgative for a patient who, while suffering from the exogenous febrile disease caused by cold, regurgitated ascarides, even though he has a high fever. If the drug, which induces the body cold, was used, he will die. If there is coldness in the stomach, the ascarides will ascend to the esophagus, a very bad sign, indeed. In this situation, Lizhong Tang (Decoction for Regulating the Middle) should be quickly adopted."

龔信曰傷寒有吐蚘者雖有大熱忌下凉藥犯之必死盖胃中有寒則蚘不安所而上膈大匈之兆也急用理中湯

51 I have said, "For the symptoms mentioned above, Lizhong Tang should be taken three to four times a day continuously, or Citri Reticulatae Pericarpium, Cinnamomi Cortex, and Polygoni multiflori Radix could be added."

論曰此證當用理中湯日三四服又連日服或理中湯加陳皮官桂白何烏

52 For a serious illness and critical symptoms, unless the patient takes the medicine three to four times a day, he cannot benefit from the full effect of the medicine; and if he takes the medicine continuously, he may recover somewhat, but not completely. Continuous taking means taking the medicine once to three times a day, and two to three days or five to six days or several months continuously. The amount of doses per day and the number of days during which the patient takes the medicine will vary according to the illness's progress.

重病危證藥不三四服則藥力不壯也又不連日服則病加於少愈也或病愈而不快也連日服者或日再服或日一服或日三服或二三日連日服或五六日連日服或數十日連日服觀其病勢圖之

Notes

1) 『*Dexiaofang*』(得效方)

The "Effective Formulas", also called the 『*Shiyi Dexiaofang*』(世醫得效方: "Effective Formulas Tested by Physicians for Generations"), compiled by Wei Yilin (危亦林) in 1345 A.D., is based on the author's family experiences as physicians for five successive generations, and in which the contents are prescriptions for children's disease, internal medicine, ophthalmology, oral disease, dentistry, bone setting, war wounds, ulcers and carbuncles.

2) 『*Yijian*』(醫鑑)

The "Mirror of Medicine", also called the 『*Yijianshu*』(醫鑑書), a comprehensive medical work by Gong Xin and Gong Tingxian; it was later supplemented by Wang Kentang (王肯堂). It deals with the theories from the time of 『*Neijing*』and 『*Nanjing*』to the Jin-Yuan (金元) dynasties' schools. It covers the methods of using acupuncture and moxibustion, and lists many prescriptions.

3) 『*Benshifang*』(本事方)

The "Effective Prescriptions", also called the 『*Leizheng Puji Benshifang*』(類證普濟本事方: "Classified Effective Prescriptions for Universal Relief"), is a work of ten volumes written by Xu Shuwei (許叔微) in the Southern Song (南宋) dynasty and published in the middle of the 12th century. This text mainly deals with common diseases related to internal medicine, listing 23 kinds of treatment with more than 300 prescriptions. At the end of each prescription, the authors' proven cases are described.

4) Xu Shuwei (許叔微)

(1079~1154 A.D.) A famous physician in the Song dynasty and a close follower of Zhang Zhongjing. Xu prepared graphic illustrations of thirty six varieties of pulse based on Zhang Zhongjing's work, and propounded the theory of using drugs in relation to the intensity of the disease. Xu was the author of several medical works, among which 『*Leizheng Puji Benshifang*』in ten volumes has been one of his most widely read.

5) 『*Haizangshu*』(海藏書)

Haizang is Wang Haogu's other name. See Wang Haogu.

6) 『*Yixue Gangmu*』(醫學綱目)

The "Compendium of Medicine", a comprehensive medical work by Lou Ying (樓英) in forty volumes. He gathered many traditional medicine treatises and descriptions to support his opinions. The scope of this work is very broad. It is well organized and the explanations to the descriptions are precise.

7) 『*Minglilun*』 (明理論)

The "Expounding on the Treatise" (1156) written by Cheng Wuji (成無己) in the Jin (金) dynasty, is a concise reference book for beginners studying the 『*Shanghanlun*』, in which the ideas related to the compatibility of ingredients are stressed.

8) 『*Danxi Xinfa*』 (丹溪心法)

The "Danxi's Experiential Therapy" was written by Zhu Zhenheng (朱震亨) in the Yuan (元) dynasty, but rearranged and edited by his disciples. In 1481 A.D., the book was reedited with supplements and corrections by Cheng Chong (程充), who added six treatises on medical theories and 100 articles dealing with various diseases, most of which are concerned with internal medicine. The author's theory that "Yang is ever excessive and yin is ever deficient" is reflected throughout the book.

9) 『*Yixue Rumen*』 (醫學入門)

The "Introduction to Medicine", a comprehensive medical work written by Li Chan in 1575. The book covers basic medical theories, explanatory diagrams of meridians, internal organs, diagnosis, acupuncture and moxibustion, herbal drugs, infection due to both exogenic and endogenic pathogens, internal medicine, gynecology, pediatrics, surgery, etc.

Discourse on the Lesser Yin Person's Interior Cold Disease Induced from the Stomach Affected by Cold

少陰人胃受寒裏寒病論

1 Zhang Zhongjing said, "The symptoms of the greater yin disease are abdominal distension with vomiting, anorexia, and worsening diarrheas with occasional abdominal pain."
張仲景曰太陰之證腹滿而吐食不下自利益甚時腹自痛

2 Abdominal distension, pain that appears time and again, vomiting and diarrheas without thirst are symptoms of the greater yin disease. Sini Tang (Frigid Extremities Decoction) or Lizhong Tang should be adopted. When abdominal distension is not reduced, or not significantly reduced, Da Chengqi Tang should be used.
腹滿時痛吐利不渴者爲太陰宜四逆湯理中湯腹滿不減減不足言宜大承氣湯

3 Diarrhea without thirst in a febrile disease caused by cold is symptomatic of the greater yin disease. It is caused by coldness in the viscera. Sini Tang should be adopted to warm the viscera.
傷寒自利不渴者屬太陰以其藏有寒故也當溫之宜用四逆湯

4 For the treatment of the greater yin pattern, accompanied by abdominal pain and diarrheas without thirst, Lizhong Tang, Lizhong Wan or Sishun Lizhong Tang or Wan also can be adopted.
太陰證腹痛自利不渴宜理中湯理中丸四順理中湯丸亦主之

5 I have said, "For the symptoms mentioned above, Lizhong Tang, Sishun Lizhong Tang and Sini Tang may be used. Since they originated in the early stage of ancient times by Zhang

Zhongjing, they are not sufficiently effective. Thus, Baikhao Ijung Tang (White Flowery Knotweed Decoction for Regulating the Middle) and Baikhao Buja Ijung Tang (White Flowery Knotweed and Aconite Decoction for Regulating the Middle) should be used. The symptom of abdominal fullness, not reduced or significantly reduced, is due to an obstinate cold pattern and indigestion. In this case, Crotonis Fructus should be used, but not Da Chengqi Tang."

論曰右證當用理中湯四順理中湯四逆湯而古方草籵藥力不具備此證當用白何烏理中湯白何烏附子理中湯腹滿不減減不足言者有痼冷積滯也當用巴豆而不當用大承氣湯

6 Zhang Zhongjing said, "If a purgative is given as a remedy for the pattern originating from yin, *pi* (qi stagnancy) will take shape. If the patient has nausea and fever as a result of a febrile disease caused by cold, and the patient feels fullness at the esophagus, but no pain, it is qi stagnancy. Banxia Xiexin Tang (Pinellia Decoction to Drain the Epigastrium) is a curative. In case adverse gas ascends from the stomach caused by a grave deficiency, the above decoction is also applicable."

張仲景曰病發於陰而反下之因作痞傷寒嘔而發熱者若心下滿不痛此爲痞半夏瀉心湯主之胃虛氣逆者亦主之

7 The incorrect application of a purgative will result in repeated diarrheas of undigested cereals several dozen times a day. Other possibilities are a gurgling sound in the abdomen, fullness and hardness at the esophagus. Nausea and restlessness are also observed. The reason for the just mentioned symptoms is a congealing of pathogenic heat, and is the adverse gas ascending from the stomach caused by a grave deficiency. Gancao Xiexin Tang (Licorice Decoction to Drain the Epigastrium) is a curative.

下後下利日數十行穀不化腹雷鳴心下痞硬乾嘔心煩此乃結熱乃胃中虛客氣上逆故也甘草瀉心湯主之

8 If a diaphoretic is used as treatment for the greater yin pattern accompanied by diarrheas with undigested cereals, abdominal distention will certainly occur. In such a case, Houpo Banxia Tang (Magnolia Bark and Pinellia Decoction) should be used.

太陰證下利清穀若發汗則必脹滿發汗後腹脹滿宜用厚朴半夏湯

9 After dispelling the febrile disease caused by cold through perspiration, Shengjiang Xiexin Tang (Fresh Ginger Decoction to Drain the Epigastrium) suits the following symptoms and signs: uneasiness of the stomach, fullness and hardness in the epigastrium, water stagnancy below the costal margin, and diarrhea with a gurgling sound in the abdomen.

汗解後胃不和心下痞硬脇下有水氣腹中雷鳴下利者生薑瀉心湯主之

10 After taking the purgative, the patient who had a febrile disease caused by cold had continuing diarrheas, fullness and hardness in the epigastrium. After the adoption of Xiexin Tang

(Drain the Epigastrium Decoction) and other purgatives, continuous diarrheas occurred. Lizhong Tang was then given to stop the diarrheas, but the diarrheas became more serious. Chishizhi Yuyuliang Tang (Halloysite and Limonite Decoction) will be the curative.

傷寒下利心下痞硬服瀉心湯後以他藥下之利不止與理中湯利益甚赤石脂禹餘粮湯主之

11 I have said, "For the above-mentioned, the pattern originating from yin, for which a purgative is given as a remedy, is the same disease which results from the stomach with a grave deficiency. Huoxiang Zhengqi San should be used rather than purgation with Rhei Radix et Rhizoma. Ephedrae Herba and Rhei Radix et Rhizoma are the drugs for a greater yin person, not the lesser yin person. Thus, it is impossible to adopt Ephedrae Herba and Rhei Radix et Rhizoma for a lesser yin person's disease, whether exterior or interior pattern, to induce diaphoresis and purgative. A lesser yin person's disease with watery diarrheas and undigested food in the stool indicates that the congestion will be spontaneously cured. For watery diarrheas with undigested food in the stool of the greater yin disease, the following is recommended: Gwakhyang Jeonggi San, Hyangsa Yangwi Tang (Nourish the Stomach Decoction with Auklandia and Amomum) or Gangchul Gwanjung Tang (Decoction for Relieving the Middle with Zingiberis Rhizoma Recens and Atractylodis Rhizoma Alba) to warm the stomach and lower yin. For lesser yin disease, if watery diarrhea with undigested food in the stool appears, the following should be adopted: Gwangye Buja Ijung Tang (Cinnamon Bark and Aconite Decoction for Regulating the Middle) to invigorate the Spleen and lower yin."

論曰病發於陰而反下之云者病發於胃弱當用藿香正氣散而反用大黃下之之謂也麻黃大黃自是太陰人藥非少陰人藥則少陰人病無論表裏麻黃大黃汗下元非可論少陰人病下利淸穀者積滯自解也太陰證下利淸穀者當用藿香正氣散香砂養胃湯薑朮寬中湯溫胃而降陰少陰證下利淸穀者當用官桂附子理中湯健脾而降陰

12 Huoxiang Zhengqi San, Xiangsha Liujunzi Tang (Six-gentlemen Decoction with Auklandia and Amomum), Kuanzhong Tang and Suhe Yuan are the variations of Xiexin Tang created by Zhang Zhongjing. It is comparable to that brilliant blue which comes from indigo blue. Ah! Although the blue is brilliant by itself, it would not be so were it not for the indigo blue. How can the blue be so blue?

藿香正氣散香砂六君子湯寬中湯蘇合元皆張仲景瀉心湯之變劑也此所謂靑於藍者出於藍噫靑雖自靑若非其藍靑何得靑

13 Zhang Zhongjing said, "If a patient with *yindu* (yin type inflammatory swelling) of the febrile disease caused by cold had a bluish face and aching as if the patient were suffering a severe beating with sticks, within five days, the pattern is curable. After seven days, it is difficult to cure."

張仲景曰傷寒陰毒之病面靑身痛如被杖五日可治七日不治

14 Li Chan said, "When the disease of the three yin meridians becomes severe, it must change into yin type inflammatory swelling. The symptoms are coldness in the limbs, vomiting, diarrheas, no thirst, curling up while sleeping, and, in more serious cases, a sore throat, speaking incoherently in a state of unconsciousness, headaches, morbid perspiration on the head, intraocular pain, shying from light, a dark-green face, lips and nails, and severe ache of the body as if beaten by a club. This symptom includes a green, white or black face, coldness in the limbs, and somnolence."

李梴曰三陰病深必變爲陰毒其證四肢厥冷吐利不渴靜踡而臥甚則咽痛鄭聲加以頭痛頭汗眼睛內痛不欲見光面脣指甲靑黑身如被杖又此證面靑白黑四肢厥冷多睡

15 I have said, "The above symptoms should be treated with Renshen Guizhi Tang or Insam Buja Ijung Tang."

論曰右證當用人蔘桂皮湯人蔘附子理中湯

16 Zhang Zhongjing said, "When a febrile disease caused by cold attacks straight into the yin meridian, in the beginning, there is no headache, no fever and no thirst, but there is intolerance to cold, curling up while sleeping, heaviness, a tendency to fall asleep, bluish lips, cold limbs, and either a feeble and expiring pulse or a hiding pulse. For the above condition, Sini Tang should be used. 'Sini' means cold limbs."

張仲景曰傷寒直中陰經初來無頭痛無身熱無渴怕寒踡臥沈重欲眠脣靑厥冷脈微而欲絶或脈伏宜四逆湯四逆者四肢逆冷也

17 Once I treated a lesser yin person with dry cholera, obstruction and rejection (dysuria and constipation with incessant vomiting) induced by cold attacking straight into the yin meridian. It was during the height of the hot summer weather. The lesser yin person's face color was sometimes green or white and also had four or five pellet-sized spots. His daily activities were almost as usual, but when he sat in the room, he leaned against the wall with general weakness and a tendency towards drowsiness. When he was asked of the cause, he said that he had had watery diarrhea one or two times several days before, after experiencing constipation for two days. Besides that, there were no other problems. Being asked of his diet, he said he had been eating barley meal. When he was treated with Badou Ruyi Dan (Pills for Alleviation with Crotonis Fructus), sweat originating from the Renzhong point immediately covered his face, and he had loose stools one or two times after an hour and a half. I found that his green watery diarrhea was accompanied with some dregs when I saw his diarrhea at sunset. He had diarrheas ten or several more times at night. The next day, from early morning to nightfall, he had diarrheas ten or more times containing grains of barley like swollen yellow beans. Since his disease was induced by indigestion, I did not allow him to eat the following three days, except for one or two bowls of water boiled with burned rice every day. On the early morning of the third day, his face looked somewhat bright, and his body showed general coldness.

While sitting, his head and neck fell two to three inches from the ground, and he could not lift his head. His condition worsened. Examining the patient in detail, I found that his limbs, bladder, flank, abdomen were all cold as ice. The entire lower abdomen was hard as stone; however, the heat from his chest and abdomen upward to the Zhongwan region felt as if it could cauterize hands. His condition was a sight! On the early morning of the fifth day, there was an outbreak of vomiting of clear froth containing a bud of rice, after which the disease subsided considerably. He began to eat several bowls of thin rice gruel and took rice gruel in the next day. Since the patient was living in a poor mountain village, it was difficult for him to take the drugs that would warm the stomach and regulation. There was another lesser yin person who had diarrheas several times a day, and his diarrhea was like still clear water. He also had whole abdominal edema. At the beginning, he was treated with Gyebugwakjin Ijung Tang (Decoction of Regulating the Middle with Cinnamomi Cortex, Aconiti Lateralis Radix Praeparata, Agastachis Herba, and Citri Reticulatae Pericarpium), in addition to 7.5g of Ginseng Radix and Cinnamomi Cortex each, and 3.75g to 7.5g of Aconiti Lateralis Radix Praeparata four times a day. A few days later, it was taken three times a day for ten or more days. There was watery diarrhea with undigested food in the stool. He had bowel movements 30 to 40 times continuously over a three day period, and the edema markedly decreased. There was another lesser yin child who had green watery diarrheas with a dark-green face and exhaustion to the point of near-sleep. He was treated with Doksam Tang (Decoction with a Heavy Dose of Ginseng Radix), in addition to 7.5g of Zingiberis Rhizoma recens, 3.75g of Citri Reticulatae Pericarpium and 3.75g of Amomi Fructus. It was taken three or four times a day. After several days, he had diarrheas ten or more times, and was relieved by profuse sweating. It is considered that if the lesser yin person with dry cholera and obstruction and rejection had perspired at the Renzhong point, then he is on his way to being out of danger. When the patient with indigestion has massive diarrheas, he is further along in being saved from danger. When the patient vomits spontaneously, then he is saved from danger immediately. Not taking rice gruel or rice, but taking water boiled with burned rice or thin rice gruel is the best way of supporting healthy qi and inhibiting the pathogens. For the patient with indigestion to take warm water boiled with burned rice is good not only for digestion, but it can also be a substitute for regular foods. Though food is not ingested for two to four days, there is no need to worry.

論曰嘗治少陰人直中陰經乾霍亂關格之病時屬中伏節候少陰人一人面部氣色或靑或白如彈丸圈四五點成團起居如常而坐於房室中倚壁一身委靡無力而但欲寐問其這間原委則曰數日前下利淸水一二行仍爲便閉至今爲兩晝夜別無他故云問所飮食則曰食麥飯云急用巴豆如意丹一半時刻其汗自人中穴出而達於面上下利一二度時當日暮觀其下利則靑水中雜穢物而出終夜下利十餘行翌日平明至日暮又十餘行下利而淸穀麥粒皆如黃豆大其病爲食滯故連三日絶不穀食日所食但進好熟冷一二碗至第三日平明病人面色則無不顯明而一身皆冷頭頸墜下去地二三寸而不能仰擧病證更重計出無聊仔細點檢病人一身則手足膀胱腰腹皆如冰冷臍下全腹硬堅如石而胸腹上中元熱氣熏騰灸手可熱最爲可觀至第五日平朝一發吐淸沫而淸沫中雜米穀一朵而出自此病勢大減因進米

飲聯服數碗其翌日因爲粥食此病在窮村故未暇溫胃和解之藥其後又有少陰人一人日下利數次而仍下淸水全腹浮腫初用桂附藿陳理中湯倍加人蔘官桂二錢附子或二錢或一錢日四服數日後則日三服至十餘日遂下利淸穀連三日三四十行而浮腫大減又少陰人小兒一人下利靑水面色靑黯氣陷如睡用獨蔘湯加生薑二錢陳皮一錢砂仁一錢日三四服數日後下利十餘行大汗解盖少陰人霍亂關格病得人中汗者始免危也食滯大下者次免危也自然能吐者快免危也禁進粥食但進好熟冷或米飲者扶正抑邪之良方也宿滯之彌留者得好熟冷乘熱溫進則消化無異於飲食雖絕食二三四日不必爲慮

18 Zhang Zhongjing said, "The symptoms and signs of the lesser yin disease are in general a feeble and weak pulse and a tendency for the patient to always fall asleep."
張仲景曰少陰病脈微細但欲寐

19 In case of the febrile disease caused by cold, if the patient cannot vomit and experiences fidgetiness, somnolence and diarrheas with thirst for five to six days, it will become the lesser yin disease. If the urine is clean, Sini Tang should be adopted.
傷寒欲吐不吐心煩但欲寐五六日自利而渴者屬少陰小便色白宜四逆湯

20 In case of the lesser yin disease, Fuzi Tang (Aconite Decoction) is suitable for pain all over the body, cold limbs and arthralgia with a deep pulse.
少陰病身體痛手足寒骨節痛脈沈者附子湯主之

21 In case of diarrhea, abdominal distension, and pain all over the body, we should warm the interior first and then treat the exterior. For warming the interior conditions, Sini Tang should be adopted. For treating the exterior conditions, Guizhi Tang should be adopted.
下利腹脹滿身體疼痛先溫其裏乃攻其表溫裏宜四逆湯攻表宜桂枝湯

22 I have said, "The above symptoms should be treated with Gwangye Buja Ijung Tang."
論曰右證當用官桂附子理中湯

23 Zhang Zhongjing said, "Mahuang Fuzi Xixin Tang (Ephedra, Aconiti Accessory Root, and Asari Herba Decoction) act as curatives for a patient in the initial stages of the lesser yin disease with a fever and a deep pulse."
張仲景曰少陰病始得之反發熱脈沈者麻黃附子細辛湯主之

24 Lesser yin disease, the first or second day: When the patient has no abnormal sensation in the mouth and has chills over the back, Fuzi Tang should be adopted.
少陰病一二日口中和背惡寒宜附子湯

25 The reason why Mahuang Fuzi Gancao Tang (Ephedra, Aconiti Accessory Root, and Licorice Decoction) was adopted to induce light perspiration on the second or third day in the lesser yin disease is that there were no symptoms or signs during this period. "No symptoms and signs" means an absence of vomiting, diarrhea and cold limbs.

少陰病二三日用麻黃附子甘草湯微發之以二三日無證故微發汗也無證謂無吐利厥證也

26 If a patient has diarrhea with undigested cereals, a deep and slow pulse, a lightly flushed face and light perspiration, his illness will be gone following a period of vertigo and perspiration. The patient will then experience a light coldness in the limbs. This is caused by the deficiency of the lower portion, which can be seen from the symptom of *daiyang* (wearing yang) on the face.

下利脈沈而遲其人面小赤身有微汗下利清穀必鬱冒汗出而解病人必微厥所以然者其面戴陽下虛故也

27 The lesser yin disease with a slender, deep and speedy pulse would indicate that the disease is at the interior. Diaphoresis is prohibited for a patient having lesser yin disease that has cold-ness in the limbs, but without perspiration. If a diaphoretic is adopted for such a case, there will be bleeding, possibly from the mouth, nose, or eyes. It is termed "Lower coldness with upper exhaustion" and is a difficult case to treat.

少陰病脈細沈數病爲在裏不可發汗少陰病但厥無汗而強發之必動其血或從口鼻或從目出是爲下厥上渴難治

28 I have said, "The greater yin disease and lesser yin disease which Zhang Zhongjing described are the same as the diarrhea of the lesser yin person with stomach qi asthenia. Greater yin disease with diarrhea is the usual symptom in serious cases, while lesser yin disease with diar-rhea is dangerous for a patient in critical condition. If a doctor considers the two diarrheas as one and he is not seriously concerned with the lesser yin disease with diarrhea, then the patient cannot avoid death. The diarrhea in the greater yin disease is the diarrhea in the large intestine, and the diarrhea in the lesser yin disease is the diarrhea in the stomach. The diar-rhea in the greater yin disease occurs when warm qi is dispelling cold qi, while the diarrhea in the lesser yin disease occurs when cold qi is suppressing warm qi."

論曰張仲景所論太陰病少陰病俱是少陰人胃氣虛弱泄瀉之證而太陰病泄瀉重證中平證也少陰病泄瀉危證中險證也人但見泄瀉同是一證而易於尋常做圖少陰病泄瀉尋常做圖則必不免死蓋太陰病泄瀉大腸之泄瀉也少陰病泄瀉胃中之泄瀉也太陰病泄瀉溫氣逐冷氣之泄瀉也少陰病泄瀉冷氣逼溫氣之泄瀉也

29 In order for the lesser yin disease to disappear naturally, there must be a lightly flushed face and light perspiration. Following a period of vertigo and perspiration, there is relief. The an-cients had seen this condition, so a patient having the lesser yin disease with only cold limbs,

but without perspiration, was forced to sweat by Ephedrae Herba. The purpose was to help the patient to spontaneous recovery. However, unexpectedly, the drug moved his blood to come out of his mouth and nose. Thus, doctors became cautious and worried. We should not make light of the use of Ephedrae Herba for the lesser yin disease. Yet for the initial one or two days, or for the initial two or three days, a patient with lesser yin disease was given Ma-huang Fuzi Gancao Tang to render light perspiration. But Ephedrae Herba is a harmful drug for the lesser yin disease. So although there are the initial symptoms for two to three days, Ephedrae Herba cannot be adopted to render perspiration. For this case, Gwangye Buja Ijung Tang should be used and Cinnamomi Ramulus can be substituted for Cinnamomi Cortex.

少陰病欲自愈則面小赤身有微汗必鬱冒汗出而解故古人有見於此少陰病但厥無汗者亦以麻黃强發汗欲其自愈而反動其血從口鼻出故於是乎始爲戒懼凡少陰病不敢輕易用麻黃而少陰病始得之一二日二三日初證以麻黃附子甘草湯微發之也然麻黃爲少陰病害藥則雖二三日初證必不可用麻黃發之也此證當用官桂附子理中湯或以桂枝易官桂

30 Since the initial symptom of the lesser yin disease can develop into a dangerous condition, we should make an early diagnosis and treatment at the initial stage of this disease to prevent the condition from worsening. Abdominal pain, spontaneous diarrhea without thirst and normal sensation in the mouth are the symptoms of the greater yin disease, while abdominal pain, spontaneous diarrhea with a feeling of thirst and with abnormal sensation in the mouth are the symptoms of the lesser yin disease. The lesser yin disease produces an aching of the body and arthralgia, which are symptomatic of the exterior pattern. Though both the exterior and interior patterns appear, the cold qi in the large intestine certainly surpasses the stomach warm qi and ascends. The greater yin disease has no aching of the body or arthralgia, which are symptomatic of the exterior pattern. This is the case in which the interior pattern appears, but the exterior pattern does not. The stomach warm qi surpasses the cold qi in the large intestine and descends.

少陰病初證因爲險證繼而爲危證此病初證早不辨證而措置則危境也凡腹痛自利無口渴口中和者爲太陰病腹痛自利而有口渴口中不和者爲少陰病少陰病有身體痛骨節痛表證此則表裏俱病而大腸寒氣必勝胃中溫氣而上升也太陰病無身體痛骨節痛表證此則裡病表不病而胃中溫氣猶勝大腸寒氣而下降也

31 Zhang Zhongjing said, "For the lesser yin disease with watery stools, pain in the epigastric region and a parched mouth, Da Chengqi Tang can be adopted."

張仲景曰少陰病自利純靑水心下痛口燥乾者宜大承氣湯

32 Zhu Gong said, "Immediate purgation is recommended for the lesser yin disease with a dry mouth and throat, and thirst. Although it does not belong to the yang brightness disease, this disease should be purged, and the slow-acting laxative also can be adopted."

朱肱曰少陰病口燥咽乾而渴宜急下之非若陽明宜下而可緩也

33 In the 『*Dongyuanshu*』[1] ("Book of Dongyuan"), Li Gao said, "The lesser yin disease should be diagnosed through the conditions of the mouth. The patient who has a normal sensation in the mouth should use warming drugs, and the patient who has a dry mouth should use purgatives. The lesser yin disease should be diagnosed by the colors of the diarrheas. The patient who has diarrhea without a greenish color should use warming drugs, and the one who has greenish diarrhea should use purgatives."

李杲東垣書曰少陰證口中辨口中和者當溫口中乾燥者當下少陰證下利辨色不靑者當溫色靑者當下

34 Li Chan said, "For dryness of the tongue and mouth or watery stool, and delirium followed by sudden difficulty in defecation, Xiao Chengqi Tang should be adopted. For bluish lips, cold limbs and dark-bluish nails, Jiangfu Tang (Ginger and Aconite Decoction) is suitable."

李梴曰舌乾口燥或下利清水譫語便閉宜小承氣湯脣靑四肢厥冷指甲靑黑宜薑附湯

35 I have said, "For watery diarrhea, Crotonis Fructus should be adopted as a purgative, and Gwangye Buja Ijung Tang as a warming drug. If there is watery stool accompanied with sudden difficulty in defecation, Crotonis Fructus should be adopted first, and then Gangchul Gwanjung Tang."

論曰下利靑水者欲下之則當用巴豆欲溫之則當用官桂附子理中湯下利靑水仍爲便閉者先用巴豆後用薑朮寬中湯

36 There once was a ten year old lesser yin boy who was always too pensive and anxious. Therefore, he experienced abdominal pain and diarrhea every one or two days. He was treated with two to four packs of Baikhao Ijung Tang (White Flowery Knotweed Decoction for Regulating the Middle), and when his condition worsened, one to two packs of Buja Ijung Tang was administered. The diarrhea was subsequently always relieved. Another time, the boy was depressed for several days. Two packs of Baikhao Ijung Tang were taken as preventive treatment, but diarrhea with watery stool persisted. He continued to take six packs of Baikhao Ijung Tang a day, but in vain. He was immediately given six packs of Buja Ijung Tang. The clear, watery stool having changed to a dark color, he took two more packs, after which the dark watery stool ceased. Afterwards, he continued to take two to three packs for recuperation. Analyzing the above case, the initial diarrhea with clear watery stool was accompanied with cholera and obstruction and rejection. In this case, there was no doubt that treatment required eliminating the obstinate cold pattern and indigestion with Crotonis Fructus. The boy got diarrhea with clear watery stool in December, in his tenth year, and on February of the next year, he got the yang collapse disease again.

嘗見少陰人十歲兒思慮耗氣每有憂愁一二日則必腹痛泄瀉一二日用白何烏理中湯二三四貼或甚則附子理中湯一二貼則泄瀉必愈矣忽一日此兒心有憂愁氣度不平數日故預治次用白何烏理中湯二貼則泄瀉因作下利靑水連用六貼靑水不止急用附子理中湯六貼靑水變爲黑水又二貼黑水泄瀉

亦愈又二三貼調理以此觀之則下利青水者病人有霍亂關格而後成此證也此證當用巴豆破積滯痼
冷自是無疑此兒十歲冬十二月有下利青水病十一歲春二月又得亡陽病

37 Zhu Gong said, "Ceaseless restlessness and coldness in the limbs is called *zangjue* (visceral shock)."

朱肱曰躁無暫定而厥者爲藏厥

38 Li Chan said, "In case of visceral shock, the patient has ceaseless restlessness, and seven to eight days after the onset of fever, he has a weak pulse, cold skin with restlessness and occasional vomiting and diarrhea with restlessness. This is induced by the shortage of the genuine visceral qi of the reverting yin. It was named visceral shock. Zhongjing was at a loss for a suitable treatment, and simply adopted cool Sini Tang. In case of the lesser yin disease, symptoms such as coldness in the limbs, vomiting, diarrhea and restlessness are difficult to cure. Sanwei Shenyu Tang is suitable."

李梴曰藏厥者發躁無休息時發熱七八日脈微膚冷而躁或吐或瀉無時暫安者乃厥陰眞藏氣絶故曰
藏厥仲景無治法而四逆湯冷飮救之又少陰病厥而吐利發躁者亦不治而三味蔘萸湯救之

39 I have said, "Lesser yin persons are at times unstably delighted, but as a result of a lack of ideas and power, they become annoyed and impatient. In the case of the febrile disease caused by cold in lesser yin disease, is the disease not due to a lack of ideas and powers, which results in symptoms such as nausea without vomiting, restlessness and tendency to fall asleep? Generally, unstable delight comes from avarice. How does a man contract the lesser yin disease from a lack of ideas and power? Why does he not have a generous mind? However, during the initial stage of febrile disease caused by cold, if a patient manifesting symptoms of nausea without vomiting, restlessness in the mind and a tendency to fall asleep is treated early, he can be saved. If the patient displays symptoms such as ceaseless restlessness and cold limbs, he is in a dangerous stage. What a pity for him! For these symptoms, he should take Shenyu Tang (Ginseng and Evodia Decoction), Sini Tang, Gwangye Buja Ijung Tang and Osuyu Buja Ijung Tang (Evodia and Aconite Decoction for Regulating the Middle)."

論曰少陰人喜好不定而計窮力屈則心煩躁也少陰病傷寒欲吐不吐心煩但欲寐者此非計窮力屈者
之病乎蓋喜好者所慾也何故至於計窮力屈而得此少陰病乎何不早用君子寬平心乎然初證傷寒欲
吐不吐心煩但欲寐者早用藥則猶可免死也其病至於躁無暫定而厥則勢在極危也豈不可憐乎此證
當用蔘萸湯四逆湯官桂附子理中湯吳茱萸附子理中湯

40 Zhu Gong said, "Coldness on the body, a deep, slender and rapid pulse, restlessness, and an inability to drink water are the manifestations of yang being kept in the exterior by excessive yin in the interior. If the patient can drink water, he does not have this disease. In reverting yin disease, if the patient wants to drink water, he will recover after frequent drinking of small amounts of water."

朱肱曰病人身冷脈沈細而疾煩躁而不飲水者陰盛隔陽也若飲水者非此證也厥陰病渴欲飲水者小
小與之愈

41 Cheng Wuji[2]) said, "*Fan* (irritability) means that the patient feels restlessness in the chest, and *zao* (restlessness) means that the qi radiates from the heat outward. If there is irritability without restlessness, or irritability first and restlessness next, the patient will be curable. If there is restlessness without irritability, or restlessness first and irritability next, the patient will be incurable. Restlessness first and irritability next is similar to the feeling of restlessness and annoyance one has after getting angry; in this case, the yang is kept in the exterior by excessive yin in the interior. Although the patient is thirsty enough to immerse himself in muddy water, he cannot drink any water at all. This action is a last-ditch attempt by the patient to replenish his qi, and can be characterized as a lamp being lit for the last time before going out."

成無己曰煩謂心中鬱煩也躁謂氣外熱躁也但煩不躁及先煩後躁者皆可治但躁不煩及先躁後煩者
皆不可治先躁後煩謂怫怫然更作躁悶此陰盛隔陽也雖大躁欲於泥水中臥但水不得入口是也此氣
欲絶而爭譬如燈將滅而暴明

42 Li Chan said, "If yang is kept in the exterior by excessive yin in the interior in a febrile disease caused by cold, the patient will experience coldness all over his body; but because of restlessness, he will want to jump into a well. He will have bluish lips and a dark face, thirst, as well as regurgitate water and pass diarrhea with black fluid. A deep, slender, and fast or impalpable pulse is a serious asthenic sign of yang being kept in the exterior by excessive yin in the interior. Pili San (Thunderbolt Powder) is suitable, but if the patient experiences cold limbs, irritability and restlessness, he will not be cured."

李梴曰傷寒陰盛隔陽其證身冷反躁欲投井中脣青面黑渴欲飲水復吐大便自利黑水六脈沈細而疾
或無脈陰盛隔陽大虛證也宜霹靂散又曰厥逆煩躁者不治

43 I have said, "For the above symptoms, Gwangye Buja Ijung Tang and Osuyu Buja Ijung Tang should be adopted; Pili San is also suitable."

論曰此證當用官桂附子理中湯吳茱萸附子理中湯或用霹靂散

44 The conditions of visceral shock and yang being kept in the exterior by excessive yin in the interior are almost the same, and both are very critical. Once facing this crisis, it is very difficult to handle it. The only way to survive this illness is to adopt Gwangye Buja Ijung Tang and Osuyu Buja Ijung Tang before these symptoms manifest themselves.

藏厥與陰盛隔陽病情大同小異俱在極危如存一髮措手難及若論此病之可治上策莫如此證未成之
前早用官桂附子理中湯吳茱萸附子理中湯

45 Generally, we have to check whether the patient has *xinfan* (fidgetiness) or not at the onset of diarrhea in a lesser yin person's disease. In case the patient has fidgetiness, he should have thirst with an abnormal sensation in the mouth. In case he has no fidgetiness, he should have no thirst with a normal sensation in the mouth. When we observe the critical conditions in a lesser yin person's disease, we have to check whether restlessness is stabilized or not. When we check whether restlessness is stable or not, we should understand the state of the patient's mind so as to see if it is stable or not. A collected mind shows that restlessness is stabilized. A restless mind shows that restlessness is unstabilized. However, in the midst of an anxious state, if the patient feels temporary comfort, the illness can be cured. For the curable patient, the administration of Zingiberis Rhizoma and Aconiti Lateralis Radix Praeparata will prove effective.

凡觀少陰人病泄瀉初證者當觀於心煩與不煩也心煩則口渴而口中不和也心不煩則口不渴而口中和也觀少陰人病危證者當觀於躁之有定無定也欲觀躁之有定無定則必占心之範圍有定無定也心之範圍綽綽者心之有定而躁之有定也心之範圍耿耿者心之無定而躁之無定也心雖耿耿忽忽猶有一半時刻綽綽卓卓則其病可治可治者用薑附而可效也

46 Generally, if a lesser yin person has diarrhea three times a day, it will be more serious than having it once or twice a day. Four to five times are certainly more serious than two to three times, and four times a day is a sign of grave illness. One day's diarrhea is milder than two day's, and two day's diarrhea is milder than three to four day's. Frequent diarrhea that persists for more than three days is frequently very serious. If an ordinary lesser yin person has diarrhea two or three times a month, he is not in a mild stage. If he has dry stool three or four times a day, he is not in a mild stage. Even though the patient has diarrhea of fluid stools containing undigested food several dozen times a day, his mouth will not be dry and his cool qi will be expelled from the exterior. If a patient has diarrhea with watery stool, he will certainly have blue water in the abdomen. If the patient has diarrhea with yellow water, it certainly will not be clear and certainly shows some dregs.

凡少陰人泄瀉日三度重於一二度也四五度重於二三度也而日四度泄瀉則太重也泄瀉一日輕於二日也二日輕於三四日也而連三日泄瀉則太重也少陰人平人一月間或泄瀉二三次則不可謂輕病人也一日間乾便三四度則不可謂輕病人也下利清穀者雖日數十行口中必不燥乾而冷氣外解也下利清水者腹中必有靑水也若下利黃水則非清水而又必雜穢物也

47 Zhang Zhongjing said, "On the seventh or eighth day of the febrile disease caused by cold, symptoms such as orange-yellowish skin, dysuria and slight abdominal distension belong to greater yin disease. Yinchenhao Tang (Virgate Wormwood Decoction) is suitable. In case of febrile disease caused by cold, if there is perspiration only over the head and neck and dysuria, the skin will turn yellowish."

張仲景曰傷寒七八日身黃如梔子色小便不利腹微滿屬太陰宜茵陳蒿湯傷寒但頭汗出餘無汗劑頸而還小便不利身必發黃

48 Li Chan said, "Infectious epidemic diseases which cause jaundice are called epidemic jaundice. This is very fatal and urgent, and Zhangdan Wan (Pills for Pestilential Jaundice) is suitable."

李梴曰天行疫癘亦能發黃謂之溫黃殺人最急宜瘴疸丸

49 I have said, "For treating the disease above, Yinchen Jupi Tang (Virgate Wormwood and Tangerine Peel Decoction), Yinchen Fuzi Tang (Virgate Wormwood and Aconite Decoction), Yinchen Sini Tang (Virgate Wormwood Decoction for Frigid Extremities), Zhangdan Wan or Badou Wan should be adopted."

論曰右證當用茵蔯橘皮湯茵蔯附子湯茵蔯四逆湯瘴疸丸或用巴豆丹

50 In the 『*Yixue Gangmu*』, we read, "*Jiexiong* (accumulation of pathogen in the chest) without high fever is caused by *shuijie* (accumulation of fluid). If there is sweating on the head only, that is *shuijiexiong* (accumulation of fluid in the chest). Xiao Banxia Tang is suitable."

醫學綱目曰但結胸無大熱者此爲水結但頭汗出名曰水結胸小半夏湯主之

51 Gong Xin said, "For accumulation of pathogen in the chest due to excessive cold without fever, one should adopt Sanwu Bai San (Powder of Three White Drugs)."

龔信曰寒實結胸無熱證者宜三物白散

52 I have said, "To treat the above symptoms, Gyeji Banha Sainggang Tang (Cinnamon Twig, Pinelliae Tuber, and Zingiberis Rhizoma Recens Decoction), Jeokbaikhao Gwanjung Tang (Decoction for Relieving the Middle with Red/White Flowery Knotweed), Sanwu Bai San or the Padu Dan should be adopted."

論曰右證當用桂枝半夏生薑湯赤白何烏寬中湯三物白散或用巴豆丹

53 In a lesser yang person's disease, hardness in the epigastrium is named the accumulation of pathogen in the chest, which is treatable. In a lesser yin person's disease, hardness in the epigastrium is named *zangjie* (accumulation of yin cold in the viscera), which is untreatable. The drugs for accumulation of fluid in the chest and *hanshijiexiong* (locked chest due to excessive cold) mentioned in the 『*Yixue Gangmu*』 and 『*Yijian*』 are almost the same as that for a lesser yin person with the greater yin disease. Those are similar to Zhang Zhongjing's Yinchenhao Tang. They do not have actual masses, but experience a sensation of fullness in the epigastrium. The symptoms of Zhang Zhongjing's Xiexin Tang are a sensation of fullness and hardness in the epigastrium due to purgation of the febrile disease caused by cold. However, a sensation of fullness and hardness in the epigastrium after the diaphoretic treatment are simply sensations in the epigastrium or above the umbilicus area; there is not an actual solid mass in the epigastrium. If a lesser yin person has a solid mass on the right side of the epigastrium, he is untreatable.

少陽人病心下結硬者名曰結胸病其病可治也少陰人病心下結硬者名曰藏結病其病不治也醫學綱目醫鑑所論水結胸寒實結胸證藥俱是少陰人太陰病而與張仲景茵蔯蒿湯證相類則此病想必非眞結硬於心下而卽痞滿於心下者也張仲景瀉心湯證傷寒下利心下痞硬汗解後心下痞硬云者亦皆痞滿於心下或臍上近處結硬也而非眞結硬於心下者也若少陰人病而心下右邊結硬則不治

54 Zhang Zhongjing asked himself, "Where there are accumulation of pathogen in the chest and accumulation of yin cold in the viscera, what are the differences and respective symptoms and signs?" He replied, "Tenderness (at the lower part of the chest and epigastrium), a pulse floating under the forefinger and deep under the middle finger are the symptoms and signs of accumulation of pathogen in the chest." And "What about accumulation of yin cold in the viscera?" he asked again. The reply was, "The symptoms and signs are similar to those of accumulation of pathogen in the chest, but with a normal intake of food and frequent loose bowels." A pulse floating under the forefinger and a feeble, deep and tense pulse under the middle finger are the symptoms and signs of accumulation of yin cold in the viscera. If the tongue's coating is white, moist and glossy, then it is considered to be a serious case. The patient used to have vital qi stagnancy in the chest. If it extends to the part near the navel and stretches to the lower abdomen and the genitals, the pattern is termed accumulation of yin cold in the viscera and may result in death.

張仲景曰病有結胸有藏結其狀如何曰按之痛寸脈浮關脈沈名曰結胸也何謂藏結曰如結胸狀飲食如故時時下利寸脈浮關脈細小沈緊名曰藏結舌上白胎滑者難治病人胸中素有痞連在臍傍引入小腹入陰筋者此名藏結死

55 Zhu Gong said, "The symptoms and signs of accumulation of yin cold in viscera are similar to those of accumulation of pathogen in the chest. Drinking and eating are as usual, there are occasional diarrhea, and a white coating on the tongue." There is a phrase for this, "Drinking and eating as usual, occasional diarrhea and white coating on the tongue. Since the pain of the abdomen and penis adjoins, he is going to die."

朱宏曰藏結狀如結胸飲食如故時時下利而舌上白胎歌曰飲食如常時下利更加舌上白胎時連臍腹痛引陰筋者此疾元來死不醫

56 I have said, "There was a lesser yin person who had a solid and hard mass in the right side of the epigastrium, and most of the drugs given were useless. After the administration of Badou Ruyi Dan, the condition worsened and was accompanied by a shaking of the head and tremors that occurred for a short time, followed by death several months later. Another lesser yin person exhibiting the same symptoms and signs used Badou Dan. He perspired all over the body except for both sides of the Renzhong point and also died one year later. After this, I observed four or five people with solid and hard mass in the epigastrium. They died within six months or a year, even though they had been treated with drugs, or received acupuncture and moxibustion. It is the accumulation of yin cold in the viscera disease and lesser yin person's disease."

論曰嘗見少陰人一人心下右邊結硬百藥無效與巴豆如意丹反劇搖頭動風有頃而止數月後死其後
又有少陰人一人有此證者用巴豆丹面上身上有汗而獨上唇人中穴左右邊無汗此人一周年後亦死
凡少陰人心下結硬有此證者目睹四五人或半年或一年鍼灸醫藥無不周至而個個無回生之望此即
藏結病而少陰人病也

57 Zhang Zhongjing said, "The period of jaundice is 18 days. After ten days, recovery should begin; but if it becomes severe, it is difficult to manage. If it is generated from the yin area, the patient should vomit. If it generates from the yang area, the patient should shiver and get feverish."

張仲景曰黃疸之病當以十八日爲期十日以上宜差反劇爲難治發於陰部其人必嘔發於陽部其人振寒而發熱

58 Every jaundice with yellow-red colored urine is induced by dampness-heat, so one must adopt the treatment against dampness-heat. Clean urine that cannot come from fever means no fever. If there are the symptoms and signs of *xuhan* (deficiency-cold type), it should be treated as *xulao* (consumption).

諸疸小便黃赤色者爲濕熱當作濕熱治小便色白不可除熱者無熱也若有虛寒證當作虛勞治

59 The patient becomes unable to sleep when accompanied by abdominal distension, a pale and yellowish face, and restlessness.

腹脹滿面萎黃躁不得睡

60 Patients with jaundice used to get fever at sunset, but have chills, which are caused by overindulgence. The urgencies in the bladder, lower abdominal distension, yellowish discoloration of the whole body, black color on the forehead, and heat sensation under the feet are the symptoms of black jaundice. The abdominal distension seems to contain fluid. There is tarry and occasionally loose stool that is caused by overindulgence. Abdominal distension is not a fluid disease; if the patient has abdominal distension, he cannot be easily cured.

黃家日晡時當發熱反惡寒此爲女勞得之膀胱急小腹滿一身盡黃額上黑足下熱因作黑疸腹脹如水狀大便黑或時溏此女勞之病非水也腹滿者難治

61 Zhu Gong said, "Yin jaundice manifests itself as restlessness, impatience, shortness of breath, nausea, and no thirst. Yinchen Jupi Tang is available. For one who has jaundice of the febrile disease caused by cold accompanied by a weak pulse and cold body, Yinchen Sini Tang showed dramatic effects. For one who has jaundice of the febrile disease caused by cold accompanied by a deep, slender, slow and weak pulse, Yinchen Fuzi Tang showed a dramatic effect."

朱肱曰陰黃煩燥喘嘔不渴宜用茵蔯橘皮湯一人傷寒發黃脈微弱身冷次第用藥至茵蔯四逆湯大效一人傷寒發黃脈沈細遲無力次第用藥至茵蔯附子湯大效

62 In the 『*Yixue Gangmu*』, we read, "A jaundice originating from dampness is accompanied by a dark yellowish discoloration, without pain on the body. A jaundice originating from heat, has a bright yellowish discoloration like orange and there is pain over the whole body."

醫學綱目曰濕家之黃色暗不明一身不痛熱家之黃如橘子一身盡痛

63 Wang Haogu said, "If one fails to adopt a diaphoretic or a diuretic, he will get jaundice."

王好古曰凡病當汗而不汗當利小便而不利亦生黃

64 Zhu Zhenheng said, "If jaundice results from food accumulation, the accumulated food should be removed by purgative. For other cases, the diuretic method should be used. Once the urine is clean, the jaundice will spontaneously disappear."

朱震亨曰黃疸因食積者下其食積其餘但利小便小便利白其黃自退

65 Li Chan said, "A patient will die if jaundice persists more than ten days and is accompanied by abdominal distension, shortness of breath, severe thirst and a dark face."

李梃曰黃疸十日以上入腹喘滿煩渴面黑者死

66 In the 『*Maijing*』[3] ("Classic of Pulse"), Wang Shuhe[4] said, "If one cannot detect a pulse near the wrist of a jaundice patient, who also has black, cold skin over the nose and mouth area, he is untreatable."

王叔和脈經曰黃家寸口脈近掌無脈口鼻冷黑色並不可治

67 I have said, "Yin jaundice is a lesser yin person's disease and should be treated with Zhu's Yinchen Jupi Tang and Yinchen Sini Tang." However, I am not sure if jaundice from over-indulgence, jaundice from heat, and jaundice treated with a diuretic are a lesser yin person's disease. Since I have no experience in treating jaundice, it is impossible to say in detail. Feeling of fullness, jaundice and edema have the same origin, and they only have different degrees of severity. If it is necessary to induce urination, Zingiberis Rhizoma, Alpiniae officinarum Rhizoma, Citri Reticulatae Pericarpium, Citri Reticulatae Pericarpium Viride, Cyperi Rhizoma, and Alpiniae oxyphyllae Fructus, etc. can promote fluent urination in a lesser yin person. Schizonepetae Herba, Saposhnikoviae Radix, Osterici Radix, Angelicae pubescentis Radix, Poria Sclerotium, and Alismatis Rhizoma etc. can promote fluent urination in a lesser yang person.

論曰陰黃卽少陰人病也當用朱氏茵陳橘皮湯茵陳四逆湯女勞之黃熱家之黃利小便之黃想或非少陰人病而余所經驗未嘗一遇黃疸而治之故未得仔細裏許然痞滿黃疸浮腫同出一證而有輕重若欲利小便則乾薑良薑陳皮青皮香附子益智仁能利少陰人小便荊芥防風羌活獨活茯苓澤瀉能利少陽人小便

Notes

1) 『*Dongyuanshu*』(東垣書)

A collection of 10 articles from various physicians including Li Gao published in 1529.

2) Cheng Wuji (成無己)

(1066~1155 A.D.) He is known for his assiduous study of Zhang Zhongjing's "Treatise on Cold-induced and Miscellaneous Diseases" and for writing several books on its comment. His 『*Zhujie Shanghanlun*』(註解傷寒論: "Commentary on the Treatise on Cold-induced Diseases", 1142 A.D.) is considered the earliest of its kind in Chinese medical literature.

3) 『*Maijing*』(脈經)

The "Classic of Pulse", written by Wang Shuhe (王叔和) in the third century, generally acknowledged as the standard work on the subject and the earliest comprehensive work dealing with pulse diagnosis now extant.

4) Wang Shuhe (王叔和)

(About 210~285 A.D.) Also called Wang Xi, versed in pulse taking, commissioner of the Imperial Academy of Medicine, and author of the 『*Maijing*』, the first comprehensive book on pulse diagnosis now extant in China. He perfected and systemized the art of pulse taking, yet emphasized the use of all four methods of diagnosis, visual inspection, audio-olfactive investigation, interrogation, and palpation and pulse diagnosis. He rearranged Zhang Zhongjing's 『*Shanghan Zabinglun*』, which contributed much towards the preservation of that important medical classic.

General Remarks on the Lesser Yin Person

少陰人泛論

1　I have said, "Fever and chills are symptomatic of the greater yang disease, while fever with no chills is symptomatic of the yang brightness disease. Although both diseases have the same symptom of fever, there are big differences in chills and the status and strength of the yang qi, which can be likened to the differences between high mountains and hills. Diarrhea with no thirst is a symptom of the greater yin disease. Diarrhea with thirst is a symptom of the lesser yin disease. Although both diseases share the symptom of diarrhea, there are big differences in thirst and the conditions of cold qi, which can be likened to the clouds in the sky and the puddles. So the symptoms of Gwakhyang Jeonggi San and Hyangsa Yangwi Tang can be thought of running horses on the plain. However, the symptoms for Doksam Palmul Tang and Gyebu Ijung Tang (Decoction for Regulating the Middle with Cinnamomi Ramulus and Aconiti Lateralis Radix Praeparata) can be thought of climbing a high mountain with a short walking stick. In case of a lesser yin person, one must distinguish whether he has yang brightness or lesser yin disease. Such diseases are very serious, like the treacherous byways of a high mountain. The patient must attempt good cultivation and take care, as though he were walking on a wide road and leaving behind a world of illusions."

論曰發熱惡寒者爲太陽病發熱不惡寒者爲陽明病太陽陽明之發熱形證一也而惡寒不惡寒之間相去遠甚而陽氣之進退强弱泰山之比岡陵也自利而不渴者爲太陰病自利而渴者爲少陰病太陰少陰之自利形證一也而渴不渴之間相去遠甚而冷氣之聚散輕重雲夢之比潴澤也是故藿香正氣散香砂養胃湯之證勢平地駿馬之病勢也獨蔘八物湯桂附理中湯之證勢太行短節之病勢也若使一天下少陰人稟賦者自知其病之陽明少陰證如太行之險路得之可畏救之不易攝身療病戒懼謹慎之道有若大路然而不迷則其庶幾乎

2   The perspiration of the greater yang disease is a sign that heat qi pushing out the cold qi. The perspiration of the yang brightness disease is a sign that cold qi is attacking heat qi. The diarrhea of the greater yin disease is a sign that warm qi is kicking out cool qi. The diarrhea of the lesser yin disease is a sign of cool qi pushing out warm qi.

太陽病汗出熱氣卻寒氣之汗出也陽明病汗出寒氣犯熱氣之汗出也太陰病下利溫氣逐冷氣之泄瀉也少陰病下利冷氣逼溫氣之下利也

3   There are two auspicious symptoms in a lesser yin person's disease. They are perspiration from the Renzhong point and the ability to drink water.

少陰人病有二吉證人中汗一吉證也能飲水一吉證也

4   There are two critical symptoms in a lesser yin person's disease. They are fever with profuse sweating and watery diarrhea.

少陰人病有二急證發熱汗多一急證也下利清水一急證也

5   There are six major symptoms in a lesser yin person's disease. The first one is the lesser yin disease; the second is the yang brightness disease; the third is yin type inflammatory swelling pattern of the greater yin disease; the fourth is the reverting yin pattern of the greater yang disease; the fifth is jaundice of the greater yin disease; and the last is the excess of the stomach and intestines of the greater yang disease.

少陰人病有六大證一曰少陰病二曰陽明病三曰太陰病陰毒證也四曰太陽病厥陰證也五曰太陰病黃疸證也六曰太陽病胃家實證也

6   Following fever with sweating, a patient's condition should improve. If it worsens, it must be the yang brightness disease. After relaxing the bowels with diarrhea, the disease should be relieved. If it gets worse after relaxing the bowels with diarrhea, it must be the lesser yin disease. Since the yang brightness and the lesser yin disease are induced by the situations in which the pathogen attacks healthy qi, we should treat the situation immediately. After chills and sweating, the illness will leave; but if the illness seems half cured, it could develop into reverting yin pattern. After abdominal pain and diarrhea, the disease will leave; but if the illness seems half cured, it could develop into the yin type inflammatory swelling disease. Since both are diseases in which healthy qi and the pathogen confront each other, we should adopt the medicine quickly. If a disease is relieved after just one bout of perspiration when the patient has fever, it is a mild condition of the greater yang disease. If indigestion is relieved after just one bout of purgation, it is a mild condition of the greater yin disease. It is not necessary to take medicine for a mild condition of the greater yang and greater yin diseases, as they become relieved naturally. However, if fever lasts for three days, even though diaphoresis is used, it could be a serious condition of the greater yang disease; and if indigestion lasts for three days, even though purgative methods are used, it could be a serious condition of the greater yin

disease. Although the serious conditions of the greater yang and greater yin diseases cannot be judged as mild cases, if the patients take two to three packs of suitable medicine, they can be relieved spontaneously. If fever lasts for six days even though a diaphoresis is used, and indigestion lasts for six days even though a purgative is used, the patient's condition belongs to the excess of the stomach and intestines and the jaundice of the greater yang and the greater yin disease. Since the excess of the stomach and intestines and the jaundice of the greater yang and the greater yin disease are induced by the blocking and congestion of healthy qi and the pathogen, the patient should take a massive dosage of medicine.

發熱汗出則病必解也而發熱汗出而病益甚者陽明病也通滯下利則病必解也而通滯下利而病益甚者少陰病也陽明少陰以邪犯正之病不可不急用藥也惡寒汗出則病必盡解也而惡寒汗出而其病半解半不解者厥陰之漸也腹痛下利則病必盡解也而腹痛下利而其病半解半不解者陰毒之漸也厥陰陰毒正邪相傾之病不可不預用藥也發熱一汗而病即解者太陽之輕病也食滯一下而病即解者太陰之輕病也太陽太陰之輕病不用藥而亦自愈也發熱三日不得汗解者太陽之尤病也食滯三日不能化下者太陰之尤病也太陽太陰之尤證已不可謂輕證而用藥二三貼亦自愈也發熱六日不得汗解食滯六日不能化下者太陽太陰之胃家實黃疸病也太陽太陰之胃家實黃疸正邪壅錮之病不可不大用藥也

7　A case of either the greater yang or greater yin disease lasting for six or seven days can develop into a dangerous or serious condition, and certainly can become a critical condition within 10 days. The yang brightness and lesser yin diseases start as serious conditions and become critical in two to three days. Therefore, one should be careful from the onset of the yang brightness and lesser yin diseases. In the case of the greater yang and greater yin diseases, the patient should be observed for approximately four to five days.

太陽太陰之病六七日或成危證或成重證而十日內必有險證陽明少陰之病自始發已爲重證而二三日內亦致險證是故陽明少陰之病不可不察於始發也太陽太陰之病不可不察於四五日間也

8　Since the developments of the greater yang and greater yin diseases are moderate and last long, there are many complications. Since the developments of yang brightness and lesser yin diseases are urgent and do not last long, there are few complications. Therefore, it is necessary to use drugs between the first and second days of the yang brightness and lesser yin diseases. It is also necessary to use drugs between the fourth and fifth days of the greater yang and greater yin diseases. Since the reverting yin of greater yang and yin type inflammatory swelling of greater yin disease can develop into the critical stage within six to seven days, one should be more careful.

太陽太陰之病病勢緩而能曠日持久故變證多也陽明少陰之病病勢急而不能曠日持久故變證少也盖陽明少陰病過一日而至二日則不可不用藥也太陽太陰病過四日而至五日則不可不用藥也太陽太陰之厥陰陰毒皆六七日之死境也尤不可不謹也

9　For the dangerous conditions of yang brightness disease and greater yang disease, Doksam

Palmul Tang and Bojung Ikgi Tang are appropriate. If the patient does not take them three or four times a day or for a few days continuously, he will not be cured. For the dangerous conditions of lesser yin disease and greater yin disease, Doksam Buja Ijung Tang and Gyebugwakjin Ijung Tang (Decoction for Regulating the Middle with Cinnamomi Ramulus, Aconiti Lateralis Radix Praeparata, Agastachis Herba, and Citri Reticulatae Pericarpium) are suitable. If he does not take them three or four times a day or for a few days continuously, he will not be cured. When the patient's condition is dangerous, he has to take the drugs four times a day. When the patient's condition is half-well, he has to take the drugs three times a day. When the patient's condition sees no change, he has to take the drugs twice a day. When a patient's condition improves slightly, he has to take the drugs three times over two days, or once one day and twice the other day. When a patient's condition gets much better, he has to take the drugs once a day. The medicine should also be taken once for two to five days. When one falls ill, one should take the medicine. If nothing is wrong, one should not take the medicine. One should take heavy medication when one has a serious problem, and mild medication for mild problems. However, if one likes to take heavy medication for mild problems and takes the drugs when nothing is wrong, his visceral qi will be weakened, and his sickness will worsen.

陽明太陽之危者獨蔘八物湯補中益氣湯可以解之而病勢危時若非日三四服而又連日服則難解也少陰太陰之危者獨蔘附子理中湯桂附藿陳理中湯可以解之而病勢危時若非日三四服而又連日服則難解也病勢極危時日四服病勢半危時日三服病勢不減則日二服病勢少減則二日三服而一日則一服一日則二服病勢大減則日一服病勢又大減則間二三四五日一服盖有病者可以服藥無病者不可以服藥重病可以重藥輕病不可以重藥若輕病好用重藥無病者好服藥臟氣脆弱益招病矣

10 Though rich foods can stimulate our appetites, if we indulge in them every day, they will prove harmful to our eating habits. Though sheepskin can protect against coldness, if we wear it every day, it will become cold. If rich foods and sheepskin can lose their effectiveness, what of medicine? The hazards of taking medicine everyday are one hundred times more harmful than no administration. Generally, if one gets sick and one's symptoms are identified, one should take the medicine. If one has no problem, though the symptoms have been identified, one should refrain from taking medicine. We can guess that taking tobacco made of opium, mercury, wild Ginseng Radix and Cervi cornu pantotrichum repeatedly will shorten lives.

膏梁雖則助味常食則損味羊裘雖則禦寒常着則攝寒膏粱羊裘猶不可以常食常着況藥乎若論常服藥之有害則反爲百倍於全不服藥之無利也盖有病者明知其證則必不可不服藥無病者雖明知其證必不可服藥歷觀於世之服鴉片烟水銀山蔘鹿茸者屢服則無不促壽者以此占之則可知矣

11 For the hematemesis of a lesser yin person, Doksam Palmul Tang should be taken. For nasopharyngeal pains, Doksam Gwangye Ijung Tang (Decoction for Regulating the Middle with Ginseng Radix and Cinnamomi Cortex) should be taken.

少陰人吐血當用獨蔘八物湯咽喉痛當用獨蔘官桂理中湯

12 I once treated a lesser yin person who had become an overeater. He began consuming twice the amount he had been eating, until one month later, his belly swelled up and he died. A lesser yin person's diabetes belongs to swelling, and is a dangerous condition. He should be treated immediately with Gunggwichongso Ijung Tang (Decoction for Regulating the Middle with Chuanxiong Rhizoma, Angelicae Gigantis Radix, Allii Fistulosi Bulbus, and Perillae Folium).

嘗見少陰人飲食倍常口味甚甘不過一月其人浮腫而死少陰人食消卽浮腫之屬而危證也不可不急治當用芎歸葱蘇理中湯

13 I once treated a lesser yin person with edema. After he had taken sliced roe liver five times, his edema was relieved. Another lesser yin person also took roe liver, and saw his vision improve and energy level increase. However, a lesser yang person with asthenia took a slice of roe liver and vomited blood until he died.

嘗見少陰人浮腫獐肝一部切片作膾一服盡連用五部其病卽效又有少陰人服獐肝一部眼力倍常眞氣湧出少陽人虛勞病服獐肝一部其人吐血而死

14 I once met a lesser yin person with general edema who had been advised by a doctor to take half a spoonful of natural salt water every day. In four or five days, his edema was greatly relieved; and one month later, the illness was cured.

嘗見少陰人浮腫有醫教以服海鹽自然汁日半匙四五日服浮腫大減一月服永爲完健病不再發

15 Once, there was a lesser yin person who had been suffering from nasopharyngeal pain for several years. A doctor advised him to take gold snake liquor, and after drinking it, he was cured. The ingredient of the liquor is a gold-colored serpent.

嘗見少陰人咽喉痛經年不愈有醫教以服金蛇酒卽效金蛇酒卽金色黃章蛇釀酒者也

16 Once, there was a lesser yin patient with dysentery. He was told to take redneck snake soup, and after eating it, he was cured. One should take the head and tail off from the redneck snake, and put it into a double silk pocket and hang it on the wooden bars of a jar. Cook the snake with five bowls of water into one bowl of soup. To prevent poisoning from direct contact with the snake's bone, it is better to put the snake into a pocket. Snake bones are toxic.

嘗見少陰人痢疾有醫教以服項赤蛇煎湯卽效項赤蛇去頭斷尾納二疊紬囊中藥缸內別設橫木懸空掛之用水五碗煎取一碗服二疊紬囊懸空掛煎者恐犯蛇骨故也蛇骨有毒

17 I witnessed that a lesser yin person with dysentery who had been cured by taking three big garlic cloves and half a spoonful of honey boiled together for three days.

嘗見少陰人痢疾有醫教以大蒜三顆清蜜半匙同煎三日服卽效

18 Once, there was a lesser yin person with a mammary abscess of open sores and pus for seven

to eight months. A doctor advised her to use a patch of wild Ginseng Radix and Ursi Fel, 0.375g each. The patient was immediately relieved. Using a patch of Ginseng Radix powder also cured another lesser yin person with whole-body swelling.

嘗見少陰人乳傍近脇有漏瘡歷七八月瘡口不合惡汁常流有醫敎以山蔘熊膽末各一分傅之卽效又
少陰人一人滿身有瘡以人蔘末塗傅卽效

19 I once saw a lesser yin person with *neiyong* (internal carbuncle) near the breast. A doctor taught her to take out pus with a heated needle. He said, "An internal carbuncle manifests itself through fever with chills, like a febrile disease caused by cold, and severe pain in the settled portion. If we identify the existence of pus through the observation of the region, we should use a heated needle."

嘗見少陰人乳傍近脇發內癰有醫敎以火鍼取膿醫曰內癰外證惡寒發熱似傷寒而有痛處也察其痛
處明知有膿則不可不用火鍼

20 I once saw a lesser yin person with *beiyong* (back carbuncle). He was told by a doctor to be operated upon with a heated knife. The doctor said, "It is good to get rid of a carbuncle with a heated knife as soon as possible. If we hesitate, then the whole back will be hardened. It is of no use to regret about it then."

嘗見少陰人背癰有醫敎以火刀裂瘡醫曰火刀裂瘡宜早也若疑訝而緩不及事則全背堅硬悔之無及

21 I witnessed a lesser yin person with hemiplegia. He was taught to take iron-enriched water and he was cured.

嘗見少陰人半身不遂病有醫敎以服鐵液水得效

22 Once I saw a lesser yin child with *funue* (chronic malaria with splenomegaly). A doctor advised him to take toasted 0.225g of finely powdered Arsenicum with the decoction of Glycyrrhizae Radix et Rhizoma in the morning when it occurred, and he was cured. The doctor said, "Yellow-din must be used and it must be toasted. The weight cannot be less or more than 0.225g. If more than 0.225g, there will be side effects. If less, it is useless. This drug was tested and used many times. If the malaria recurs after relief from this drug, we cannot use it again. If we use it again, the disease will worsen, so we may only use the drug once." According to the doctor, children who recover after one treatment and no recurrence are lesser yin children. If not, they are not lesser yin children. This medicine is only to be adopted for a lesser yin child with chronic malaria with splenomegaly, and not for ordinary malaria. When he has chills, two to three packs of Cheongung Gyeji Tang (Chuanxiong and Cinnamon Twig Decoction) should be adopted for a lesser yin person with ordinary malaria over a two-day period; he will certainly be cured. If a patient has fullness in the abdomen and constipation, though he has malaria, he may also be given Crotonis Fructus.

嘗見少陰人小兒腹瘧病有醫敎以瘧病將發之早朝用火煅金頂砒極細末六理生甘草湯調下卽效醫

曰砒藥必金頂砒然後可用而又火煆然後可用也必不可過六理而又不可不及六理也過六理則藥毒太過也不及六理則瘧不愈也此藥屢試屢驗而有一服愈後瘧又再發者又用之則其病益甚而危盖此藥可以一服不可再服云聽醫言而究其理則一服愈而瘧不再發者皆少陰人兒也一服愈而瘧又再發者皆非少陰人兒也惟少陰人兒腹瘧病難治者用此藥尋常瘧不必用此不祥之藥少陰人尋常間日瘧惡寒時用川芎桂枝湯二三貼則亦無不愈又腹中實滿而大便硬瘧發者亦可用巴豆

23 We cannot say that every drug is bad, but Arsenic trioxide for lesser yin person and Pedicellus Melo for greater yin person are the worst drugs. It is very dangerous to adopt Arsenic trioxide for every disease in the lesser yin person; it must only be used to cure malaria in the lesser yin person. However, this is a cure in name only: the medicine is actually useless, and doctors should beware. It is better to take Cinnamomi Ramulus, Ginseng Radix, and Paeoniae Radix Alba three or four times to treat malaria. Arsenic trioxide is not only useless, but hazardous as well, is it not? Pedicellus Melo is dangerous for every disease of the greater yin person, except in curing phlegm. It is thus useless, and doctors should beware. It is better to take Platycodi Radix, Liriopis seu Ophiopogonis Tuber, and Schizandrae Fructus for three or four times for removing the phlegm. Pedicellus Melo is not only useless, but hazardous as well, is it not? Those two drugs can be used externally, but not orally.

百藥莫非善藥而惟少陰人信砒藥太陰人瓜蒂藥最爲惡藥也何哉少陰人信砒藥百病用之皆殆而祇有治瘧之一能者亦有名無實不無危慮萬不如桂枝人蔘白芍藥三四服之治瘧則此非天下萬害無用之藥乎太陰人瓜蒂藥百病用之皆殆而祇有治痰涎壅塞之一能者亦有名無實不無危慮萬不如桔梗麥門冬五味子三四服之治痰涎壅塞則此非天下萬害無用之藥乎此二藥外治可用內服不可用

24 There was once a lesser yin person who had had a stroke, curled tongue and aphagia. A doctor inserted a needle into the Hegu (LI 4) point, and the patient was cured as if by miracle. We can see that acupuncture can also get wonderful results when a drug has no immediate effects. It is of the opinion that there are certain points along the four constitutions that have wondrous effects upon the qi's up-down and slow-fast flow. As physicians, we must take this into account, and I wait and hope to see future doctors who have faithful hospitality and are pleased to save their patients.

嘗見少陰人中氣病舌卷不語有醫鍼合谷穴而其效如神其他諸病之藥不能速效者鍼能速效者有之盖鍼穴亦有太少陰陽四象人應用之穴而必有升降緩束之妙繫是不可不察敬俟後之謹厚而好活人者

03-1

Twenty Three Prescriptions for the Lesser Yin Person's Disease from Zhang Zhongjing's『*Shanghanlun*』

張仲景傷寒論中少陰人病經驗設方藥二十三方

1　Cinnamon Twig Decoction (Guizhi Tang)

· Cinnamomi Ramulus 11.25g　　　　　· Paeoniae Radix Alba 7.5g

· Glycyrrhizae Radix et Rhizoma 3.75g　· Zingiberis Rhizoma recens 3 slices

· Jujubae Fructus 2 pcs.

桂枝湯

桂枝三錢白芍藥二錢甘草一錢生薑三片大棗二枚

2　Decoction for Regulating the Middle (Lizhong Tang)

· Ginseng Radix 7.5g　　　　　　· Atractylodis Rhizoma Alba 7.5g

· Zingiberis Rhizoma 7.5g

· Glycyrrhizae Radix et Rhizoma (stir-baked with adjuvant) 3.75g

理中湯

人蔘白朮乾薑各二錢灸甘草一錢

3　Ginger and Aconite Decoction (Jiangfu Tang)

· Zingiberis Rhizoma (stir-baked at high temperature) 37.5g

· Aconiti Lateralis Radix Praeparata (stir-baked at high temperature) 18.75g

Stew and take the decoction. When 18.75g of Aconiti Lateralis Radix Praeparata is used in its raw form, it is called Baitong Tang.

薑附湯

炮乾薑一兩炮附子一枚剉取五錢水煎服附子生用名曰白通湯

4 Decoction of Four Drugs for Favorable Condition and Regulating the Middle (Sishun Lizhong Tang)

· Ginseng Radix 7.5g · Atractylodis Rhizoma Alba 7.5g

· Zingiberis Rhizoma 7.5g

· Glycyrrhizae Radix et Rhizoma (stir-baked with adjuvant) 7.5g

四順理中湯

人蔘白朮乾薑炙甘草各二錢

5 Cinnamon Twig and Ginseng Decoction (Guizhi Renshen Tang)

· Glycyrrhizae Radix et Rhizoma (stir-baked with adjuvant) 6.75g

· Cinnamomi Ramulus 6.75g

· Atractylodis Rhizoma Alba 5.625g · Ginseng Radix 5.625g

· Zingiberis Rhizoma 5.625g

桂枝人蔘湯

炙甘草桂枝各一錢八分白朮人蔘乾薑各一錢五分

6 Frigid Extremities Decoction (Sini Tang)

· Glycyrrhizae Radix et Rhizoma (stir-baked with adjuvant) 22.5g

· Zingiberis Rhizoma (stir-baked at high temperature) 18.75g

· Aconiti Lateralis Radix Praeparata (crude) 1 pc.

Chop up the above ingredients and make two packs. Stew and take the decoction.

四逆湯

炙甘草六錢炮乾薑五錢生附子一枚剉分二貼水煎服

7 Magnolia Bark and Pinellia Decoction (Houpo Banxia Tang)

· Magnoliae officinalis Cortex 11.25g · Pinelliae Tuber 5.625g

· Ginseng Radix 5.625g · Glycyrrhizae Radix et Rhizoma 2.625g

· Zingiberis Rhizoma recens 7 slices

厚朴半夏湯

厚朴三錢人蔘半夏各一錢五分甘草七分五里生薑七片

8 Pinellia Powder (Banxia San)

· Pinelliae Tuber (detoxicated with ginger decoction) 7.5g

· Glycyrrhizae Radix et Rhizoma (stir-baked) 7.5g

· Cinnamomi Ramulus 7.5g

半夏散

製半夏炙甘草桂枝各二錢

9 Halloysite and Limonite Decoction (Chishizhi Yuyuliang Tang)

· Halloysitum Rubrum 9.375g   · Limonitum Cum Terra 9.375g

赤石脂禹餘粮湯

赤石脂禹餘粮各二錢五分

10 Aconite Decoction (Fuzi Tang)

· Atractylodis Rhizoma Alba 15g   · Paeoniae Radix Alba 11.25g

· Poria Sclerotium (white) 11.25g

· Aconiti Lateralis Radix Praeparata (stir-baked at high temperature) 7.5g

· Ginseng Radix 7.5g

附子湯

白朮四錢白芍藥白茯苓各三錢炮附子人蔘各二錢

11 Ephedra, Aconite, and Asarum Decoction (Mahuang Fuzi Xixin Tang)

· Ephedrae Herba 7.5g

· Asari Herba 7.5g

· Aconiti Lateralis Radix Praeparata (stir-baked at high temperature) 3.75g

麻黃附子細辛湯

麻黃細辛各二錢炮附子一錢

12 Ephedra, Aconite, and Licorice Decoction (Mahuang Fuzi Gancao Tang)

· Ephedrae Herba 11.25g   · Glycyrrhizae Radix et Rhizoma 11.25g

· Aconiti Lateralis Radix Praeparata (stir-baked at high temperature) 3.75g

麻黃附子甘草湯

麻黃甘草各三錢炮附子一錢

13 Chinese Angelica Decoction for Frigid Extremities (Danggui Sini Tang)

· Paeoniae Radix Alba 7.5g   · Angelicae Gigantis Radix 7.5g

· Cinnamomi Ramulus 5.625g   · Asari Herba 3.75g

· Tetrapanacis medulla 3.75g   · Glycyrrhizae Radix et Rhizoma 3.75g

當歸四逆湯

白芍藥當歸各二錢桂枝一錢五分細辛通草甘草各一錢

14 Pinellia Decoction to Drain the Epigastrium (Banxia Xiexin Tang)

· Pinelliae Tuber (detoxicated with ginger decoction) 7.5g

· Ginseng Radix 5.625g

· Glycyrrhizae Radix et Rhizoma 5.625g   · Scutellariae Radix 5.625g

· Zingiberis Rhizoma 3.75g   · Coptidis Rhizoma 1.875g

· Zingiberis Rhizoma recens 3 slices   · Jujubae Fructus 2 pcs.

半夏瀉心湯

製半夏二錢人蔘甘草黃芩各一錢五分乾薑一錢黃連五分生薑三片大棗二枚

15 Fresh Ginger Decoction to Drain the Epigastrium (Shengjiang Xiexin Tang)
  · Zingiberis Rhizoma recens 7.5g   · Pinelliae Tuber 7.5g
  · Ginseng Radix 5.625g   · Zingiberis Rhizoma 5.625g
  · Coptidis Rhizoma 3.75g   · Glycyrrhizae Radix et Rhizoma 3.75g
  · Scutellariae Radix 1.875g   · Jujubae Fructus 3 pcs.
  生薑瀉心湯
  生薑半夏各二錢人蔘乾薑各一錢五分黃連甘草各一錢黃芩五分大棗三枚

16 Licorice Decoction to Drain the Epigastrium (Gancao Xiexin Tang)
  · Glycyrrhizae Radix et Rhizoma 7.5g   · Zingiberis Rhizoma 5.625g
  · Scutellariae Radix 5.625g
  · Pinelliae Tuber (detoxicated with ginger decoction) 3.75g
  · Ginseng Radix 3.75g   · Jujubae Fructus 3 pcs.
  甘草瀉心湯
  甘草二錢乾薑黃芩各一錢五分製半夏人蔘各一錢大棗三枚

17 Virgate Wormwood Decoction (Yinchenhao Tang)
  · Artemisiae scopariae Herba 37.5g   · Rhei Radix et Rhizoma et Radix 18.75g
  · Gardeniae Fructus 7.5g
  Stew Artemisiae scopariae Herba in water until half of the water remains. Add the remaining two drugs and stew until the water decreases again by half. Take the decoction for two days. This is only for the patient who has difficulty in urination and whose urine is bloody. Abdominal distension will be reduced, and jaundice will disappear with urination.
  茵陳蒿湯
  茵陳一兩大黃五錢梔子二錢
  先煎茵陳減半納二味煎又減半服日二小便當利色正赤腹漸減黃從小便去也

18 Appropriate Decoction (Didang Tang)
  · Hirudo (stir-baked) 10 pcs.
  · Tabanus (stir baked, remove the legs and wings) 10 pcs.
  · Persicae Semen (with the tip) 10 pcs.
  · Rhei Radix et Rhizoma (steamed) 11.25g
  抵當湯
  水蛭炒虻蟲炒去足翅桃仁留尖各十枚大黃蒸三錢

19 Peach Pit Decoction for Purgation (Taoren Chengqi Tang)
  · Rhei Radix et Rhizoma 11.25g   · Cinnamomi Cortex 7.5g

· Natrii Sulfas 7.5g   · Glycyrrhizae Radix et Rhizoma 3.75g

· Persicae Semen (with the tip) 10 pcs.

桃仁承氣湯

大黃三錢桂心芒硝各二錢甘草一錢桃仁留尖十枚

20 Cannabis Fruit Pill (Maren Wan)

· Rhei Radix et Rhizoma (steamed) 150g   · Aurantii Fructus immaturus 75g

· Magnoliae officinalis Cortex 75g   · Paeoniae Radix Rubra 75g

· Cannabis Semen 56.25g   · Armeniacae Semen 46.875g

Make the bolus with honey, as big as an empress tree seed. Take 50 boli on an empty stomach with warm water.

麻仁丸

大黃蒸四兩枳實厚朴赤芍藥各二兩麻子仁一兩五錢杏仁一兩二錢五分

爲末蜜丸梧子大空心溫湯下五十丸

21 Purgative Method with Honey

This is used for the weak and elderly who cannot take drugs. Pour the powdered Gleditsiae Fructus into boiling honey, and from the mixture make suppositories. Insert the suppository into the anus in order to loosen the stool.

蜜導法

老人虛人不可用藥者用蜜熬入皂角末少許稔作錠子納肛門卽通

22 Decoction for Potent Purgation (Da Chengqi Tang)

· Rhei Radix et Rhizoma 15g   · Magnoliae officinalis Cortex 7.5g

· Aurantii Fructus immaturus 7.5g   · Natrii Sulfas 7.5g

First stew Aurantii Fructus immaturus and Magnoliae officinalis Cortex with two large glasses of water, and then stew until one glass of water remains. Remove the dregs and add Rhei Radix et Rhizoma et Radix. Stew the remaining amount and remove the dregs. Add Natrii Sulfas and boil it again. Take it while it is warm.

大承氣湯

大黃四錢厚朴枳實芒硝各二錢水二大盞

先煎枳朴至一盞乃下大黃煎至七分去滓入芒硝再一沸溫服

23 Decoction for Mild Purgation (Xiao Chengqi Tang)

· Rhei Radix et Rhizoma 15g   · Magnoliae officinalis Cortex 5.625g

· Aurantii Fructus immaturus 5.625g

Chop up the three drugs and make a pack. Stew it and take the decoction.

小承氣湯

大黃四錢厚朴枳實各一錢五分

剉作一貼水煎服

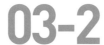

Thirteen Prescriptions and Six Other Prescriptions Containing Crotonis Fructus for the Lesser Yin Person's Disease Mentioned in the Writings of Famous Doctors in the Song, Yuan and Ming Dynasties

宋元明三代醫家著述中
少陰人病經驗行用要藥十三方巴豆藥六方

1　Decoction of Ten Powerful Tonics (Shiquan Dabu Tang)

- Ginseng Radix 3.75g
- Paeoniae Radix Alba 3.75g
- Atractylodis Rhizoma Alba 3.75g
- Glycyrrhizae Radix et Rhizoma (stir-baked with adjuvant) 3.75g
- Astragali Radix 3.75g
- Cinnamomi Cortex 3.75g
- Angelicae Gigantis Radix 3.75g
- Chuanxiong Rhizoma 3.75g
- Poria Sclerotium (white) 3.75g
- Rehmanniae Radix praeparata 3.75g
- Zingiberis Rhizoma recens 3 slices
- Jujubae Fructus 2 pcs.

This prescription from Wang Haogu's 『*Haizangshu*』 is for consumptive patients. In accordance with results from recent studies, Poria Sclerotium (white) and Rehmanniae Radix praeparata should be excluded from this prescription, and Amomi Fructus and Citri Reticulatae Pericarpium should be added.

十全大補湯

人蔘白朮白芍藥灸甘草黃芪肉桂當歸川芎白茯苓熟地黃各一錢生薑三片大棗二枚
此方出於王好古海藏書中治虛勞〇今考更定此方當去白茯苓熟地黃當用砂仁陳皮

2　Tonify the Middle to Augment the Qi Decoction (Buzhong Yiqi Tang)

- Astragali Radix 5.625g
- Glycyrrhizae Radix et Rhizoma (stir-baked with adjuvant) 3.75g
- Ginseng Radix 3.75g
- Atractylodis Rhizoma Alba 3.75g

· Angelicae Gigantis Radix 2.625g   · Citri Reticulatae Pericarpium 2.625g

· Cimicifugae Rhizoma 1.125g   · Bupleuri Radix 1.125g

· Zingiberis Rhizoma recens 3 slices   · Jujubae Fructus 2 pcs.

This prescription from Li Gao's 『*Dongyuanshu*』 is for patients suffering from exhaustion, asthenia, fever, irritability, spontaneous perspiration and weariness. In accordance with results from recent studies, the dosage of Astragali Radix should be increased to 11.25g, Cimicifugae Rhizoma and Bupleuri Radix should be excluded, and Agastachis Herba and Perillae Folium must be added.

補中益氣湯

黃芪一錢五分灸甘草人蔘白朮各一錢當歸陳皮各七分升麻柴胡各三分生薑三片大棗二枚

此方出於李杲東垣書中治勞倦虛弱身熱而煩自汗倦怠○今考更定此方黃芪當用三錢而當去升麻柴胡當用藿香紫蘇葉

3   Decoction of Cyperus and Amomum with Six Noble Ingredients (Xiangsha Liujunzi Tang)

· Cyperi Rhizoma 3.75g   · Atractylodis Rhizoma Alba 3.75g

· Poria Sclerotium (white) 3.75g   · Pinelliae Tuber 3.75g

· Citri Reticulatae Pericarpium 3.75g   · Magnoliae officinalis Cortex 3.75g

· Amomi Fructus rotundus 3.75g   · Ginseng Radix 1.875g

· Glycyrrhizae Radix et Rhizoma 1.875g   · Aucklandiae Radix 1.875g

· Amomi Fructus 1.875g   · Alpiniae oxyphyllae Fructus 1.875g

· Zingiberis Rhizoma recens 3 slices   · Jujubae Fructus 2 pcs.

This prescription, from Gong Xin's 『*Yijian*』 ("Mirror of Medicine") is for patients with loss of appetite, slowness of digestion and fullness of stomach after meal. In accordance with results from recent studies, Poria Sclerotium (white) should be excluded from this prescription, and Polygoni multiflori Radix Alba must be added.

香砂六君子湯

香附子白朮白茯苓半夏陳皮厚朴白豆蔻各一錢人蔘甘草木香縮砂益智仁各五分生薑三片大棗二枚

此方出於龔信醫鑑書中治不思飲食食不下食後倒飽○今考更定此方當去白茯苓當用白何首烏

4   Powder of Qi-Normalizing with Costus Root (Muxiang Shunqi San)

· Linderae Radix 3.75g   · Cyperi Rhizoma 3.75g

· Citri Reticulatae Pericarpium Viride 3.75g   · Citri Reticulatae Pericarpium 3.75g

· Magnoliae officinalis Cortex 3.75g   · Aurantii Fructus 3.75g

· Pinelliae Tuber 3.75g   · Amomi Aucklandiae Radix 1.875g

· Amomi Fructus 1.875g   · Cinnamomi Cortex 1.125g

· Zingiberis Rhizoma 1.125g

· Glycyrrhizae Radix et Rhizoma (stir-baked with adjuvant) 1.125g

· Zingiberis Rhizoma recens 3 slices   · Jujubae Fructus 2 pcs.

These prescriptions, from Gong Xin's 『*Wanbing Huichun*』[1] ("Recovery from All Ailments")

is for patients who have been attacked by qi. This disease occurs when a person is fighting and is so overwhelmed by anger that he loses consciousness. The above drug should be taken, after Zingiberis Rhizoma recens decoction is administered and the patient regains consciousness.

木香順氣散

烏藥香附子靑皮陳皮厚朴枳殼半夏各一錢木香縮砂各五分桂皮乾薑灸甘草各三分生薑三片大棗二枚
此方出於龔信萬病回春書中治中氣病中氣者與人相爭暴怒氣逆而暈倒也先以薑湯救之甦後用此藥

5　Storax Pill (Suhexiang Yuan)

· Atractylodis Rhizoma Alba 75g	· Aucklandiae Radix 75g
· Aquilariae Lignum Resinatum 75g	· Moschus 75g
· Caryophylli Flos 75g	· Benzoinum 75g
· Lignum Santali Albi 75g	· Chebulae Fructus 75g
· Cyperi Rhizoma 75g	· Piperis Longi Fructus 75g
· Rhinoceri cornu 75g	· Cinnabaris 75g
· Olibanum 37.5g	· Borneolum 37.5g

(Use half of the Cinnabaris for coating the boli. Mix Storax oil with Benzoinum paste) Make the above drugs into powder and mix them with the Benzoinum paste and honey. Pound 1000 times in a mortar. Make 40 boli from 37.5g of the resulting mixture. Two or three boli should be taken with spring water or warm water. This prescription from the 『*Jufang*』[2] ("Formularies of the Bureau of People's Welfare Pharmacies") is for patients suffering from all manner of qi-related diseases: qi attack, reversed flow of qi, stagnation of qi, pain due to qi disorders. In the 『*Benshifang*』 ("Effective Prescriptions") by Xu Shuwei said, "This prescription should be used for the cases, where excessive joy impairs yang, sudden anger impairs yin, and melancholy results from stuffiness, which, if serious, reverses the flow of qi. If used for apoplexy, many patients will die." In the 『*Dexiaofang*』, Wei Yilin said, "The patient who is affected by wind has a floating pulse, fever and abundant expectoration in the mouth. The patient who is attacked by qi has a deep and sinking pulse, cold body, and dry mouth." In accordance with results from recent studies, Moschus, Rhinoceri cornu, Cinnabaris, Borneolum, and Olibanum should be excluded from this prescription, and Agastachis Herba, Foeniculi Fructus, Cinnamomi Cortex, Faeces Trogopterorum, and Rhizoma Corydalidis must be added.

蘇合香元

白朮木香沈香麝香丁香安息香白檀香訶子皮香附子蓽撥犀角朱砂各二兩朱砂半爲衣蘇合油入安
息香膏內乳香龍腦各一兩
右細末用安息香膏並煉蜜搜和千搗每一兩分作四十丸每取二三丸井華水或溫水下治一切氣疾中
氣上氣氣逆鬱氣痛此方出於局方許叔微本事方曰凡人暴喜傷陽暴怒傷陰憂愁怫意氣多厥逆當
用此藥若槩作中風治多致殺人○危亦林得效方曰中風脈浮身溫口多痰涎中氣脈沈身涼口無痰涎
○今考更定此方當去麝香犀角朱砂龍腦乳香當用藿香茴香桂皮五靈脂玄胡索

6　Agastache Powder to Rectify the Qi (Huoxiang Zhengqi San)

- Agastachis Herba 5.625g
- Perillae Folium 3.75g
- Magnoliae officinalis Cortex 1.875g
- Arecae Pericarpium 1.875g
- Atractylodis Rhizoma Alba 1.875g
- Citri Reticulatae Pericarpium 1.875g
- Pinelliae Tuber 1.875g
- Glycyrrhizae Radix et Rhizoma 1.875g
- Platycodi Radix 1.875g
- Angelicae dahuricae Radix 1.875g
- Poria Sclerotium (white) 1.875g
- Zingiberis Rhizoma recens 3 slices
- Jujubae Fructus 2 pcs.

This prescription, from Gong Xin's 『*Yijian*』 is for patients affected by cold. In accordance with results from recent studies, Platycodi Radix, Angelicae dahuricae Radix, and Poria Sclerotium (white) should be excluded from this prescription, while Cinnamomi Cortex, Zingiberis Rhizoma, and Alpiniae oxyphyllae Fructus must be added.

藿香正氣散

藿香一錢五分紫蘇葉一錢厚朴大腹皮白朮陳皮半夏甘草桔梗白芷白茯苓各五分生薑三片大棗二枚

此方出於龔信醫鑑書中治傷寒〇今考更定此方當去桔梗白芷白茯苓當用桂皮乾薑益智仁

7　Cyperus and Perilla Leaf Powder (Xiangsu San)

- Cyperi Rhizoma 11.25g
- Perillae Folium 9.375g
- Citri Reticulatae Pericarpium 5.625g
- Atractylodis Rhizoma 3.75g
- Glycyrrhizae Radix et Rhizoma 3.75g
- Zingiberis Rhizoma recens 3 slices
- Allii Fistulosi Bulbus 2 stems

This prescription, from Wei Yilin's 『*Dexiaofang*』 is for patients suffering from four seasons' epidemic febrile diseases. In the 『*Jufang*』, we read, "Once upon a time, there was an old man. He gave this prescription to a man. There were many patients who suffered from epidemic febrile disease in that city. Everyone who took that medicine recovered."

香蘇散

香附子三錢紫蘇葉二錢五分陳皮一錢五分蒼朮甘草各一錢生薑三片蔥白二莖

此方出於危亦林得效方書中治四時瘟疫〇局方曰昔有一老人授此方與一人令其合施城中大疫服此皆愈

8　Cinnamon Twig and Aconite Decoction (Guizhi Fuzi Tang)

- Aconiti Lateralis Radix Praeparata (stir-baked at high temperature) 11.25g
- Cinnamomi Ramulus 11.25g
- Paeoniae Radix Alba 7.5g
- Glycyrrhizae Radix et Rhizoma (stir-baked with adjuvant) 3.75g
- Zingiberis Rhizoma recens 3 slices
- Jujubae Fructus 2 pcs.

This prescription from Li Chan's 『*Yixue Rumen*』 is for patients with continuous sweating and stiffness of the limbs.

桂枝附子湯

炮附子桂枝各三錢白芍藥二錢灸甘草一錢生薑三片大棗二枚

此方出於李梴醫學入門書中治汗漏不止四肢拘急難以屈

9　Virgate Wormwood Decoction for Frigid Extremities (Yinchen Sini Tang)

· Artemisiae scopariae Herba 37.5g

· Aconiti Lateralis Radix Praeparata (stir-baked at high temperature) 3.75g

· Zingiberis Rhizoma (stir-baked at high temperature) 3.75g

· Glycyrrhizae Radix et Rhizoma (stir-baked with adjuvant) 3.75g

This prescription cures yin jaundice with incessant cold sweating.

茵蔯四逆湯

茵蔯一兩炮附子炮乾薑灸甘草各一錢

治陰黃病冷汗不止

10　Virgate Wormwood and Aconite Decoction (Yinchen Fuzi Tang)

· Artemisiae scopariae Herba 37.5g

· Aconiti Lateralis Radix Praeparata (stir-baked at high temperature) 3.75g

· Glycyrrhizae Radix et Rhizoma (stir-baked with adjuvant) 3.75g

This prescription cures yin jaundice with cold body.

茵蔯附子湯

茵蔯一兩炮附子灸甘草各一錢

治陰黃病身冷

11　Virgate Wormwood and Tangerine Peel Decoction (Yinchen Jupi Tang)

· Artemisiae scopariae Herba 37.5g　　· Citri Reticulatae Pericarpium 3.75g

· Atractylodis Rhizoma Alba 3.75g　　· Pinelliae Tuber 3.75g

· Zingiberis Rhizoma recens 3.75g

This prescription cures yin jaundice with asthma, vomiting and no thirst. The above three prescriptions originate from Zhu Gong's 『*Huorenshu*』 ("Book for Saving Life").

茵蔯橘皮湯

茵蔯一兩陳皮白朮半夏生薑各一錢

治陰黃病喘嘔不渴右三方出於朱肱活人書中

12　Decoction of Three Drugs including Ginseng and Evodia (Sanwei Shenyu Tang)

· Evodiae Fructus 11.25g　　· Ginseng Radix 7.5g

· Zingiberis Rhizoma recens 4 slices　　· Jujubae Fructus 2 pcs.

This prescription cures reverting yin pattern with vomiting of frothy sputum, lesser yin pattern with cold limbs, irritability and restlessness, and yang brightness pattern with a tendency to vomit after eating.

三味蔘萸湯

吳茱萸三錢人蔘二錢生薑四片大棗二枚

治厥陰證嘔吐涎沫少陰證厥冷煩躁陽明證食穀欲嘔皆妙

13 Thunderbolt Powder (Pili San)

· Aconiti Lateralis Radix Praeparata 1 pc

Bake it well at high temperature and bury it in cold ashes for 30 minutes. Take out from the ashes and cut it into many pieces. Stew them with 3.75g of old tea leaves in one glass of water until six-tenths of the liquid remains. Remove the dregs, add half a spoonful of honey and take it when it cools down. After a short time, the patient's irritability will cease, and he will fall asleep and perspire. Recovery follows. This prescription is for patients whose yang is kept in the exterior by excessive yin in the interior. The above two prescriptions originate from Li Chan's 『*Yixue Rumen*』.

霹靂散

附子一枚

炮過以冷灰培半時取出切半枚細剉入臘茶一錢水一盞煎至六分去渣入熟蜜半匙放冷服之須臾躁止得睡汗出差治陰盛隔陽證右二方出於李梴醫學入門書中

14 Warm and White Pills (Wenbai Yuan)

· Aconiti Radix (stir-baked at high temperature) 93.75g

· Evodiae Fructus 18.75g	· Platycodi Radix 18.75g
· Bupleuri Radix 18.75g	· Apori graminei Rhizoma 18.75g
· Asteris Radix 18.75g	· Coptidis Rhizoma 18.75g

· Zingiberis Rhizoma (stir-baked at high temperature) 18.75g

· Cinnamomi Cortex 18.75g	· Rubiae Radix (stir-baked) 18.75g

· Poria Sclerotium (red) 18.75g

· Gleditsiae Spina (stir-baked with adjuvant) 18.75g

· Magnoliae officinalis Cortex 18.75g	· Ginseng Radix 18.75g

· Crotonis Fructus Pulveratum 18.75g

Pound the above drugs and make pills with honey as big as an empress tree seed. Take three to seven pills with the decoction of Zingiberis Rhizoma recens. This prescription from the 『*Jufang*』 is for patients with abdominal mass, hypochondriac lump, jaundice, abdominal distention, ten types of disease due to water retention, nine types of heart-related pain, eight types of disease due to hypochondriac obstruction, five types of gonorrhea and chronic malaria. In the 『*Yijian*』, Gong Xin says, "This medicine is for patients who have an abdominal mass as though pregnant, weight loss, fatigue, and sometimes extreme mood swings as if insane. This drug will bring spontaneous relief. When used for chronic diseases, it will cause the patient to discharge stool containing worm-, snake- or pus-like elements."

溫白元

川烏炮二兩五錢吳茱萸桔梗柴胡石菖蒲紫菀黃連乾薑炮肉桂川椒炒赤茯苓皂角灸厚朴人蔘巴豆

霜各五錢右爲末煉蜜和丸梧子大薑湯下三丸或五丸至七丸此方出於局方治積聚癥癖黃疸鼓脹十
種水氣九種心痛八種痞塞五種淋疾遠年瘧疾○龔信醫鑑曰婦人腹中積聚有似懷孕羸瘦困弊或歌
哭如邪祟服此藥自愈久病服之則皆瀉出蟲蛇惡膿之物

15 Pills for Pestilential Jaundice (Zhangdan Wan)

- Artemisiae scopariae Herba 37.5g
- Gardeniae Fructus 37.5g
- Rhei Radix et Rhizoma 37.5g
- Natrii Sulfas 37.5g
- Armeniacae Semen 22.5g
- Dichroae Radix 15g
- Carapax Trionycis 15g
- Crotonis Fructus Pulveratum 15g
- Sojae Semen Praeparatum 7.5g

Pound the drugs into a powder and make the pills with rice cake as big as an empress tree seed. Three to five pills are to be taken with warm water. This prescription from Wei Yilin's 『*Dexiaofang*』 is also called Yinchen Wan. It cures epidemic febrile diseases, endemic malaria, jaundice, and dampness-heat disease.

瘴疸丸

茵蔯梔子大黃芒硝各一兩杏仁六錢常山鱉甲巴豆霜各四錢豆豉二錢

右爲末蒸餅和丸梧子大每三丸或五丸溫水送下此方出於危亦林得效方書中一名茵蔯丸治時行瘟
疫及瘴瘧黃疸濕熱病

16 Pills for Removing Stagnancy of Indigested Food with Sparganium (Sanling Xiaoji Wan)

- Sparganii Rhizoma 26.25g
- Curcumae Rhizoma 26.25g
- Massa Medicata Fermentata 26.25g
- Foeniculi Fructus 18.75g
- Crotonis Fructus (with skin, stir-baked with rice and then remove the rice) 18.75g
- Citri Reticulatae Pericarpium Viride 18.75g
- Citri Reticulatae Pericarpium 18.75g
- Caryophylli Flos (skin) 11.25g
- Alpiniae oxyphyllae Fructus 11.25g

Pound the drugs into a powder and make the pasted pills with vinegar as big as an empress tree seed. 30~40 pills are taken with the decoction of Zingiberis Rhizoma recens. This prescription from 『*Dongyuanshu*』 written by Li Gao, treats the patient who suffers from indigestion induced by raw and cold food, with a stuffness-fullness sensation.

三稜消積丸

三稜蓬朮神麴各七錢巴豆和皮入米同炒黑去米青皮陳皮茴香各五錢丁香皮益智仁各三錢

右爲末醋糊和丸梧子大薑湯下三四十丸此方出於李杲東垣書中治生冷物不消滿悶

17 Secretly Prescribed Pills for Removing Stagnancy (Mifang Huazhi Wan)

- Sparganii Rhizoma 18g
- Curcumae Rhizoma (roasted in hot ashes with Sparganii Rhizoma) 18g
- Pinelliae Tuber (fermented) 9.375g
- Aucklandiae Radix 9.375g
- Caryophylli Flos 9.375g
- Citri Reticulatae Pericarpium Viride 9.375g

· Citri Reticulatae Pericarpium (only pink portion) 9.375g

· Coptidis Rhizoma 9.375g

· Crotonis Fructus (preserve in vinegar for one night and stew until dried) 22.5g

Pound the drugs into a powder with Mume Fructus and some wheat flour and make pasted pills as big as an oat. Take five to ten pills. In order to facilitate bowel movement, take with hot water. To eliminate abdominal mass, taken with the decoction of Citri Recitulatae Pericarpium. To bine the bowels, take with cold water. This prescription originated from 『*Danxi Xinfa*』 written by Zhu Zhenheng. It regulates the flow of all kinds of qi, removes all kinds of abdominal mass and makes the obstinate chronic abdominal mass spontaneously. It quickly removes the mass whether the mass appeared suddenly or a short time ago. It has the function of clearing blockage by using natural laws and has the wonder of reinforcing and reducing by regulating yin and yang.

秘方化滯丸

三稜蓬朮並煨各四錢八分半夏麴木香丁香靑皮陳皮並去白黃連各二錢五分巴豆肉醋浸一宿熬乾六錢右爲末以烏梅末入麵少許煮作糊和丸黍米大每服五七丸至十丸欲通利則以熱湯下欲磨積則陳皮湯下欲止泄則飮冷水此方出於朱震亨丹溪心法書中理一切氣化一切積久堅沈痼磨之自消暴積乍留導之立去奪造化有通塞之功調陰陽有補瀉之妙

18 Powder of Three White Drugs (Sanwu Bai San)

· Platycodi Radix 11.25g

· Bulbus Fritillariae Cirrhosae 11.25g

· Crotonis Fructus (remove husk, stew the seeds and mash to form a greasy pulp) 3.75g

Pound the drugs into a powder, mix 2g of the drugs with hot water and have the patient take it. If the patient is weak, the dosage should be reduced by half. In case the patient vomits or loose stool is desired, give a cup of hot rice gruel. In case of ceaseless diarrhea, a cup of cold rice gruel should be given.

三物白散

桔梗貝母各三錢巴豆去皮心熬研如脂一錢

右爲末和勻白湯和服半錢弱人減半或吐或利不利進熱粥一碗利不止進冷粥一碗

19 Pills for Alleviation (Ruyi Dan)

· Aconiti Radix (stir-baked at high temperature) 30g

· Arecae Semen 18.75g

· Ginseng Radix 18.75g	· Bupleuri Radix 18.75g
· Evodiae Fructus 18.75g	· Rubiae Radix 18.75g
· Poria Sclerotium (white) 18.75g	· Zingiberis Rhizoma recens 18.75g
· Coptidis Rhizoma 18.75g	· Asteris Radix 18.75g
· Magnoliae officinalis Cortex 18.75g	· Cinnamomi Cortex 18.75g

· Angelicae Gigantis Radix 18.75g   · Platycodi Radix 18.75g

· Gleditsiae Spina 18.75g   · Acori graminei Rhizoma 18.75g

· Crotonis Fructus Pulveratum 9.375g

Pound the drugs into powder and make pills with honey as big as an empress tree seed and coat with Cinnabaris. Take five to seven pills with warm water. It can cure all kinds of epidemic febrile diseases and possessedness. The above two prescriptions originated from Li Chan's 『*Yixue Rumen*』.

如意丹

川烏炮八錢檳榔人蔘柴胡吳茱萸川椒白茯苓白薑黃連紫菀厚朴肉桂當歸桔梗皂角石菖蒲各五錢 巴豆霜二錢五分

右爲末煉蜜和丸梧子大朱砂爲衣每五丸或七丸溫水下專治瘟疫及一切鬼祟右二方出於李梴醫學 入門書中

I have said that the above six prescriptions originated from the experiments of ancient doctors, and all of them use the effectiveness of Crotonis Fructus. The purposes of its use are not different from one another. Generally, in a lesser yin person's disease, it must be used. Do not use the drug in an imprudent manner, nor be afraid of using it. I have set down my experiences with these six prescriptions. Someone who knows the principles well will obtain good results, but it is not to be used in an imprudent manner.

論曰右巴豆六方卽古人之各自置方各自經驗而此六方同是一巴豆之力則所用亦無異而同歸於一 也盖巴豆少陰人病之必不可不用而又不可輕用必不可浪用而又不可疑用之藥故聯錄六方備述經 驗昭明其理者欲其用之必中而不敢輕忽也

Notes

1) 『*Wanbing Huichun*』(萬病回春)

The "Recovery from All Ailments", a comprehensive medical work consisting of eight volumes by Gong Tingxian, published in 1587. The book describes in detail numerous diseases and patterns. It explains treatments and prescriptions in detail. This work was a great influence on later practitioners.

2) 『*Jufang*』(局方)

The "Formularies of the Bureau of People's Welfare Pharmacies", 『*Taiping Huimin Heji Jufang*』(太平惠民和劑局方), or simply 『*Heji Jufang*』(和劑局方), compiled by Chen Shiwen (陳師文) and others, in 1151 A.D.. It is a ten volume work dividing 788 oft-used and effective prescriptions into fourteen categories.

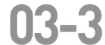

Twenty Four Newly Formulated Prescriptions for the Lesser Yin Person's Disease

新定少陰人病應用要藥二十四方

1 Astragalus, Cinnamon Twig, and Aconite Decoction (Hwanggi Gyeji Buja Tang)
  · Cinnamomi Ramulus 11.25g   · Astragali Radix 11.25g
  · Paeoniae Radix Alba 7.5g   · Angelicae Gigantis Radix 3.75g
  · Glycyrrhizae Radix et Rhizoma (stir-baked with adjuvant) 3.75g
  · Aconiti Lateralis Radix Praeparata (stir-baked at high temperature) 3.75~7.5g
  · Zingiberis Rhizoma recens 3 slices
  · Jujubae Fructus 2 pcs.
  黃芪桂枝附子湯
  桂枝黃芪各三錢白芍藥二錢當歸灸甘草各一錢炮附子一錢或二錢薑三片棗二枚

2 Ginseng, Cinnamon Twig, and Aconite Decoction (Insam Gyeji Buja Tang)
  · Ginseng Radix 15g   · Cinnamomi Ramulus 11.25g
  · Paeoniae Radix Alba 7.5g   · Astragali Radix 7.5g
  · Angelicae Gigantis Radix 3.75g
  · Glycyrrhizae Radix et Rhizoma (stir-baked with adjuvant) 3.75g
  · Aconiti Lateralis Radix Praeparata (stir-baked at high temperature) 3.75~7.5g
  · Zingiberis Rhizoma recens 3 slices
  · Jujubae Fructus 2 pcs.
  人蔘桂枝附子湯
  人蔘四錢桂枝三錢白芍藥黃芪各二錢當歸灸甘草各一錢炮附子一錢或二錢薑三片棗二枚

3 Aconite Decoction for Ascending Yang and Replenishing Qi (Seungyang Ikgi Buja Tang)

· Ginseng Radix 7.5g   · Cinnamomi Ramulus 7.5g

· Paeoniae Radix Alba 7.5g   · Astragali Radix 7.5g

· Polygoni multiflori Radix 3.75g   · Cinnamomi Cortex 3.75g

· Angelicae Gigantis Radix 3.75g

· Glycyrrhizae Radix et Rhizoma (stir-baked with adjuvant) 3.75g

· Aconiti Lateralis Radix Praeparata (stir-baked at high temperature) 3.75~7.5g

· Zingiberis Rhizoma recens 3 slices

· Jujubae Fructus 2 pcs.

升陽益氣附子湯

人蔘桂枝白芍藥黃芪各二錢白何首烏官桂當歸灸甘草各一錢炮附子一錢或二錢薑三片棗二枚

4 Ginseng, Cinnamon Bark, and Aconite Decoction (Insam Gwangye Buja Tang)

· Ginseng Radix 18.75~37.5g   · Cinnamomi Cortex 11.25g

· Astragali Radix 11.25g   · Paeoniae Radix Alba 7.5g

· Angelicae Gigantis Radix 3.75g

· Glycyrrhizae Radix et Rhizoma (stir-baked with adjuvant) 3.75g

· Aconiti Lateralis Radix Praeparata (stir-baked at high temperature) 7.5~9.375g

· Zingiberis Rhizoma recens 3 slices

· Jujubae Fructus 2 pcs.

The above four prescriptions are used for yang collapse, which is a critical disease. If the yang collapse patient's urine is clean and fluent, there is a possibility of recovery. The patient should take 3.75g of Aconiti Lateralis Radix Praeparata twice a day. If he is in critical condition, with reddish and difficult urination, then there is little chance for recovery. The patient should take 7.5g of Aconiti Lateralis Radix Praeparata two or three times a day. However, in general, before facing the critical condition, 3.75g of Aconiti Lateralis Radix Praeparata should be taken. The same amount is also used when the patient is no longer in critical condition. If the patient is nursing himself, 3.75g of Aconiti Lateralis Radix Praeparata should be taken twice a day.

人蔘官桂附子湯

人蔘五錢或一兩官桂黃芪各三錢白芍藥二錢當歸灸甘草各一錢炮附子二錢或二錢五分薑三片棗二枚

右四方皆亡陽危病藥也亡陽病人小便白而多危有餘地則用附子一錢日再服小便赤而少危無餘地則用附子二錢日二三服病在將危用一錢病在免危用一錢病在調理亦一錢日再服

5 Decoction for Ascending Yang and Replenishing Qi (Seungyang Ikgi Tang)

· Ginseng Radix 7.5g   · Cinnamomi Ramulus 7.5g

· Astragali Radix 7.5g   · Paeoniae Radix Alba 7.5g

· Polygoni multiflori Radix 3.75g   · Cinnamomi Cortex 3.75g

· Angelicae Gigantis Radix 3.75g

· Glycyrrhizae Radix et Rhizoma (stir-baked with adjuvant) 3.75g

· Zingiberis Rhizoma recens 3 slices

· Jujubae Fructus 2 pcs.

升陽益氣湯

人蔘桂枝黃芪白芍藥各二錢白何首烏官桂當歸灸甘草各一錢薑三片棗二枚

6 Tonify the Middle to Augment the Qi Decoction (Bojung Ikgi Tang)

· Ginseng Radix 11.25g   · Astragali Radix 11.25g

· Glycyrrhizae Radix et Rhizoma (stir-baked with adjuvant) 3.75g

· Atractylodis Rhizoma Alba 3.75g   · Angelicae Gigantis Radix 3.75g

· Citri Reticulatae Pericarpium 3.75g   · Pogostemonis Herba 1.125~1.875g

· Perillae Folium 1.125~1.875g   · Zingiberis Rhizoma recens 3 slices

· Jujubae Fructus 2 pcs.

補中益氣湯

人蔘黃芪各三錢灸甘草白朮當歸陳皮各一錢藿香蘇葉各三分或各五分薑三片棗二枚

7 Astragalus and Cinnamon Twig Decoction (Hwanggi Gyeji Tang)

· Cinnamomi Ramulus 11.25g   · Paeoniae Radix Alba 7.5g

· Astragali Radix 7.5g   · Polygoni multiflori Radix 3.75g

· Angelicae Gigantis Radix 3.75g

· Glycyrrhizae Radix et Rhizoma (stir-baked with adjuvant) 3.75g

· Zingiberis Rhizoma recens 3 slices   · Jujubae Fructus 2 pcs.

黃芪桂枝湯

桂枝三錢白芍藥黃芪各二錢白何烏當歸灸甘草各一錢薑三片棗二枚

8 Chuanxiong and Cinnamon Twig Decoction (Cheongung Gyeji Tang)

· Cinnamomi Ramulus 11.25g   · Paeoniae Radix Alba 7.5g

· Chuanxiong Rhizoma 3.75g   · Atractylodis Rhizoma 3.75g

· Citri Reticulatae Pericarpium 3.75g

· Glycyrrhizae Radix et Rhizoma (stir-baked with adjuvant) 3.75g

· Zingiberis Rhizoma recens 3 slices

· Jujubae Fructus 2 pcs.

川芎桂枝湯

桂枝三錢白芍藥二錢川芎蒼朮陳皮灸甘草各一錢薑三片棗二枚

9 Powder of Chuanxiong, Chinese Angelica, Cyperus, and Perilla Leaf Powder (Gunggwi Hy-angso San)

· Cyperi Rhizoma 7.5g   · Perillae Folium 3.75g

· Chuanxiong Rhizoma 3.75g   · Angelicae Gigantis Radix 3.75g

· Atractylodis Rhizoma 3.75g　　　　· Citri Reticulatae Pericarpium 3.75g

· Glycyrrhizae Radix et Rhizoma (stir-baked with adjuvant) 3.75g

· Allii Radix 5 stems

· Zingiberis Rhizoma recens 3 slices

· Jujubae Fructus 2 pcs.

芎歸香蘇散

香附子二錢紫蘇葉川芎當歸蒼朮陳皮灸甘草各一錢葱白五莖薑三片棗二枚

10 Agastache Powder to Rectify the Qi (Gwakhyang Jeonggi San)

· Agastachis Herba 5.625g　　　　· Perillae Folium 3.75g

· Atractylodis Rhizoma 1.875g　　　· Atractylodis Rhizoma Alba 1.875g

· Pinelliae Tuber 1.875g　　　　　· Citri Reticulatae Pericarpium 1.875g

· Citri Reticulatae Pericarpium Viride 1.875g · Arecae Pericarpium 1.875g

· Cinnamomi Ramulus 1.875g　　　· Zingiberis Rhizoma 1.875g

· Alpiniae oxyphyllae Fructus 1.875g

· Glycyrrhizae Radix et Rhizoma (stir-baked with adjuvant) 1.875g

· Zingiberis Rhizoma recens 3 slices　· Jujubae Fructus 2 pcs.

藿香正氣散

藿香一錢五分紫蘇葉一錢蒼朮白朮半夏陳皮靑皮大腹皮桂皮乾薑益智仁灸甘草各五分薑三片棗二枚

11 Decoction of Eight Noble Ingredients (Palmul Gunja Tang)

· Ginseng Radix 7.5g　　　　　　· Astragali Radix 3.75g

· Atractylodis Rhizoma Alba 3.75g　· Paeoniae Radix Alba 3.75g

· Angelicae Gigantis Radix 3.75g　· Chuanxiong Rhizoma 3.75g

· Citri Reticulatae Pericarpium 3.75g

· Glycyrrhizae Radix et Rhizoma (stir-baked with adjuvant) 3.75g

· Zingiberis Rhizoma recens 3 slices

· Jujubae Fructus 2 pcs.

If Polygoni multiflori Radix is substituted for Ginseng Radix in this prescription, it is named Baikhao Gunja Tang. If one uses 3.75g of both Ginseng Radix and Astragali Radix, and adds 37.5g of Ginseng Radix and 3.75g of Astragali Radix and Cinnamomi Ramulus to the remaining drugs, it is named Sibjeon Daibo Tang. If one uses 3.75g each of Ginseng Radix and Astragali Radix, it is named Doksam Palmul Tang.

八物君子湯

人蔘二錢黃芪白朮白芍藥當歸川芎陳皮灸甘草各一錢薑三片棗二枚

本方以白何首烏易人蔘則名曰白何烏君子湯本方用蔘芪各一錢加白何烏官桂各一錢則名曰十全大補湯本方用人蔘一兩黃芪一錢則名曰獨蔘八物湯

12 Decoction of Eight Ingredients with Cyperus (Hyangbuja Palmul Tang)

· Cyperi Rhizoma 7.5g · Angelicae Gigantis Radix 7.5g

· Paeoniae Radix Alba 7.5g · Atractylodis Rhizoma Alba 3.75g

· Polygoni multiflori Radix 3.75g · Chuanxiong Rhizoma 3.75g

· Citri Reticulatae Pericarpium 3.75g

· Glycyrrhizae Radix et Rhizoma (stir-baked with adjuvant) 3.75g

· Zingiberis Rhizoma recens 3 slices

· Jujubae Fructus 2 pcs.

I once obtained good results in treating a woman who had a dry throat and parched tongue with a mild headache as a consequence of her anxiety impairing her Spleen.

香附子八物湯

香附子當歸白芍藥各二錢白朮白何烏川芎陳皮灸甘草各一錢薑三片棗二枚

嘗治婦人思慮傷脾咽乾舌燥隱隱有頭痛神效

13 Cinnamon Twig, Pinellia, and Ginger Decoction (Gyeji Banha Sainggang Tang)

· Zingiberis Rhizoma recens 11.25g · Cinnamomi Ramulus 7.5g

· Pinelliae Tuber 7.5g · Paeoniae Radix Alba 3.75g

· Atractylodis Rhizoma Alba 3.75g · Citri Reticulatae Pericarpium 3.75g

· Glycyrrhizae Radix et Rhizoma (stir-baked with adjuvant) 3.75g

This prescription cures vomiting brought on by deficiency-cold and accumulation of water in the chest.

桂枝半夏生薑湯

生薑三錢桂枝半夏各二錢白芍藥白朮陳皮灸甘草各一錢

治虛寒嘔吐水結胸等證

14 Nourish the Stomach Decoction with Auklandia and Amomum (Hyangsa Yangwi Tang)

· Ginseng Radix 3.75g · Atractylodis Rhizoma Alba 3.75g

· Paeoniae Radix Alba 3.75g

· Glycyrrhizae Radix et Rhizoma (stir-baked with adjuvant) 3.75g

· Pinelliae Tuber 3.75g · Cyperi Rhizoma 3.75g

· Citri Reticulatae Pericarpium 3.75g · Zingiberis Rhizoma 3.75g

· Crataegi Fructus 3.75g · Amomi Fructus 3.75g

· Amomi Fructus rotundus 3.75g · Zingiberis Rhizoma recens 3 slices

· Jujubae Fructus 2 pcs.

香砂養胃湯

人蔘白朮白芍藥灸甘草半夏香附子陳皮乾薑山查肉砂仁白豆蔻各一錢薑三片棗二枚

15 Decoction for Relieving the Middle with Red/White Flowery Knotweed (Jeokbaikhao Gwanjung Tang)

· Polygoni multiflori Radix Alba 3.75g   · Polygoni multiflori Radix Rubra 3.75g

· Alpiniae officinarum Rhizoma 3.75g   · Zingiberis Rhizoma 3.75g

· Citri Reticulatae Pericarpium Viride 3.75g · Citri Reticulatae Pericarpium 3.75g

· Cyperi Rhizoma 3.75g   · Alpiniae oxyphyllae Fructus 3.75g

· Jujubae Fructus 2 pcs.

This prescription is for patients experiencing exhaustion in all four limbs, difficulty in urination, impotency and the strong possibility of edema. If Magnoliae officinalis Cortex, Aurantii Fructus immaturus, Aucklandiae Radix, and Arecae Pericarpium, 1.875g each, are added, it will promote the normal flow of qi in the meridian. After the appearance of an edema, one should calm the patient for 100 days and give him two packs of this prescription every day; the edema will disappear. If Ginseng Radix is substituted for Polygoni multiflori Radix Rubra in this prescription, it is named Insam Baikhao Gwanjung Tang. If Angelicae Gigantis Radix is substituted for Polygoni multiflori Radix Rubra in this prescription, it is named Danggwi Baikhao Gwanjung Tang. There is an old prescription that consists of Zingiberis Rhizoma, Alpiniae officinarum Rhizoma, Citri Reticulatae Pericarpium Viride, and Citri Reticulatae Pericarpium in equal dosage. When it is made into pills or a decoction, it is named Kuan-zhong Tang. I have treated lesser yin person experiencing discomfort in urination, impotency, general exhaustion and weakness with the above, and obtained good results in all cases. In the case where 3.75g each of Faeces Trogopterorum and Alpiniae oxyphyllae Fructus are added to the Kuanzhong Wan, it will relieve the abdominal pain miraculously.

赤白何烏寬中湯

白何烏赤何烏良薑乾薑靑皮陳皮香附子益智仁各一錢棗二枚

治四體倦怠小便不快陽道不興將有浮腫之漸者用之本方加厚朴枳實木香大腹皮各五分則又有通氣脈之功力雖浮腫已成者安心靜慮一百日而日再服則自無不效之理本方以人蔘易赤何烏則名曰人蔘白何烏寬中湯以當歸易赤何烏則名曰當歸白何烏寬中湯○古方有乾薑良薑靑皮陳皮等分作湯丸名曰寬中湯嘗治少陰人小便不快陽道不興四體倦怠無力者用之必效百發百中又寬中丸本方加五靈脂益智仁各一錢則治腹痛神效

16 Garlic and Honey Decoction (Sanmil Tang)

· Polygoni multiflori Radix Alba 3.75g   · Atractylodis Rhizoma Alba 3.75g

· Paeoniae Radix Alba 3.75g   · Cinnamomi Ramulus 3.75g

· Artemisiae scopariae Herba 3.75g   · Leonurus japonicus Houtt 3.75

· Halloysitum Rubrum 3.75g   · Papaveris Fructus 3.75g

· Zingiberis Rhizoma recens 3 slices   · Jujubae Fructus 2 pcs.

· Garlic 5 roots   · Honey: half of a spoon

This prescription treats dysentery.

蒜蜜湯

白何烏白朮白芍藥桂枝茵蔯益母草赤石脂罌粟殼各一錢薑三片棗二枚大蒜五根淸蜜半匙

治痢疾

17 Paste of Chicken and Ginseng (Gyesam Go)

· Ginseng Radix 37.5g   · Cinnamomi Cortex 3.75g

· Chicken 1

Stew and take the decoction. It may be flavored with black pepper and honey. This prescription has a long tradition of treating malaria and dysentery miraculously. I once cured a case of chronic malaria, first using Crotonis Fructus as a purgative drug, and then Gyesam Go for several days. It also cured chronic malaria. Often, a cinnamon core is substituted for Cinnamomi Cortex.

鷄蔘膏

人蔘一兩桂皮一錢鷄一首濃煎服或以胡椒淸蜜助滋味無妨

此方自古有方治瘧疾痢疾神效嘗治久瘧先用巴豆通利大便後數三日連用鷄蔘膏快效桂皮或以桂心代用

18 Pellet of Croton (Padu Dan)

· Crotonis Fructus 1 grain (remove husk)

Take a half-grain or whole grain of Crotonis Fructus with warm water. While the other drugs are being stewed, Crotonis Fructus can directly affect the stomach and intestine. After the effect of Crotonis Fructus has almost cleared, the decoction is taken and it will go together with Crotonis Fructus. This will clear the contents in the stomach and intestines and raise the normal qi. After defecation, take Crotonis Fructus continuously. A whole grain can induce diarrhea, while a half-grain can eliminate retained stool.

巴豆丹

巴豆一粒去殼

取粒溫水吞下全粒或半粒仍煎湯藥以煎藥時刻巴豆獨行腹胃間太半用力然後服湯藥則湯藥可以與巴豆同行通快腹胃升提其氣也再煎湯藥大便通後又連服之巴豆全粒下利半粒化積

19 Ginseng and Tangerine Peel Decoction (Insam Jinpi Tang)

· Ginseng Radix 37.5g   · Zingiberis Rhizoma recens 3.75g

· Amomi Fructus 3.75g   · Citri Reticulatae Pericarpium 3.75g

· Jujubae Fructus 2 pcs.

If Zingiberis Rhizoma (stir-baked at high temperature) is substituted for Zingiberis Rhizoma recens and 3.75g of Cinnamomi Cortex is added in this prescription, it will warm the stomach and expel the cold more efficiently. I once treated a baby, only several months old, who had chronic infantile convulsions due to yin type inflammatory swelling. I administered the drug for several days, and the infant recovered. However, I did not subsequently have the baby take the medicine continuously, and he suffered a relapse from which he never recovered.

人蔘陳皮湯

人蔘一兩生薑砂仁陳皮各一錢棗二枚

本方以炮乾薑易生薑又加桂皮一錢則尤有溫胃逐冷之力以本方嘗治未周年小兒陰毒慢風連服數日病快愈矣病愈後更不服藥再發不治

20 Ginseng and Evodia Decoction (Insam Osuyu Tang)

· Ginseng Radix 37.5g   · Evodiae Fructus 11.25g

· Zingiberis Rhizoma recens 11.25g   · Paeoniae Radix Alba 3.75g

· Angelicae Gigantis Radix 3.75g   · Cinnamomi Cortex 3.75g

人蔘吳茱萸湯

人蔘一兩吳茱萸生薑各三錢白芍藥當歸官桂各一錢

21 Cinnamon Bark and Aconite Decoction for Regulating the Middle (Gwangye Buja Ijung Tang)

· Ginseng Radix 11.25g   · Atractylodis Rhizoma Alba 7.5g

· Zingiberis Rhizoma (stir-baked at high temperature) 7.5g

· Cinnamomi Cortex 7.5g   · Paeoniae Radix Alba 3.75g

· Citri Reticulatae Pericarpium 3.75g

· Glycyrrhizae Radix et Rhizoma (stir-baked with adjuvant) 3.75g

· Aconiti Lateralis Radix Praeparata (stir-baked at high temperature) 3.75~7.5g

官桂附子理中湯

人蔘三錢白朮炮乾薑官桂各二錢白芍藥陳皮灸甘草各一錢炮附子一錢或二錢

22 Evodia and Aconite Decoction for Regulating the Middle (Osuyu Buja Ijung Tang)

· Ginseng Radix 7.5g   · Atractylodis Rhizoma Alba 7.5g

· Zingiberis Rhizoma (stir-baked at high temperature) 3.75g

· Cinnamomi Cortex 7.5g   · Paeoniae Radix Alba 3.75g

· Citri Reticulatae Pericarpium 3.75g

· Glycyrrhizae Radix et Rhizoma (stir-baked with adjuvant) 3.75g

· Evodiae Fructus 3.75g   · Foeniculi Fructus 3.75g

· Psoraleae Fructus 3.75g

· Aconiti Lateralis Radix Praeparata (stir-baked at high temperature) 3.75~7.5g

吳茱萸附子理中湯

人蔘白朮炮乾薑官桂各二錢白芍藥陳皮灸甘草吳茱萸小茴香破故紙各一錢炮附子一錢或二錢

23 White Flowery Knotweed and Aconite Decoction for Regulating the Middle (Baikhao Buja Ijung Tang)

· Polygoni multiflori Radix Alba 7.5g   · Atractylodis Rhizoma Alba (stir-baked) 7.5g

· Paeoniae Radix Alba (stir-baked to just dry) 7.5g

· Cinnamomi Ramulus 7.5g

· Zingiberis Rhizoma (stir-baked at high temperature) 7.5g

· Citri Reticulatae Pericarpium 3.75g

· Glycyrrhizae Radix et Rhizoma (stir-baked with adjuvant) 3.75g

· Aconiti Lateralis Radix Praeparata (stir-baked at high temperature) 3.75g

白何烏附子理中湯

白何首烏白朮炒白芍藥微炒桂枝炮乾薑各二錢陳皮灸甘草炮附子各一錢

24 White Flowery Knotweed Decoction for Regulating the Middle (Baikhao Ijung Tang)

· Polygoni multiflori Radix Alba 7.5g   · Atractylodis Rhizoma Alba 7.5g

· Paeoniae Radix Alba 7.5g   · Cinnamomi Ramulus 7.5g

· Zingiberis Rhizoma (stir-baked at high temperature) 7.5g

· Citri Reticulatae Pericarpium 3.75g

· Glycyrrhizae Radix et Rhizoma (stir-baked with adjuvant) 3.75g

If you have Ginseng Radix, use it; if none is available, use Polygoni multiflori Radix Alba instead. The properties and flavor of Polygoni multiflori Radix Alba and Ginseng Radix are similar, but compared to Polygoni multiflori Radix Alba, Ginseng Radix is lacking in cooling and dispersing properties. Its warming and tonifying properties, however, are superior, so there are differences between the two. In case of a critical pattern or a dangerous disease, if it is not possible to use more than 7.5g of Ginseng Radix, then Polygoni multiflori Radix Alba should be used instead. Since there have been few cases of the use of Polygoni multiflori Radix Alba in prescriptions of the past, and also because the medicine remains so unfamiliar, Polygoni multiflori Radix Alba is rarely used. This medicine, however, should not be ignored as a tonifying drug. An old prescription, Heren Yin, is used with 18.75g of Polygoni multiflori Radix Alba to treat malaria. The drugs below for a lesser yin person should be prepared as follows. Aconiti Lateralis Radix Praeparata should be stir-baked at high temperature; Glycyrrhizae Radix et Rhizoma should be stir-baked with adjuvant; Zingiberis Rhizoma should be stir-baked at high temperature or used raw; Astragali Radix should be stir-baked with adjuvant or used raw.

白何首烏理中湯

白何烏白朮白芍藥桂枝炮乾薑各二錢陳皮灸甘草各一錢

有人蔘則用人蔘無人蔘則用白何烏○白何烏與人蔘性味相近而清越之力不及溫補之力過之不無異同之處險病危證人蔘二錢以上不可全恃白何烏代用古方經驗不多藥材生疎故也然此一味必不可遺棄於補藥中而古方何人飲用白何烏五錢治瘧病右少陰人藥諸種附子炮用甘草灸用乾薑炮用或生用黃芪灸用或生用

25 If a person falls ill in a remote or secluded place, it is better to use a simple recipe than to leave him untreated. For yang brightness disease, though it is a simple recipe, we can use Astragali Radix, Cinnamomi Ramulus, Ginseng Radix, and Paeoniae Radix. For lesser yin disease, though it is a simple recipe, we can use Aconiti Lateralis Radix Praeparata, Paeoniae Radix, Ginseng Radix, and Glycyrrhizae Radix et Rhizoma. For greater yang disease, though it is a simple recipe, we can use Perillae Folium, Allii Radix, Astragali Radix, and Cinnamomi Ramulus. For greater yin disease, though it is a simple recipe, we can use Atractylodis Rhizoma Alba, Zingiberis Rhizoma, Citri Reticulatae Pericarpium, and Pogostemonis Herba. If the complete prescription is not available, use a simple recipe first. If the complete prescription is available, one should not hesitate to treat the patient. We must only use the drugs appropriate to that prescription; to use inappropriate drugs is unacceptable.

窮巷僻村病起倉卒雖單方猶百勝於束手無策陽明病雖單黃芪桂枝人蔘芍藥亦可用少陰病雖單附子芍藥人蔘甘草亦可用太陽病雖單蘇葉葱白黃芪桂枝亦可用太陰病雖單白朮乾薑陳皮藿香亦可用爲先用單方而一邊求得全方則必無救病失機之理然當用全方中所有之藥不當用全方中所無之藥

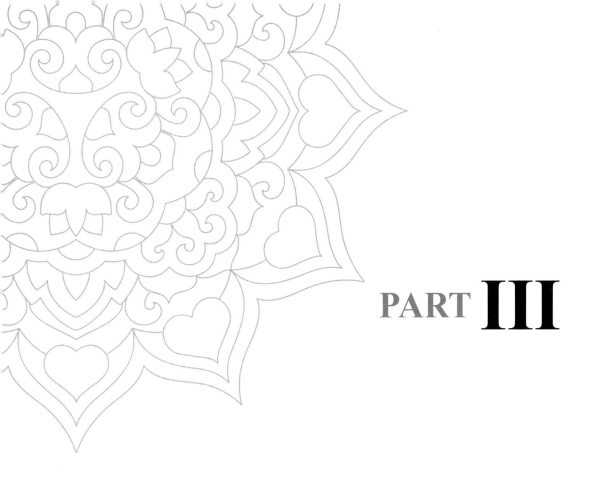

PART III

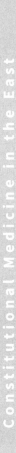

Constitutional Medicine in the East

01

Discourse on the Soyang (Lesser Yang) Person's Exterior Cold Disease Induced from the Spleen Affected by Cold

少陽人脾受寒表寒病論

1 Zhang Zhongjing said, "For the symptoms and signs of the greater yang disease such as a floating and tense pulse, fever, chills, aching of the body and restlessness without sweating, Da Qinglong Tang (Big Blue Dragon Decoction) is suitable."
張仲景曰太陽病脈浮緊發熱惡寒身痛不汗出而煩躁者大靑龍湯主之

2 I have said, "Symptoms and signs such as fever, chills, aching of the body, a floating and tense pulse, and irritability and restlessness without sweating are related to the lesser yang person's exterior cold disease induced from the Spleen affected by cold. For this disease, Da Qinglong Tang should not be adopted, but rather Hyeongbang Paidok San (Schizonepeta and Saposhnikovia Powder for Toxin-Vanquishing) should be used."
論曰發熱惡寒脈浮緊身痛不汗出而煩躁者卽少陽人脾受寒表寒病也此證不當用大靑龍湯當用荊防敗毒散

3 Zhang Zhongjing said, "The symptoms and signs of the lesser yang disease are bitterness in the mouth, a parched throat and vertigo."
張仲景曰少陽之爲病口苦咽乾目眩

4 Vertigo and bitterness in the mouth with a parched tongue belong to the lesser yang disease.
眩而口苦舌乾者屬少陽

5 Bitterness in the mouth, deafness and fullness in the chest are the symptoms and signs of the febrile disease caused by wind of the lesser yang disease.

口苦耳聾胸滿者少陽傷風證也

6 Bitterness in the mouth, a parched throat, vertigo, deafness and fullness in the chest and costal region, or alternate attacks of chills and fever and nausea are the symptoms of the lesser yang disease. Avoid using an emetic or purgative rather; regulate with Xiao Chaihu Tang (Minor Bupleurum Decoction).

口苦咽乾目眩耳聾胸脇滿或往來寒熱而嘔屬少陽忌吐下宜小柴胡湯和之

8 The lesser yang disease mentioned by Zhang Zhongjing with the symptoms of bitterness in the mouth, a parched throat, fullness in the chest and the costal region or alternate attacks of chills and fever is the disease in which the lesser yang person's Kidney yin qi is besieged by the evil heat, and the Spleen yin qi is blocked by the evil heat. As a result, the Spleen yin qi cannot descend to connect with the Kidney yin, and congeals in the vertebra to become an obstinate disease. Vomiting is due to the ascending of the exogenous evil cold surrounding the internal heat, and the alternate attacks of chills and fever are due to the Spleen yin qi going down occasionally, even though on the whole, the Spleen yin qi cannot go down when it tries. Bitterness in the mouth, a parched throat, vertigo and deafness are due to the yin qi's descent being blocked in the vertebra. This induces chills without fever and deafness. Bitterness in the mouth, a parched throat and vertigo are ordinary symptoms; however, deafness indicates a serious condition. The agitation in the chest and the costal region develops into an accumulation of pathogen in the chest. Fullness of the costal region is not a serious condition, however, fullness in the chest is a serious symptom. The ancients treated this kind of disease with diaphoretics, emetics and purgatives. These types of treatments caused deteriorated cases such as delirium, and are dangerous. Therefore, Zhang Zhongjing designed Xiao Chaihu Tang to clear away phlegm and to eliminate sputum, and tried to regulate it evenly by mixing up warm and cold drugs together in order to prevent aggravating the disease and achieve spontaneous relief. Speaking from the perspective of the diaphoretic, emetic and purgative methodology, this decoction must be valued as an excellent drug. Xiao Chaihu Tang, however, is not a prescription that can regulate the functional relations of the internal organs and prevent the illness from getting worse. This illness is as tragic today as it was in the past. How can Xiao Chaihu Tang be applied to deafness, sensation of fullness in the chest and the symptoms induced by the evil wind? Is Gong Xin's Jingfang Baidu San not the most suitable prescription for a lesser yang person's exterior cold disease? To treat the above symptoms, if the interior heat is cleared out and the exterior yin is lowered, the phlegm and fluid that has been retained will be dispersed spontaneously and an accumulation of pathogen in the chest will not form. Clearing away phlegm and eliminating sputum are not helpful in lowering yin and dispersing phlegm; it might even cause an accumulation of pathogen in the chest to mutate into another disease.

張仲景所論少陽病口苦咽乾胸脇滿或往來寒熱之證即少陽人腎局陰氣爲熱邪所陷而脾局陰氣爲

熱邪所壅不能下降連接於腎局而凝聚脊間膠固囚滯之病也此證嘔者外寒包裹熱而挾疾上逆也寒熱往來者脾局陰氣欲降未降而或降故寒熱或往或來也口苦咽乾目眩耳聾者陰氣囚滯脊間欲降未降故但寒無熱而至於耳聾也口苦咽乾目眩者例證也耳聾者重證也胸脅滿者結胸之漸也脅滿者猶輕也胸滿者重證也古人之於此證用汗吐下三法則其病輒生譫語壞證病益危險故仲景變通之而用小柴胡湯清痰燥痰溫冷相雜平均和解欲其病不轉變而自愈此法以汗吐下三法論之則可謂近善而巧矣然此小柴胡湯亦非平均和解病不轉變之藥則從古斯今得此病者真是寒心矣耳聾脅滿傷風之病豈可以小柴胡湯擬之乎噫後來龔信所製荊防敗毒散豈非少陽人表寒病三神山不死藥乎此證清裹熱而降表陰則痰飲自散而結胸之證預防不成也清痰而燥痰則無益於陰降痰散延拖結胸將成而或別生奇證也

7　I have said, "Xiao Chaihu Tang should not be used; instead, we ought to use Hyeongbang Paidok San, Hyeongbang Dojeok San (Schizonepeta and Saposhnikovia Powder for Treating Dark Urine), and Hyeongbang Sabaik San (Schizonepeta and Saposhnikovia Powder for Expelling Lung-heat)."

論曰此證不當用小柴胡湯當用荊防敗毒散荊防導赤散荊防瀉白散

9　Zhu Gong said, "If a patient perspires in droplets above the waist, and perspires but a little from the waist down, he will not recover."

朱肱曰凡發汗腰以上雖淋漓而腰以下至足微潤則病終不解

10　I have said, "In the lesser yang person's disease, whether exterior or interior disease, the patient can be relieved after there is perspiration on the palms of the hands and the soles of the feet. If there is no sweating on the palms and soles, he will not recover, even though he might be sweating all over his body."

論曰少陽人病無論表裹病手足掌心有汗則病解手足掌心不汗則雖全體皆汗而病不解

11　In the lesser yang person's exogenous febrile disease caused by cold, some patients get well after repeated pain with sweating. This disease is not a case of repeated pain with sweating induced by repeated invasion of wind and cold. Originally, the disease is the same as the disease of a lesser yang person with symptoms of headache, stiff neck, alternate attacks of chills and fever, deafness, and a sensation of fullness in the chest. If the exogenous pathogen is deeply congealed, the disease will be relieved after three bouts of pain. Whether sweating for the first, second or third time, we have to apply two packs of Hyeongbang Paidok San or Hyeongbang Dojeok San or Hyeongbang Sabaik San a day until the symptoms disappear. Afterwards, we must apply ten or more packs to prevent a relapse.

少陽人傷寒病有再痛三痛發汗而愈者此病非再三感風寒而再痛發汗三痛發汗也少陽人頭痛腦強寒熱往來耳聾胸滿尤甚之病元來如此表邪深結至於三痛然後方解也無論初痛再痛三痛用荊防敗毒散或荊防導赤散荊防瀉白散每日二貼式至病解而用之病解後又用十餘貼如此則自無後病而完健

12 Zhang Zhongjing said, "A lesser yang disease with the following symptoms, such as a clammy body with perspiration, hardness and fullness in the epigastrium, a referred pain below the costal margin, nausea with shortness of breath, and no chills may indicate that the interior pattern is still dominating, even after the exterior pattern is gone. Shizao Tang (Ten Jujubes Decoction) can be taken. If the decoction's purgative action is in vain, the patient will experience abdominal distension and general edema of the whole body."

張仲景曰少陽證漐漐汗出心下痞硬滿引脇下痛乾嘔短氣不惡寒表解裏未和也宜十棗湯若合下不下令人脹滿遍身浮腫

13 When a purgative is given to the patient whose exterior pattern caused by cold has not been cleared away, he will feel pain in a part of the diaphragm because of compression, and fullness and hardness in the chest. This indicates that an accumulation of pathogen in the chest is taking shape. Da Xianxiong Tang (Major Decoction for Pathogens Stuck in the Chest) will be the curative.

傷寒表未解醫反下之膈內拒痛手不可近心下滿而硬痛此爲結胸宜大陷胸湯

14 Though the patient is thirsty for water, he will still regurgitate any ingested water; this is called *shuini* (water regurgitation). Wuling San (Five-Ingredient Powder with Poria Sclerotium) will be the curative.

渴欲飲水水入即吐名曰水逆五苓散主之

15 Du Ren[1]) said, "The domination of the interior pattern manifests itself in the phlegm and the pathogenic dryness congealing in the middle-*jiao*. Its symptoms include headaches, retching and sweating. These are due to the phlegm in the diaphragm. Without Shizao Tang, one cannot heal this illness."

杜壬曰裏未和者盖痰與燥氣壅於中焦故頭痛乾嘔汗出痰隔也非十棗湯不治

16 Gong Xin said, "Hardness and pain in the epigastrium (which one cannot even touch), thirst, delirium, constipation, and a deep and forceful pulse are due to the major accumulation of phlegm-heat in the chest. Da Xianxiong Tang as a purgative should be adopted. If the patient becomes more irritated after taking the drug, he will die. The minor accumulation of phlegm-heat in the chest manifests itself only in the epigastrium. Xiao Xianxiong Tang (Minor Decoction for Pathogens Stuck in the Chest) should be used."

龔信曰心下硬痛手不可近燥渴譫語大便實脈沈實有力爲大結胸大陷胸湯下之反加煩燥者死小結胸正在心下按之則痛宜小陷胸湯

17 I have said, "The above three patterns that Zhang Zhongjing mentioned are all accumulations of pathogen in the chest. The tenderness in the chest, thirst and delirium are the most serious symptoms along with an accumulation of pathogen in the chest. Regurgitating any

ingested water, feeling of fullness in the epigastrium, retching and shortness of breath are secondary ones. Generally, an accumulation of pathogen in the chest induces vomiting just after drinking medicine or water. Only the powder of Euphorbia Kansui Radix taken with saliva, and drinking some warm water to rinse the mouth will not cause the patient to vomit. I had an experience curing an accumulation of pathogen in the chest. The patient took the powder of Euphorbia Kansui Radix with warm water. The patient vomited until the sixth time and his bowels relaxed. On the second day, he vomited water again, so he took Euphorbia Kansui Radix and was cured after one bout of diarrhea. Since an accumulation of pathogen in the chest is generally a serious disease, we should use Euphorbia Kansui Radix and Hyeongbang Dojeok San to stop it. When there are only symptoms of retching and shortness of breath, but no vomiting of drugs, we do not have to use Euphorbia Kansui Radix. If we use Hyeongbang Dojeok San with Poria Sclerotium and Rhizoma Alismatis, 3.75g each, two or three packs a day, then the patient will be cured. Thirst and delirium are signs of the most dangerous conditions. Immediately apply Euphorbia Kansui Radix and take three or four packs of Jihwang Baikho Tang (White tiger decoction with Rehmannia) to stop it. The patient must then take Jihwang Baikho Tang every day. Zhang Zhongjing said, 'When a purgative is to be given to a patient whose exterior pattern caused by cold has not been cleared away', the necessary purgative is Da Chengqi Tang, not Xianxiong Tang or Shizao Tang. Using Euphorbia Kansui Radix is better than using either Shizao Tang or Xianxiong Tang. For an accumulation of pathogen in the chest, we generally use 1.125g of Euphorbia Kansui Radix, and for the major accumulation of pathogen in the chest, we use 1.875g of Euphorbia Kansui Radix. Gamsu Cheonil Dan (Tianyi pills with Euphorbia Kansui Radix) also can be adopted. For curing a patient with symptoms of thirst, delirium and irritability with restlessness to death mentioned by Gong Xin, the delirium will disappear through purgation with Shizao Tang; Baihu Tang will cure irritability with restlessness.

論曰右張仲景所論三證皆結胸病而膈內拒痛手不可近燥渴譫語者結胸之最尤甚證也飲水水入即吐心下痞硬滿乾嘔短氣者次證也凡結胸病皆藥湯入口輒還吐惟甘遂末入口口涎含下因以溫水嗽口而下則藥不還吐嘗治結胸用甘遂散溫水調下五次輒還吐至六次不還吐而下利一度其翌日又水還吐又用甘遂一次快通利而病愈凡結胸無非險證當先用甘遂仍煎荊防導赤散以壓之乾嘔短氣而藥不還吐者不用甘遂但用荊防導赤散加茯苓澤瀉各一錢二三服又連日服而亦病愈燥渴譫語者尤極險證也急用甘遂仍煎地黃白虎湯三四貼以壓之又連日服地黃白虎湯張仲景曰傷寒表未解醫反下之云者以大承氣湯下之之謂也非十棗陷胸下之之謂也然十棗陷胸不如單用甘遂或用甘遂天一丸結胸甘遂末例用三分大結胸用五分龔信所論燥渴譫語煩燥死者若十棗湯下後因以譫語證治之連用白虎湯則煩燥者必無不治之理

18 Euphorbia Kansui Radix is a drug for removing the accumulation of fluid in the chest in the exterior cold disease. Gypsum Fibrosum is a drug for relaxing the bowels in the interior heat disease. For the exterior disease, Euphorbia Kansui Radix can be used, but not Gypsum Fibrosum. For the interior disease, Gypsum Fibrosum can be used, but not Euphorbia Kansui

Radix. For symptoms such as waving of hands and feet, thirst and diarrhea, Gypsum Fibrosum should be used. For symptoms such as arthralgia with numbness, cold knees and constipation, Euphorbia Kansui Radix should be used.

甘遂表寒病破水結之藥也石膏裡熱病通大便之藥也表病可用甘遂而不可用石膏裡病可用石膏而不可用甘遂然揚手擲足引飲泄瀉證用石膏痺風膝寒大便不通證用甘遂

19 There are symptoms, such as hardness and fullness in the lower abdomen in the exogenous febrile disease caused by cold in the lesser yin person, and the accumulation of pathogens in the epigastrium in the exogenous febrile disease caused by cold in the lesser yang person. These two symptoms are both due to the struggle, lasting for several days, between the healthy qi and the pathogen induced by the deficiency of the exterior qi of both yin and yang, and the unevenness of the interior qi.

少陰人傷寒病有小腹硬滿之證少陽人傷寒病有心下結胸之證此二證俱是表氣陰陽虛弱正邪相爭累日不決之中裡氣亦秘澁不和而變生此證也

20 In his 『*Shanghan Shiquanlun*』[2] (Ten Pieces of Advice on Exogenous Febrile Disease"), Li Zijian[3] said, "When there is abdominal pain in the exogenous febrile disease caused by cold which belongs to the heat pattern, be careful in giving drugs of a warm nature." He said, "We should differentiate the yin and yang patterns when the patient shows symptoms of spontaneous diarrhea in the exogenous febrile disease caused by cold. Do not make thoughtless prescriptions for taking drugs of warm nature or anti-diarrheal drugs."

李子建傷寒十勸論曰傷寒腹痛亦有熱證不可輕服溫煖藥又曰傷寒自利當觀陰陽證不可例服溫煖及止瀉藥

21 Zhu Zhenheng said, "For the yang pattern of the exogenous febrile disease caused by cold with symptoms and signs such as fever, fast pulse, restlessness with thirst and spontaneous diarrhea, Chailing Tang (Decoction of Bupleuri Radix and Poria Sclerotium) should be adopted."

朱震亨曰傷寒陽證身熱脈數煩渴引飲大便自利宜柴苓湯

22 The Banryongsan elder said, "A lesser yang person with symptoms of fever, headache and diarrhea should be treated with Jeorycong Chajconja Tang (Polyporus and Plantain Seed Decoction) and Hyeongbang Sabaik San. The symptoms of chills, abdominal pain and diarrhea should be treated by Hwalseok Gosam Tang (Talcum and Sophora Decoction) and Hyeongbang Jihwang Tang (Schizonepeta, Saposhnikovia, and Rehmannia Decoction). These diseases are called *mangyin* (yin collapse) disease."

盤龍山老人論曰少陽人身熱頭痛泄瀉當用猪苓車前子湯荊防瀉白散身寒腹痛泄瀉當用滑石苦參湯荊防地黃湯此病名謂之亡陰病

23 If a lesser yang person has a fever, headache and diarrhea, his diarrhea may stop for no reason one to four days later. However, if his fever and headache are not relieved, and he becomes constipated, then his condition is dangerous, and he will become delirious.

少陽人身熱頭痛泄瀉一二日或三四日而泄瀉無故自止身熱頭痛不愈大便反秘者此危證也距譫語不遠

24 If a patient barely has a bowel movement in the twenty four hours following diarrhea or has of a small amount of loose bowels three to five times in one day. And he still has the symptoms of fever and headache, this indicates constipation. If these symptoms occur before delirium, delirium will occur a few days later. If these symptoms occur after delirium, endogenous wind stirring will occur.

泄瀉後大便一晝夜間艱辛一次滑利或三四五次小小滑利身熱頭痛因存者此便秘之兆也譫語前有此證則譫語當在數日譫語後有此證則動風必在咫尺

25 If a lesser yang person vomits suddenly, there will be some strange symptoms. We should apply Hyeongbang Paidok San immediately. If the patient has a fever, a headache and diarrhea, Gypsum Fibrosum will be suitable for these symptoms. If the patient displays symptoms of chills, headache and diarrhea, Coptidis Rhizoma and Sophorae flavescentis Radix will be suitable.

少陽人忽然有吐者必生奇證也當用荊防敗毒散以觀動靜而身熱頭痛泄瀉者用石膏無疑身寒頭痛泄瀉者用黃連苦參無疑

26 I once treated a lesser yang baby under a year of age. He vomited suddenly, and then had diarrhea, fever, headache, waving of his hands and feet, rolling his body. He also experienced thirst and diarrhea several times. After taking six packs of Hyeongbang Sabaik San for two days, the diarrhea stopped, and the fever and headache were gone, too. He took six more packs and fully recovered.

嘗見少陽人兒生未一周年忽先一吐而後泄瀉身熱頭痛揚手擲足轉輾其身引飲泄瀉四五六次無度數者用荊防瀉白散日三貼兩日六貼然後泄瀉方止身熱頭痛清淨又五六貼而安

27 A lesser yang person displaying symptoms of fever, headache, waving of hands and feet and thirst are in a serious danger. Though he has diarrhea, we must use Gypsum Fibrosum. Whether he has diarrhea or not, we must use Hyeongbang Sabaik San with Coptidis Rhizoma and Trichosanthis Semen, 3.75g each, or use Jihwang Baikho Tang.

少陽人身熱頭痛揚手擲足引飲者此險證也雖泄瀉必用石膏無論泄瀉有無當用荊防瀉白散加黃連瓜蔞各一錢或地黃白虎湯

28 If a lesser yang person has symptoms of fever and headache, his condition is no more than a mild one; but if he also has diarrhea, he is in danger. We must use Hyeongbang Sabaik

San two or three times per a day. Once the symptoms such as fever and headache are cleared away, then he can be saved.

凡少陽人有身熱頭痛則已非輕證而兼有泄瀉則危險證也必用荊防瀉白散日二三服又連日服身熱頭痛清淨然後可免危險

29 If a lesser yang person has symptoms of chills, abdominal pains and diarrhea three to five times a day, he should take Hwalseok Gosam Tang. If he displays symptoms of chills and abdominal pains without diarrhea for two or three days, or has one bout of diarrhea, he should take Hwalseok Gosam Tang or Sukjihwang Gosam Tang (Rehmanniae Radix Praeparata and Sophora Root Decoction).

少陽人身寒腹痛泄瀉一晝夜間三四五次者當用滑石苦蔘湯身寒腹痛二三晝夜間無泄瀉或艱辛一次泄瀉者當用滑石苦蔘湯或用熟地黃苦蔘湯

30 I have seen a lesser yang person who had been suffering from continuous abdominal pain, and he was cured after taking sixty packs of Liuwei Dihuang Tang (Decoction of Six Drugs with Rehmanniae Radix Praeparata). I also have seen a lesser yang person who had had abdominal pain for more than ten years. Each time, it had lasted five to six, three to four, or one or two months; and each time it occurred, he took ten or more packs of Hwalseok Gosam Tang to stop the pain. During those periods where he experienced no pain, the patient tried to calm himself down and avoid sorrow and anger. He subsequently recovered within a year. I also have seen a lesser yang boy who always had indigestion and a feeling of hardness and fullness in the abdomen. He sometimes had abdominal pain and lumbago, and, later, facial paralysis occurred. From the start, he took two hundred packs of Dokhwal Jihwang Tang (Rehmannia and Pubescent Angelica Decoction) and tried to ease his mind by avoiding sorrow and anger. He subsequently recovered his health within one hundred days.

嘗見少陽人恒有腹痛患苦者用六味地黃湯六十貼而病愈又見少陽人十餘年腹痛患苦一次起痛則或五六個月或三四個月一二個月叫苦者每起痛臨時急用滑石苦蔘湯十餘貼不痛時平心靜慮恒戒哀心怒心如此延拖一周年而病愈又見少陽人小年兒恒有滯證痞滿間有腹痛腰痛又有口眼喎斜初證者用獨活地黃湯一百日內二百貼服使之平心靜慮恒戒哀心怒心一百日而身健病愈

31 An ancient doctor said, "There is no headache that is due to cold, and there is no abdominal pain that is due to heat." However, this is not true. Why? Since the lesser yin person originally has excessive cold inside, his headache also cannot be induced by heat, but by cold. Since the lesser yang person originally has excessive heat inside, his abdominal pain also cannot be induced by cold, but by heat. Another ancient doctor also said, "Too much perspiration causes yang collapse, and too much purgation causes yin collapse." That is true. Why? Although the lesser yin's nature is cold, because his yang is defeated and expelled by the yin excess, the defeated yang outwardly induces fever and profuse sweating. This is called the yang collapse disease. Conversely, although the lesser yang's nature is heat, because his yin is de-

feated and forced inwardly by the yang excess, the defeated yin inwardly induces an aversion to cold and diarrhea. This is called the yin collapse disease. If there is no drug administration, or no emergency management, the patient will die.

古醫有言頭無冷痛腹無熱痛此言非也何謂然耶少陰人元來冷勝則其頭痛亦自非熱痛而即冷痛也少陽人元來熱勝則其腹痛亦自非冷痛而即熱痛也古醫又言汗多亡陽下多亡陰此言是也何謂然耶少陰人雖則冷勝然陰盛格陽敗陽外遁則煩熱而汗多也此之謂亡陽病也少陽人雖則熱勝然陽盛格陰敗陰內遁則畏寒而泄下也此之謂亡陰病也亡陽亡陰病非用藥必死也不急治必死也

32 The yang collapse implies that the yang descends instead of ascends. The yin collapse implies that the yin ascends instead of descends. Due to the excessive yin expelling yang out of the upper part of the body, the yang is inhibited by yin and cannot ascend to the diaphragm and descend to the large intestine and circulate outside the bladder. As a result, fever with restlessness over the back and sweating occurs. The fever and sweating are not induced by an overabundance of yang. This is the so-called state of ice within and charcoal outside, and is the sign of dying yang. Due to excessive yang expelling yin out of the lower part of the body, yin is obstructed by yang and cannot descend to the bladder and ascend to the paravertebral musculature of the back and circulate inside the diaphragm. As a result, the stomach and intestine become averse to cold, and diarrhea occurs. The aversion to cold and diarrhea are not induced by an overabundance of yin. This is the so-called state of charcoal within and ice outside, and is the sign of dying yin.

亡陽者陽不上升而反爲下降則亡陽也亡陰者陰不下降而反爲上升則亡陰也陰盛格陽於上則陽爲陰抑不能上升於胸膈下陷大腸而外遁膀胱故背表煩熱而汗出也煩熱而汗出者非陽盛也此所謂內冰外炭陽將亡之兆也陽盛格陰於下則陰爲陽壅不能下降於膀胱上逆背膂而內遁膈裏故腸胃畏寒而泄下也畏寒而泄下者非陰盛也此所謂內炭外冰陰將亡之兆也

33 A lesser yin patient will definitely be cured if his yang qi ascends and induces perspiration on the Renzhong point on the first day. If his perspiration does not cease on the second or third day and he is not cured, there is no doubt that the yang cannot ascend and is exhausted. A lesser yang patient will definitely be cured if his yin qi descends and induces diarrhea, with sweat on the palms and soles on the first day. If there is continuous diarrhea in the second or third day and no sign of recovery, there is no doubt that the yin cannot descend and is exhausted. Generally, a doctor who understands the medical theories can predict the symptoms of yang collapse and yin collapse before they occur. Those diseases are easy to perceive on the first and second day, and on the third day it is as clear as daylight, so that even those less knowledgeable can discern the symptoms. On the fourth day, it is somewhat late; and on the fifth day, the patient will be in the dangerous state. Therefore, the drugs must be taken before the second or third day.

少陰人病一日發汗陽氣上升人中穴先汗則病必愈也而二日三日汗不止病不愈則陽不上升而亡陽無疑也少陽人病一日滑利陰氣下降手足掌心先汗則病必愈也而二日三日泄不止病不愈則陰不下

降而亡陰無疑也凡亡陽亡陰證明知醫理者得病前可以預執證也得病一二日明白易見也至于三日
則雖愚者執證亦明若觀火矣用藥必無過二三日矣四日則晚矣五日則臨危也

34 If a lesser yin person who is usually restless with profuse perspiration falls ill, he will certainly
get yang collapse. A lesser yang person who usually has a cold body with frequent diarrhea
falls ill, he will certainly get yin collapse. It is advisable for those who are susceptible to yang
collapse or yin collapse to take the preventive drugs reinforcing yin or yang. It is very difficult
to save a patient who contracts yang collapse or yin collapse and whose condition has become
dangerous.

少陰人平居裡煩汗多者得病則必成亡陽也少陽人平居表寒下多者得病則必成亡陰也亡陽亡陰人
平居預治補陰補陽可也不可至於亡陽亡陰得病臨危然後救病也

35 For a lesser yin person, the recovery from the disease shows itself through sweating on the
Renzhong point first. Then with one bout of sweating, the patient feels his chest refreshed
and becomes active. However, in yang collapse, sweating occurs on and off on the Renzhong
point, and after several bouts of sweating, the patient feels restlessness in the chest and the
qi becomes depressed. For a lesser yang person, the recovery from the disease shows itself
through sweating on the palms and soles first. With one round of diarrhea, the exterior qi
becomes clear and refreshes the mind. In yin collapse, there is no sweating on the palms and
soles, and after several rounds of diarrhea, the exterior qi becomes cold and dizziness occurs.

少陰人病愈之汗人中先汗而一次發汗胸膈壯快而活潑亡陽之汗人中或汗或不汗屢次發汗胸膈悶
燥而下陷也少陽人病愈之泄手足掌心先汗而一次滑泄表氣清寧而精神爽明亡陰之泄手足掌心不
汗屢次泄利表氣溯寒而精神鬱冒

36 Both an excess of the stomach and intestine of the lesser yin person and an accumulation
of pathogen in the chest of the lesser yang person are produced by the conflicts between
healthy qi and the pathogen, and those of yin and yang as well. They become dangerous as
time passes. The yang collapse in the lesser yin person and the yin collapse in the lesser yang
person are produced by the conflicts between healthy qi and the pathogen, and the conflicts
between yin and yang which are unable to match each other. They are already serious at the
onset and become dangerous later. We can liken these cases to war. During the first day's
battle, the enemy defeats our army and we lose a number of troops. During the second and
third day's battle, our army is again defeated, with yet more losses. If we analyzed those three
day's battles, we would surmise that the fourth and fifth day's battles would lead to the loss
of all remaining troops. In the same way, we must not tarry in administering the medication
after the illness's third day.

少陰人胃家實病少陽人結胸病止邪陰陽相敵而相格故日久而後危證始見也少陰人亡陽病少陽人
亡陰病正邪陰陽不敵而相格故初證已為險證繼而因為危證矣譬如用兵合戰交鋒初一日合戰正兵
為邪兵所敗折正兵幾許兵數二日又戰又敗又折幾許數三日又戰又敗又折幾許數以三日交鋒觀之

則將愈益戰而愈益敗愈益折矣若四日復戰五日復戰則正兵之全軍覆沒可知矣所以用藥必無過三
日也

37   I call myself the Banryongsan elder because of my residence near this hill. Thus, the phrases "I have said" in this book are uttered by the Banryongsan elder. When writing about yin collapse and yang collapse, I cite myself as the Banryongsan elder to emphasize that yang collapse and yin collapse are the most dangerous diseases whose study is worthwhile.

盤龍山老人者李翁所居地有盤龍山故李翁自謂盤龍山老人也此書中論曰二字無非盤龍山老人之
論而此章特舉盤龍山老人者盖亡陽亡陰最是險病而人必尋常視之易於例治故別以盤龍山老人提
舉驚呼而警覺之也

38   There was not much experience or medications for the yin collapse disease previously, although Li Zijian and Zhu Danxi[4]'s books mention it a little; however, neither physician's experiences are clear or conclusive. It may be that death came so quickly that it was difficult to obtain knowledge and experience.

亡陰證古醫別無經驗用藥頭話而李子建朱震亨書中若干論及之然自無明的快驗盖此病從古以來
殺人孟浪甚速未暇經驗獵得裡許故也

39   Zhang Zhongjing said, "Before the greater yang disease evanesces, it changes into the lesser yang disease. Then the following symptoms and signs such as hardness and fullness below the costal region, retching, anorexia, and alternate attacks of chills and fever appear. If the pulse is deep and tense before an emetic or purgative is adopted, Xiao Chaihu Tang will be the curative. When delirium appears after the adoption of an emetic, purgative, or diaphoretic, it means that the Xiao Chaihu Tang patterns disappear and are followed by something worse. Therapy should be done according to the relevant diagnosis."

張仲景曰太陽病不解轉入少陽者脇下硬滿乾嘔不能食往來寒熱者尚未吐下脈沈緊者與小柴胡湯
若已吐下發汗譫語柴胡證證罷此爲壞病依壞法治之

40   The exogenous febrile disease caused by cold with a tight and slender pulse, headache and fever would indicate that the pattern is in the lesser yang disease. Diaphoresis is prohibited, as its adoption will cause delirium.

傷寒脈弦細頭痛發熱者屬少陽不可發汗發汗則譫語

41   I once treated a lesser yang person suffering from the exogenous febrile disease caused by cold and who exhibited symptoms of mania and delirium. It was the Qingming (Pure Brightness: fifth solar term) season in 1875. He got the febrile disease caused by cold and had more chills than fever. Four to five days later, dyspnea and shortness of breath were noted in the afternoon. At that time, I lacked experience. I only knew that the lesser yang person should be treated with Liuwei Dihuang Tang (Six-Ingredient Decoction Containing Rehmannia), so I

dared not use any other drugs. After taking a pack of Liuwei Dihuang Tang, his shortness of breath was cured, but several days later, the symptoms such as mania, delirium and shortness of breath recurred. He took a pack of Liuwei Dihuang Tang again, and there was a slight improvement for the shortness of breath. He then experienced continuous mania for three days and shortness of breath again in the afternoon, so he was given Liuwei Dihuang Tang. There was no relief for his shortness of breath, however, and shortly after the endogenous wind stirring; the patient developed a curled tongue, a closed mouth, and difficulty in speech. I thereupon found out that Liuwei Dihuang Tang was ineffective and gave him a pack of Baihu Tang immediately. I fed the patient through the nose to the throat using a bamboo tube. The curled tongue and closed mouth persisted, but he gave off mild bowel sounds. After taking three packs of the drugs continuously, he gave loud bowel sounds like breaking wind. Three men helped him to take the drugs, and even they could not handle the patient due to his strength. Like this, he continued taking 300g of Gypsum Fibrosum from noon till midnight. Later, the patient's abdomen got fuller, and opisthotonos developed. After the opisthotonos, the patient sweated and slept. At dawn the next day, the patient took a pack of Baihu Tang. After sunrise, he passed loose stool and recovered. Later, he contracted an eye disease, and it, too, was cured after the application of Gypsum Fibrosum and Phellodendri Cortex 3.75g each twice a day, for seven or eight days. At the time, I had yet to understand the importance of examining stool and did not consider the duration of constipation. After reflecting on the case, I concluded that the constipation from the exterior cold disease had resulted in this disease.

嘗治少陽人傷寒發狂譫語證時則乙亥年清明節候也少陽人一人得傷寒寒多熱少之病四五日後午末辰刻喘促短氣伊時經驗未熟但知少陽人應用藥六味湯最好之理故不敢用他藥而祗用六味湯一貼病人喘促卽時頓定又數日後病人發狂譫語喘促又發又用六味湯一貼則喘促雖少定而不如前日之頓定矣病人發狂連三日午後喘促又發又用六味湯喘促署不少定有頃舌卷動風口噤不語於是而始知六味湯之無能爲也急煎白虎湯一貼以竹管吹入病人鼻中下咽而察其動靜則舌卷口噤之證不解而病人腹中微鳴仍以兩爐煎藥荏苒灌鼻數三貼後病人腹中大鳴放氣出焉三人扶持病人竹管吹鼻灌藥而病人氣力益屈强三人扶持之力幾不能支當矣又荏苒灌鼻自未申時至亥子時凡用石膏八兩末境病人腹中大脹角弓反張之證出焉角弓反張後少頃得汗而睡翌日平明病人又服白虎湯一貼日出後滑便一次而病快愈愈後有眼病用石膏黃柏末各一錢日再服七八日後眼病亦愈伊時未知大便驗法故不察大便之秘閉幾日然想必此病人先自表寒病得病後有大便秘閉而發此證矣

42 Later, a lesser yang person who had the febrile disease caused by cold with more fever than chills got *yangdu* (yang type inflammatory swelling) with eruptions due to his eating pheasant as suggested by others. I prescribed three packs of Baihu Tang, but the patient only took half a pack. Several days later, delirium occurred and turned very serious. When I was asked to see the patient again, I noticed that he was in a coma and showed signs of the endogenous wind stirring. He also exhibited symptoms of deafness, delirium, and white coating on the tongue. Later, at my house, I found that there were only 600g of Gypsum Fibrosum and

37.5g of Talcum in the drug box, so I immediately decocted 37.5g of Gypsum Fibrosum and 3.75g of Talcum and gave it to him. I did the same the following day. He had no bowel movement for but a day, and on the third day, I decided to refrain from giving him Gypsum Fibrosum - his family was worried about the side effects of the heavy doses. On the fourth day, his family hurriedly asked me to see the patient again. I found that the patient had had no bowel movement for two nights and one day, and he was speaking incoherently and could not drink water due to trismus. I decocted 75g of Gypsum Fibrosum and forced him to take it. Half of the decoction was regurgitated, and after a while, he could move his jaw; his speech, however, was still unclear. I continued to give him 37.5g of Gypsum Fibrosum. Since I was worried that he might have an endogenous wind stirring which would make him unable to swallow in the afternoon, and in order to prevent that situation, I gave the medicine to him in the morning. He afterwards continued to take the medicine for five to six days, and the total amount of Gypsum Fibrosum that he had taken was 530g. For the last several days, he had mania and his speech became loud, and his illness was relieved. Several months later, the patient was able to walk in the house garden.

其後又有少陽人一人得傷寒熱多寒少之病有人敎服雉肉湯仍成陽毒發斑余敎服白虎湯連三貼而其人只服半貼數日後譫語而病重病家惶急顛倒往觀則病人外證昏憒已有動風之漸而耳聾譫語舌上白胎藥囊祗有石膏一斤滑石一兩而無他藥故急煎石膏一兩滑石一錢頓服而其翌日又服石膏一兩滑石一錢此兩日則大便皆不過一晝夜至于第三日病家以過用石膏歸咎故一日不用石膏矣至于第四日病家惶急顛倒往觀則病人大便秘閉兩夜一晝而語韻不分明牙關緊急水飲不入急煎石膏二兩艱辛下咽而半吐半下咽少頃牙關開而語韻則不分明如前又連用石膏一兩其翌日則以午後動風藥不下咽之慮故預爲午前用藥以備動風而又五六日用之前後用石膏凡十四兩而末境發狂數日語韻宏壯而病愈數月然後方出門庭

43 Later, another lesser yang person who first suffered from headache, fever and exterior cold disease for eight or nine days came to my house. After he had taken Coptidis Rhizoma, Trichosanthis Semen, Osterici Radix, and Saposhnikoviae Radix etc., there had been a little improvement, but his later mania persisted for three days. His family regarded it as a common disease and did not pay much attention to it; they only used Coptidis Rhizoma and Trichosanthis Semen. After the delirium continued for several days, the patient began to take one pack of Jiwhang Baikho Tang. The next afternoon, the endogenous wind stirred, and I immediately decocted three packs of Dihuang Baihu Tang to prevent serious endogenous wind stirring, but they were difficult to swallow. The day after, he took Baihu Tang with 37.5g of Gypsum Fibrosum before noon to prevent endogenous wind stirring. After continuing treatment for three days more, the patient could stand and sit, urinate and defecate by himself; his health was much improved. Unfortunately, his illness worsened due to incomplete treatments, and in the end, he could not be saved. It is regrettable that this patient took two packs of Baihu Tang only in the morning to prevent from the endogenous wind stirring, but did not continue to take medications in the afternoon, too. According to the above three

patients'cases, for mania and delirium, Baihu Tang should be given not only once before noon to prevent endogenous wind stirring, but five to ten additional doses per day. It would be better not to wait for the delirium to occur, but to administer when the mania shows itself. It is better to observe and detect the signs of oncoming mania rather than wait for mania to occur.

其後又有少陽人一人初得頭痛身熱表寒病八九日其間用黃連瓜蔞羌活防風等屬病勢少愈而永不快袪矣仍爲發狂三日病家以尋常例證視之而祗用黃連瓜蔞等屬又譫語數日始用地黃白虎湯一貼其翌日午後動風急煎地黃白虎湯連三貼救急而艱辛下咽其翌日則白虎湯加石膏一兩午前用之以備動風而連三日用之病人自起坐立能大小便病勢比前快蘇快壯矣不幸病加於少愈慮不周於完治此人竟不救恨則午前祗用白虎湯二貼以備動風而午後全不用藥以繼之也以此三人病觀之則發狂譫語證白虎湯非但午前用藥以備動風而已矣日用五六貼七八貼十餘貼以晝繼夜則好矣不必待譫語後而用藥發狂時當用藥可也不必待發狂後而用藥發狂前早察發狂之漸可也

44 Later, there was a seventeen year old lesser yang girl who had previously suffered from a lack of vital energy and abdominal pain due to indigestion. One day, she suddenly had a headache, chills with fever and indigestion. A doctor prescribed her three Suhe Yuan and ordered her to take them with a ginger decoction. She then had diarrhea over ten times a day for more than ten days. The patient felt seriously thirsty, and had insomnia and occasional delirium. It was November 23, 1875. I prescribed Rehmanniae Radix and Gypsum Fibrosum, 225g each, and 113g of Anemarrhenae Rhizoma for that night. The diarrhea decreased by half in frequency. The next day, I prescribed two packs of Hyeongbang Jihwang Tang and added 15g of Gypsum Fibrosum to be taken orally. She then slept soundly and had smooth urination that day. It is clear that the pharmaceutical power of this decoction is ten times more effective than Zhimu Baihu Tang (White Tiger Decoction with Anemarrhenae Rhizoma), so I proceeded to use it for several days, twice in the day and twice at night. The diarrhea ceased completely, but she was sweating over the preauricular region. Suddenly, the delirium turned into mania. Her family stopped her treatment for two days out of fear, and she lapsed into a dangerous state. She had no perspiration over the head, but had dysuria, oliguria, coldness of the mouth and lips, and was unconscious. These symptoms were sinister signs. I was forced to use Hyeongbang Jihwang Tang and added 37.5g of Gypsum Fibrosum, ten packs a night, to be taken orally. The patient urinated three bowls at night. Mania persisted, but she regained consciousness. The next day, she took six packs, and four to six packs continuously for the next five days. The mania disappeared, and the patient fell asleep easily, if somewhat fitfully. After taking three to four packs a day for five days continuously, she had sweat in the preauricular region and fell asleep within half an hour, and was able to take rice gruel. Afterwards, I added 3.75g of Gypsum Fibrosum to the decoction, for two packs a day. When she had no bowel movement, I added 15g of Gypsum Fibrosum. By the 23rd of December, her critical condition had stabilized, and she was able to stand up in the room. She had taken a total of 1687.5g of Gypsum Fibrosum for a month. Later, she walked for a mile

to see me on the fifteenth of next January. She continued to take Hyeongbang Jihwang Tang with 3.75g of Gypsum Fibrosum added until March.

其後又有一少陽人十七歲女兒素證間有悖氣食滯腹痛矣忽一日頭痛寒熱食滯有醫用蘇合元三介薑湯調下仍爲泄瀉日數十行十餘日不止引飮不眠間有譫語證時則己亥年冬十一月二十三日也卽夜用生地黃石膏各六兩知母三兩其夜泄瀉度數減半其翌日用荊防地黃湯加石膏四錢二貼連服安睡而能通小便荊防地黃湯二貼藥力十倍於知母白虎湯可知矣於是每日用此藥四貼晝二貼連服夜二貼連服數日用之泄瀉永止頭部兩鬢有汗而病兒譫語證變爲發狂證病家驚惑二晝夜疑不用藥病勢遂危頭汗不出小便秘結口嚙冰片不省人事爻象可惡矣勢無奈何以不得已之計一夜間用荊防地黃湯加石膏一兩連十貼灌口其夜小便通三碗狂證不止然知人看面稍有知覺其翌日又用六貼連五日日用四五六貼發狂始止夜間或霎時就睡然不能久睡便覺又日用三四貼連五日頭頂兩鬢有汗而能半時刻就睡稍進粥飮少許其後每日荊防地黃湯加石膏一錢日二貼用之大便過一日則加四錢至于十二月二十三日始得免危能起立房室中一朔內凡用石膏四十五兩新年正月十五日能行步一里地而來見我其後又連用荊防地黃湯加石膏一錢至于新年三月

45 I have said, "The lesser yang person's diseases are mainly due to the fire-heat; thus, it progresses rapidly. The initial symptoms must not be taken lightly. Generally, if a lesser yang person has a headache from the exterior disease, and constipation from the interior disease, he is already in a serious condition. Only one to three packs of inappropriate medications for a serious disease can kill the patient; and if one to three packs, normally suitable medication for a critical condition, are not used, the patient cannot be saved, either."

論曰少陽人病以火熱爲證故變動甚速初證不可輕易視之也凡少陽人表病有頭痛裏病有便秘則已爲重病也重病不當用之藥一二三貼誤投則必殺人險病危證當用之藥一二三貼不及則亦不救命

Notes

1) Du Ren (杜任)

He is cited in the 『*Yixue Gangmu*』(醫學綱目), but he has not been identified.

2) 『*Shanghan Shiquanlun*』(傷寒十卷論)

The "Ten Pieces of Advice on Exogenous Febrile Disease", written by Li Zijian.

3) Li Zijian (李子建)

A famous physician in the Song dynasty, and author of the 『*Shanghan Shiquanlun*』. Little is known about him except that he studied Zhang Zhongjing (張仲景)'s works and concluded that febrile diseases were not as dangerous to people as mediocre doctors who gave out erroneous prescriptions.

4) Zhu Danxi (朱丹溪)

Danxi is Zhu Zhenheng's other name. See Zhu Zhenheng.

Discourse on the Lesser Yang Person's Interior Febrile Disease Induced from the Stomach Affected by Heat

少陽人胃受熱裏熱病論

1 Zhang Zhongjing said, "In the greater yang disease, after eight to nine days, the patient has fever and chills with malaria, but more fever than chills. If there is a feeble pulse and chills, they are the symptom of a deficiency both in yin and yang. For such a case, neither a diaphoretic, nor a purgative, nor an emetic should be used. A flushed face, which indicates the color of heat, and an itchy skin caused by a lack of light perspiration, signifies that the pattern is not gone. Guima Geban Tang (Half Cinnamon Twig and Half Ephedra Decoction) will disperse the remaining pattern."

張仲景曰太陽病八九日如瘧狀發熱惡寒熱多寒少脈微而惡寒者此陰陽俱虛不可更發汗更下更吐面色反有熱色者未欲解也不能得小汗出身必痒宜桂麻各半湯

2 In the greater yang disease, when the patient has fever with chills like malaria, but more fever than chills, with a feeble pulse, it is a disease of yang collapse. A diaphoretic should not be adopted if there is no itching. Guipi Geban Tang (Half Cinnamon Twig and Half Maidservant Decoction) can be adopted.

太陽病似瘧發熱惡寒熱多寒少脈微弱者此亡陽也身不痒不可發汗宜桂婢各半湯

3 I have said, "In this pattern, if stool is passed within twenty four hours, Hyeongbang Sabaik San should be used. If not, Jihwang Baikho Tang should be used."

論曰此證大便不過一晝夜而通者當用荊防瀉白散大便過一晝夜而不通者當用地黃白虎湯

4 Zhang Zhongjing said, "For the yang brightness pattern, Zhuling Tang (Polyporus Decoction) is suitable when there is dysuria and a floating pulse with thirst."

張仲景曰陽明證小便不利脈浮而渴猪苓湯主之

5 A combination of the three yang diseases displays symptoms such as headaches, a dirty face, delirium and incontinence. It manifests itself through fever both in the interior and the exterior. When there is spontaneous perspiration, restlessness with thirst, abdominal pain and a heavy feeling in movement, Baihu Tang can be adopted.
三陽合病頭痛面垢譫語遺尿中外俱熱自汗煩渴腹痛身重白虎湯主之

6 I have said, "The yang brightness pattern is the only apparent fever with no chills. A combination of the three yang diseases means that the greater yang, lesser yang and yang brightness diseases are simultaneously complicated. For this case, we should use Zhuling Tang and Baihu Tang. The ancient prescription of Zhuling Tang is no better than the recent practice of prescribing Jeoryeong Chajeonja Tang. Similarly, the ancient Baihu Tang is no better than the new prescription of Jihwang Baikho Tang. If the yang brightness disease has symptoms such as dysuria and constipation, it is suitable to use Jihwang Baikho Tang."
論曰陽明證者但熱無寒之謂也三陽合病者太陽少陽陽明證俱有之謂也此證當用猪苓湯白虎湯然古方猪苓湯不如新方猪苓車前子湯之俱備古方白虎湯不如新方地黃白虎湯之全美矣若陽明證小便不利者兼大便秘燥則當用地黃白虎湯

7 Zhu Gong said, "Yang syncope is the disease which shows fever and headache, and looks like yang pattern externally in the initial stage, with syncope not appearing until the fourth or fifth day. Syncope is suddenly accompanied with fever within half a day. There never is syncope until the heat qi is localized deeply. It is a serious fever if the fever suddenly occurs when syncope is mild. The pulse can only be detected when pressed deeply, and the pulse is slippery. This means that there is a fever inside which may lead to symptoms, including drinking large amounts of water, waving of hands and feet, restlessness with insomnia, constipation, reddish urine and coma. Baihu Tang should be used."
朱肱曰陽厥者初得病必身熱頭痛外有陽證至四五日方發厥厥至半日却身熱蓋熱氣深方能發厥若微厥却發熱者熱甚故也其脈雖伏按之滑者爲裡熱或飲水或揚手擲足或煩燥不得眠大便秘小便赤外證多昏憒用白虎湯

8 I have said, "For the interior febrile disease of the lesser yang person, Jihwang Baikho Tang would be the best drug. Before adopting this decoction, we must monitor a patient's bowel movements. If he has not passed anything for one day, we may use it; if he has not passed anything for two days, we must use it. Generally, if a lesser yang person cannot pass stool for one day, his stomach-heat has been already congealed. If there was no bowel movement for two days in the lesser yang person, he has a serious fever. If there is no bowel movement within three days and nights, his condition is dangerous. It is reasonable to adopt the drug when the patient has had no bowel movement for over a day or two. One should not, how-

ever, allow this constipation to last a third day and night; and if there is delirium and constipation, do not let the symptoms persist for more than one day and night."

論曰少陽人裡熱病地黃白虎湯爲聖藥而用之者必觀於大便之通不通也大便一晝夜有餘而不通則可用也二晝夜不通則必用也凡少陽人大便一晝夜不通則胃熱已結也二晝夜不通則熱重也三晝夜不通則危險也一晝夜八九辰刻二晝夜恰好用之無至三晝夜之危險若譫語證便秘則不可過一晝夜

9 If the stomach of a lesser yang person receives the heat, his feces will be dry. If his Spleen receives the cold, diarrhea will be induced. If there is yin collapse with diarrhea for two to three days and constipation for one day and night, the clean yin will be exhausted, and the patient's condition will be in danger. If there is the stomach-heat pattern with constipation for three days and nights and perspiration, the clean yang will be exhausted, and the patient's condition will be in danger.

少陽人胃受熱則大便燥也脾受寒則泄瀉也故亡陰證泄瀉二三日而大便秘一晝夜則清陰將亡而危境也胃熱證大便三晝夜不通而汗出則清陽將竭而危境也

10 If a lesser yang person with constipation takes three to four packs of Baihu Tang, he will recover, though he will not have had any bowel movement that day. If he takes two to three packs continuously the next day, he will certainly have a bowel movement.

少陽人大便不通病用白虎湯三四服當日大便不通者將爲融會貫通大吉之兆也不必疑惑而翌日又服二三貼則必無不通

11 When attempting to identify a lesser yang person's disease, whether it is the exterior or interior pattern, and whether aggravated or relieved, it is important that one examines the stool. If the feces are dry at first and loose later, and there is no difficulty in bowel movement, the lesser yang person is in good health. If his bowel movements cease after passing a large amount of loose stool, once or twice, his illness will be relieved. Ordinarily, smooth stool, once or twice, indicates that the patient's condition has not changed. No bowel movement for more than one day and night, or small amount of loose stools three to five times for one day and night indicates that his stool will be constipated. This stool indicates a bad prognosis, which we must prevent.

少陽人表裏病結解必觀於大便而少陽人大便頭燥尾滑體大而疏通者平時無病者之大便也其次大滑便一二次快滑泄廣多而止者有病者之病快解之大便也其次一二次尋常滑便者有病者病勢不加之大便也其次或過一晝夜有餘不通或一晝夜間三四五次小小滑利者將澁之候也非好便也宜預防

12 At the onset of the lower abdomen cold pattern of the lesser yin person's interior cold disease, symptoms such as borborygmus and diarrhea are easily detected, and a treatment should be adopted as early as possible. At the onset of the chest-phrenic fever pattern of the lesser yang person's interior febrile disease, symptoms such as restlessness in the chest cannot be easily detected, and a treatment is usually adopted at a later stage. If a lesser yang person

had marked restlessness in the chest that can be easily identified, it is very difficult to treat, because such a symptom indicates that his condition is already serious. Generally, for the exterior disease of the lesser yang person, we can easily understand that headache is one of the initial symptoms. If there are other symptoms, such as thirst and reddish urine, we must be cautious; and if there are other symptoms, such as diarrhea and waving of hands and feet, we must practice prudence here, as well. As for the interior disease of the lesser yang person, it is clear that no bowel movement for more than one day and night belongs to the initial symptom of the interior disease. If a patient has had no bowel movement for more than three days and nights, he is in danger. A patient, who suffers from diseases such as back carbuncle, brain carbuncle, swollen lips, diphtheria and laryngopharyngeal disease, is already in danger from onset. The macule due to yang type inflammatory swelling, multiple erysipelas and jaundice also indicates a dangerous condition from onset. The illnesses of the face, eyes, mouth, nose and teeth are serious when they occur. Generally, Hyeongbang Paidok San should be used for headache induced by the exterior disease, and Baikho Tang should be used for the interior disease of a lesser yang person who has had no bowel movement for more than one day and night.

少陰人裏寒病臍腹冷證受病之初已有腹鳴泄瀉之機驗而其機甚顯則其病執證易見而用藥可早也少陽人裏熱病胸膈熱證受病之初雖有胸煩悶燥之機驗而其機不甚顯則執證難見而用藥太晚也若使少陽人病胸煩悶燥之驗顯然露出使人可覺則其病已險而難爲措手矣凡少陽人表病有頭痛則自是表病明白易見之初證也若復引飲小便赤則可畏也泄瀉揚手擲足則大畏也少陽人裡病大便過一晝夜有餘而不通則自是裏病明白易見之初證也若復大便過三晝夜不通則危險矣背癰腦疽脣瘇纏喉風咽喉等病受病之日已爲危險證也陽毒發斑流注丹毒黃疸等病受病之日已爲險證也面目口鼻牙齒之病成病之日皆爲重證也凡少陽人表病有頭痛證則必用荊防敗毒散裏病有大便過一晝夜不通證則用白虎湯

13 Wang Haogu said, "There are three types of thirst disease whose names are *xiaoke* (polydipsia), *xiaozhong* (polyphagia), and *xiaoshen* (polyuria). Restlessness in the chest and reddish tongue and lips are caused by the ascending heat qi. This thirst, called polydipsia, is characterized by an imbibing of a large amount of fluids and frequent urination in small quantities, and belongs to the upper-*jiao*. Hyperphagia, over-appetite, and emaciation are caused by the accumulation of heat in the middle-*jiao*. This results in a thirst in which the restlessness in the chest is mild, urination is frequent, and the urine tastes sweet; it belongs to the middle-*jiao* This thirst is called polyphagia, and is characterized by emaciation of the thigh and knee joint, soreness and pain in the joints, drinking small amounts of water, and a large quantity of turbid urine. These are all caused by the latency of the heat in the lower-*jiao*. This disease is called polyuria, and one symptom is a leakage of sperm without sexual intercourse induced by the over-consumption of five mineral stones that causes the exhaustion of the essential qi and the remainder of mineral heat. This thirst is called *qiangzhong* (persistent erection). Polydipsia is mild, polyphagia is serious, and polyuria even more so. The persistent erection is

a fatal disease where death is welcome relief."

王好古曰渴病有三曰消渴曰消中曰消腎熱氣上騰胸中煩燥舌赤脣紅此渴引飲常多小便數而少病屬上焦謂之消渴熱蓄於中消穀善飢飲食倍常不生肌肉此渴亦不甚煩小便數而甛病屬中焦謂之消中熱伏於下腿膝枯細骨節痠疼飲水不多隨卽尿下小便多而渴病屬下焦謂之消腎又有五石過度之人眞氣旣盡石勢獨留陽道興强不交精泄謂之强中消渴輕也消中甚焉消腎尤甚焉若强中則其斃可立而待也

14 Zhu Zhenheng said, "Baihu Tang should be adopted for diabetes involving the upper-*jiao*, which manifests itself as a red and fissured tongue, and polyposia with severe thirst. Huanglian Zhudu Wan (Pills of Coptidis Rhizoma and Pig Stomach) should be adopted for diabetes involving the middle-*jiao*, whose symptoms include polyposia with emaciation, spontaneous perspiration, constipation and frequent urination. Liuwei Dihuang Tang should be adopted for diabetes stemming from the lower-*jiao*, whose symptoms are restlessness with much drinking of water, oily urine, and dry and thin legs."

朱震亨曰上消者舌上赤裂大渴引飲白虎湯主之中消者善食而瘦自汗大便硬小便數黃連猪肚丸主之下消者煩燥引飲小便如膏腿膝枯細六味地黃湯主之

15 In the 『*Yixue Gangmu*』, we read, "Polyposia with thirst is diabetes involving the upper-*jiao*. Polyposia with polyphasia is diabetes involving the middle-*jiao*; and thirst with frequent and oily urination is diabetes involving the lower-*jiao*."

醫學綱目曰渴而多飲爲上消消穀善飢爲中消渴而尿數有膏油爲下消

16 Wei Yilin said, "If a person overindulgent in sensual pleasures takes a mineral stone while his essential qi is already exhausted and only the evil heat remains, he will display symptoms of polyphagia, emaciation, oily urine, and persistent erection with spontaneous ejaculation. This is the most serious type among the three diabetic diseases."

危亦林曰因耽嗜色慾或服丹石眞氣旣脫熱邪獨盛飲食如湯消雪肌膚日削小便如膏油陽强興盛不交精泄三消之中最爲難治

17 I have said, "Diabetes is induced by a person's own mean and narrow mind. A hard, hasty, shallow and unoriginal mind makes it difficult for the large intestine qi to ascend. Hence, gradually, the qi is exhausted, and the disease is formed. If the clean yang in the stomach ascends and cannot nourish the head, face and four limbs, diabetes involving the upper-*jiao* will be formed. If the clean yang in the large intestine ascends and cannot nourish the stomach, diabetes involving the middle-*jiao* will be formed. Originally, diabetes involving the upper-*jiao* was serious, but diabetes involving the middle-*jiao* is twice as serious as diabetes involving the upper-*jiao*. Diabetes involving the middle-*jiao* is a dangerous disease, but diabetes involving the lower-*jiao* is twice as dangerous as diabetes involving the middle-*jiao*. Yanggyeok Sanhwa Tang (Decoction for Cooling the Diaphragm and Dispersing Fire)

should be used for diabetes involving the upper-*jiao*, Indongdeung Jigolpi Tang (Honeysuckle Stem and Lycium Root Bark Decoction) should be used for diabetes involving the middle-*jiao*, and Sukjihwang Gosam Tang (Rehmanniae Radix Praeparata and Sophora Root Decoction) should be used for diabetes involving the lower-*jiao*. Sufferers should be generous and broad-minded. To be generous means to be slow-paced, and as a result, a person's clean yang will ascend and flow. To be narrow-minded means to be in a hurry; his clean yang will be exhausted in the lower part."

論曰消渴者病人胸次不能寬闊闊達而陋固膠小所見者淺所欲者速計策鶻突意思艱乏則大腸淸陽上升之氣自不快足日月耗困而生此病也胃局淸陽上升而不快足於頭面四肢則成上消病大腸局淸陽上升而不快足於胃局則成中消病上消自爲重證而中消倍重於上消中消自爲險證而下消倍險於中消上消宜用凉膈散火湯中消宜用忍冬藤地骨皮湯下消宜用熟地黃苦參湯尤宜寬潤其心不宜膠小其心寬潤則所欲必緩淸陽上達膠小則所欲必速淸陽下耗

18 Stable emotion with a peaceful mind will raise the yang qi and spread this qi to the face, head and limbs. This qi is called primordial qi and clean yang. The exertion of the mind will lower and concentrate the yang qi. This will lead to the stagnated heat on the face, head, and limbs. This qi is called the fire qi and the consuming yang.

平心靜思則陽氣上升輕淸而充足於頭面四肢也此元氣也淸陽也勞心焦思則陽氣下陷重濁而鬱熱於頭面四肢也此火氣也耗陽也

19 Wei Yilin said, "Since diabetes must try to prevent the formation of carbuncles, it is advisable to take the root, stem, flower or leaf of the Lonicerae Caulis without consideration of amounts."

危亦林曰消渴須防發癰疽忍冬藤不拘多少根莖花葉皆可服

20 Li Gao said, "If a diabetic patient is able to eat food, he will get a carbuncle on the nape and back in the late stages; and if a patient cannot eat food, he will have abdominal distension or tympanites."

李杲曰消渴之疾能食者末傳必發腦疽背瘡不能食者必傳中滿鼓脹

21 In the 『*Dongui Uibang Yuchui*』[1] ("Classified Collection of Eastern Medical Prescriptions"), we read, "Diabetes can lead to carbuncles, fluid imbalance or total blindness."

東醫醫方類聚曰消渴之病變成發癰疽或成水病或雙目失明

22 I have said, "Carbuncles and optic diseases are developed from diabetes involving the middle-*jiao*. Since diabetes involving the middle-*jiao* is already dangerous, we should treat it when it is still involving the upper-*jiao*. In the case of diabetes involving the middle-*jiao*, we should treat it immediately. Diabetes involving the lower-*jiao* may be regarded as virtually fatal."

論曰癰疽眼病皆是中消之變證也中消自爲險證則上消當早治也中消必急治也下消則濱死

23 Wang Haogu said, "One child sweated at night for seven years. He took many drugs, but did not experience any improvement. He took Liangge San (Powder for Cooling the Diaphragm) for three days, and then he recovered from his illness."
王好古曰一童子自嬰至童盜汗七年諸藥不效服凉膈散三日病已

24 I have said, "If the lesser yang person's large intestine clean yang flows up to the stomach and nourishes the head, face and limbs, there will be no sweating. The sweating of the lesser yang person is induced by the weakness of yang. Here, recovery by Liangge San means that the disease is diabetes involving the upper-*jiao*, and is but a mild case."
論曰少陽人大腸淸陽快足於胃充溢於頭面四肢則汗必不出也少陽人汗者自是陽弱也而服凉膈散病已則此病卽上消而其病輕也

25 In the 『*Dongui Uibang Yuchui*』, we read, "Generally, the diabetic patient drinks water frequently, and certainly has symptoms such as dizziness and cold back with vomiting. These symptoms are caused by his asthenia."
東醫醫方類聚曰夫渴者數飲水其人必頭面眩背寒而嘔因虛故也

26 Gong Xin said, "Generally, yin deficiency pattern shows chills and fever every day in the afternoon, which is relieved after slight sweating. If we treat it as malaria, it cannot be cured."
龔信曰凡陰虛證每日午後惡寒發熱至晚亦得微汗而解誤作瘧治多致不救

27 Sun Simiao[2], in his 『*Qianjinfang*』[3] ("Essential Prescriptions Worth a Thousand Gold Pieces") said, "There are three things which diabetes should avoid: drinking, overindulging in sensual pleasures and eating salty food and noodles. If he avoids them, he may recover from his illness without taking drugs."
孫思邈千金方書曰消渴宜愼者有三一飲酒二房勞三鹹食及麫能愼此三者雖不服藥亦可自愈

28 I have said, "Even though the ascending qi of the interior yang is exhausted in diabetes involving the upper-*jiao* and diabetes involving the middle-*jiao*, their descending qi of the exterior yin is still strong; so though the diseases are dangerous, the patient can manage for a long time. Afternoon fever and insatiable thirst show yin deficiency, and the two with a cold back and vomiting indicates that their yin and yang of both the exterior and interior are totally exhausted. Their condition is in as much danger as though they were suffering diabetes involving the lower-*jiao*. However, if they can maintain good psychosomatic cultivation and proper administration of drugs, six to seven out of ten will stay alive. If, however, they neglect psychosomatic cultivation and simply rely upon the drugs, they will be unable to cure the patient. Dokhwal Jihwang Tang (Decoction of Rehmanniae Radix Praeparata with Angelicae Pubescentis Radix) and Sibimi Jihwang Tang (Decoction of Twelve Drugs Containing Rehmanniae Radix Praeparata) should be adopted."

論曰上消中消裏陽升氣雖則虛損表陰降氣猶恃完壯故其病雖險猶能歲月支撐者以此也若夫陰虛午熱飲水背寒而嘔者表裏陰陽俱爲虛損所以爲病尤險與下消畧相輕重然能善攝身心服藥則十之六七尙可生也不善攝身心服藥則百之百必死也此證當用獨活地黃湯十二味地黃湯

29 In the undivided third line of the Xu (需) in the 『*Ijing*』[4] ("Classic of Changes"), we read, "The third line of the Xu, undivided, shows its subject in the mud (close by the stream). He thereby invites the approach of the enemy." It says in the Great Symbolism, "'He is waiting in the mud.' This tells us that calamity is close at hand in the outer trigram. 'He himself invites the approach of the enemy' tell us that if he be reverent and careful, he will not be bested." If we say, quoting the meaning above, "Though a patient has afternoon fever caused by yin deficiency, cold back and vomiting, which is dangerous, his death will depend upon other factors. If he cleans and purifies his mind, respects his body and takes the proper medicine, he will recover."

易之需九三爻辭曰需于泥致寇至象曰需于泥災在外也自我致寇敬慎不敗也以此意而傲之曰陰虛午熱背寒而嘔其病雖險然死尙在外也能齋戒其心恭敬其身又服好藥不死也

Notes

1) 『*Dongui Uibang Yuchui*』(東醫醫方類聚)

The "Classified Collection of Eastern Medical Prescriptions". King Sejong (世宗) of the Joseon dynasty ordered his officers to gather all the traditional medical books and to compile a comprehensive medical work for the sake of medical practice improvement. It comprises 266 volumes.

2) Sun Simiao (孫思邈)

(581~682 A.D.) A prominent physician of the Tang dynasty and author of the 『*Qianjin Yaofang*』(千金要方: "Essential Prescriptions Worth a Thousand Gold Pieces", 652 A.D.) and 『*Qianjin Yifang*』(千金翼方: "Supplement to Prescriptions Worth a Thousand Gold Pieces", 682 A.D.), which are considered a collection of the medical achievements before the 7th century.

3) 『*Qianjinfang*』(千金方)

The "Essential Prescriptions Worth a Thousand Gold Pieces", also called the 『*Beiji Qianjin Yaofang*』(備急千金要方: "Essential Prescriptions Worth a Thousand Gold Pieces for Emergencies") or 『*Qianjin Yaofang*』, compiled by Sun Simiao (孫思邈) at the end of the seventh century in thirty volumes. This text gives a general introduction, deals with the prescriptions of various clinical branches, diet, pulse taking, acupuncture, etc.

4) 『*Ijing*』(易經)

The "Classic of Changes", an ancient Chinese text that is one of the Five Classics of Confucianism. The uniqueness of 『*Ijing*』 is in its presentation of 64 symbolic hexagrams that, if properly understood and interpreted, are said to contain profound meanings applicable to daily life. Throughout the ages, the 『*Ijing*』 enthusiasts have claimed that the book is a means of understanding, and even controlling, future events.

147

General Remarks
on the Lesser Yang Person

少陽人泛論

1 For the lesser yang person's disease, there are five major symptoms: stroke, hematemesis, vomiting, abdominal pain, and indigestion with a feeling of fullness. All of these five symptoms have the same cause, and there are different degrees of each symptom. Another group of five symptoms is edema, dyspnea, accumulation of pathogen in the chest, dysentery and alternate attacks of chills and fever with fullness in the chest and costal region. These all have the same cause, but different intensities in expression.

少陽人病中風吐血嘔吐腹痛食滯痞滿五證同出一屬而自有輕重浮腫喘促結胸痢疾寒熱往來胸脅滿五證同出一屬而自有輕重

2 There is no way to cure the hemiplegia or monoplegia of the upper limbs induced by stroke in a lesser yang person. If the stroke is severe, the patient will die, and if it is mild, he can survive. Since there is no guarantee the patient will recover, he should take drugs from time to time and hope for the best.

少陽人中風半身不遂一臂不遂末如何之疾也重者必死輕者猶生間以服藥安而復之待其自愈而不可期必治法之疾也

3 If a lesser yang person has hematemesis, he must control his hard and irritable temper; not fight with others; eat a simple diet; take the proper drug, and cultivate himself like a Buddhist. After 100 days, his illness will somewhat improve; after 200 days, it will be much improved; one year later, he will have all but recovered; and three years later, he will have fully recovered. If he does not follow this direction, the illness will recur. If this happens, all prior efforts will have been in vain, and the patient must begin anew. If he follows the directions

for ten or twenty years, he will have a long life.

少陽人吐血者必蕩滌剛愎偏急與人並駈爭塗之淡食服藥修養如釋道一百日則可以少愈二百日則可以大愈一周年則可以快愈三周年則可保其壽凡吐血調養失道則必再發再發則前功皆歸於虛地若再發者則又自再發日計數一百日少愈一周年快愈若十年二十年調養則必得高壽

4 Generally, a lesser yang person will sometimes experience slight bleeding in the nasal cavity or in the sputum. Even though it is slight, it is still hematemesis. If there is bleeding in the mouth and cold phlegm, though there be no vomiting, it still belongs to vomiting. A young man contracting this illness will die shortly. This is caused by negligence. These two symptoms are very serious and dangerous, so the patient must take medicine. After ridding the patient of the root of his illness, his life can be saved.

凡少陽人間有鼻血少許或口鼻間痰涎中有血雖細微皆吐血之屬也又口中暗有冷涎逆上者雖不嘔吐亦嘔吐之屬也少年有此證者多致夭折以其等閑任置故也此二證必在重病險病之列不可不預防服藥永除病根然後可保無虞

5 A stroke is so serious in nature that we cannot expect to cure it; hematemesis, however, is milder, and the patient's chances of recovery are high. These two diseases can be cured first, by taking care of oneself, and second, by taking medicine. However, for symptoms such as vomiting, abdominal pain and indigestion with a feeling of fullness, a patient must take medicine as well as care of himself, if he expects to recover.

中風受病太重故治法不可期必吐血受病猶輕故治法可以期必中風吐血調養爲主服藥次之嘔吐以下腹痛食滯痞滿服藥調養則其病易愈

6 For stroke and vomiting, Dokhwal Jihwang Tang should be adopted; and for hematemesis, Sibimi Jihwang Tang.

中風嘔吐宜用獨活地黃湯吐血宜用十二味地黃湯

7 Edema is a disease that has to be treated quickly. If not, the patient will be in danger. The more quickly he takes medicine, the more easily he will recover; if not, he will die. From outward appearances, this disease seems to progress slowly and not pose much of a threat to a person's health, but it is not so. It must be treated within four or five days, and must not last more than ten days. In the beginning, the patient of edema takes Moktong Daian Tang (Decoction for Greatly Stabilizing with Akebiae Caulis) or Hyeongbang Jihwang Tang added Akebiae Caulis, then once more afterwards. In six or seven days, the edema will be cured. Following recovery, he must take one or two packs of the above decoction (Hyeongbang Jihwang Tang added Akebiae Caulis) every day for 100 days, to clean the urine and to prevent the disease from recurring. If it recurs, recovery will prove difficult. After the relief from edema, the patient should not take much food. If he takes too much, the disease will recur. In cases of edema, reddish urine is a sign of malignancy. If the urine is clean, the edema will

be successfully treated, but if it is red, edema will occur.

浮腫爲病急治則生不急治則危用藥早則容易愈也用藥不早則孟浪死也此病外勢平緩似不速死故人必易之此病實是急證四五日內必治之疾謨不可以十日論之也浮腫初發當用木通大安湯或荊防地黃湯加木通日再服則六七日內浮腫必解浮腫解後百日內必用荊防地黃湯加木通二三錢每日一二貼用之以清小便以防再發再發難治浮腫初解飲食尤宜忍飢而小食若如平人大食則必不免再發大畏小便赤也小便清則浮腫解小便赤則浮腫結

8 If a lesser yang person who has diabetes involving the middle-*jiao* has abdominal distension, he will definitely develop tympanites, which is incurable. A lesser yang person with tympanites, just as a lesser yin person with *zangjie* (accumulation of yin cold in the viscera), dies within five months to a year. In a lesser yin person with accumulation of yin cold in the viscera, though his exterior yang warm qi is almost exhausted, his interior yin warm qi stands out strongly. In a lesser yang person with tympanites, though his interior yang cool qi is almost exhausted, his exterior yin cool qi stands out strongly. Both may live with their respective disease for quite a long time before dying.

少陽人中消者腹脹則必成鼓脹鼓脹不治少陽人鼓脹病如少陰人藏結病皆經歷五六七八月或周年而竟死盖少陰人藏結表陽溫氣雖在幾絕裏陰溫氣猶恃完壯少陽人鼓脹裏陽清氣雖在幾絕表陰清氣猶恃完壯故皆經歷久遠而死也

9 For shortness of breath due to a febrile disease caused by cold in a lesser yang person, first, 0.375g of Cinnabaris should be used with warm water, and just after decocted Schizonepetae Herba, Saposhnikoviae Radix, and Trichosanthis Semen, etc. should be taken. There is no time to wait for the decoction.

少陽人傷寒喘促宜先用靈砂一分溫水調下因煎荊防瓜蔞等藥用之則必無煎藥時刻遲滯救病

10 Since the effect of Cinnabaris is very strong, it must not be used many times. The medicine is good for emergencies only. It must be boiled into soup. After the stomach and intestine are filled with it, it can tonify and invigorate yin and yang.

靈砂藥力急迫可以一再用而不可屢用盖救急之藥敏於救急而已藥必湯服然後充滿腸胃能爲補陰補陽

11 When compared to accumulation of pathogen in the chest, dysentery is regarded as a mild disease. However, when dysentery is close in seriousness to edema, it is regarded as a serious disease. When compared to abdominal pain, vomiting is a deteriorated case. However, when vomiting is close in seriousness to stroke, it is regarded as a malignant disease.

痢疾之比結胸則痢疾爲順證也而痢疾之謂重證者以其浮腫相近也嘔吐之比腹痛則嘔吐爲逆證也而嘔吐之謂惡證者以其距中風不遠也

12 For dysentery in a lesser yang person, Hwanglyeon Cheongjang Tang (Decoction for Clear-

ing the Intestines with Coptidis Rhizoma) should be adopted.

少陽人痢疾宜用黃連淸腸湯

13 There is a type of malaria which has a three-day cycle of one day on and two days off in a lesser yang person: it is malaria with general debility. It must be treated slowly, not hastily. When the malaria is off, the patient should take two packs of Dokhwal Jihwang Tang during the morning and the evening. When it starts again, he should take two packs of Hyeongbang Paidok San continuously when he feels chilly. If the patient accepts the standard of taking 40 packs of Dokhwal Jihwang Tang and 20 packs of Hyeongbang Paidok San within a month, the disease will be cured.

少陽人瘧病有間兩日發者卽勞瘧也可以緩治不可急治此證瘧不發日用獨活地黃湯二貼朝暮服瘧發日預煎荊防敗毒散二貼待惡寒發作時二貼連服一月之內以獨活地黃湯四十貼荊防敗毒散二十貼爲準的則其瘧必無不退之理

14 For the lesser yang person, the swelling inside the throat and outside the neck and cheeks is called diphtheria. In two or three days, it will kill the patient. Swelling in the raphe of the upper lip is called swollen lips. Swelling that looks like hulled millet around both sides of the raphe is also dangerous. When the above two diseases are still mild in the initial stage, the patient should take Yanggyeok Sanhwa Tang and Yangdok Baikho Tang (White Tiger Decoction for Yang Type Inflammatory Swelling). If serious, nasal fumigation with mercury should be adopted. If there is perspiration over the neck and cheeks after fumigation into the nose, the patient will be cured. If there is no fumigant, he should take a pill mixed with 0.5625g of Calomelas, Olibanum, Myrrha, and Euphorbia Kansui Radix, 1.875g each, with starch at once.

少陽人內發咽喉外腫項頰者謂之纏喉風二三日內殺人最急又上脣人中穴瘇謂之脣瘇凡人中左右逼近處一指許發瘇雖微如粟粒亦危證也此二證始發而輕者當用凉膈散火湯陽毒白虎湯重者當用水銀熏鼻方一炷熏鼻而項頰汗出則愈若倉卒無熏鼻藥則輕粉末一分五里乳香沒藥甘遂末各五分和勻糊丸一服盡

15 If a lesser yang child eats much, but remains thin, he should take Luhui Feier Wan (Children's Weight-gaining Pills with Aloe) or Indongdeung Jigolpi Tang.

少陽人小兒食多肌瘦宜用蘆薈肥兒丸忍冬藤地骨皮湯

16 I once observed a lesser yang person with *duzhong* (poisonous swelling) on his shoulder. He had no sensation of heat when boiled sesame oil was poured on the swelling and the skin and flesh was burnt. A doctor taught him to place a piece of bull's horn on the coal and let the smoke into the swelling. The poisonous pus was flushed and the swelling cured.

嘗見少陽人肩上有毒瘇火熬香油灌瘡肌肉焦爛而不知其熱有醫敎以牛角片置火炭上燒而熏之烟入瘡口毒汁自流其瘇立愈

17　I once observed a seventy year old lesser yang person who had a carbuncle on the nape of his neck. A doctor had told him to patch it with a powdered swellfish's egg, and he recovered immediately. Since swellfish's eggs are very poisonous, pigs or dogs die immediately when they eat them. When they are hung in a tree, birds do not dare eat them.

嘗見少陽人七十老人發腦疽有醫敎以河豚卵作末傅之其疽立愈河豚卵至毒彘犬食之則立死掛於林木間烏鵲不敢食

18　I once treated a lesser yang person with a carbuncle resembling a serpent's head. A swellfish's egg was made into powder; a small amount was placed on the adhesive plaster, and the dressing was changed daily. After five or six days, we could see the effects: new flesh had grown quickly, but there was too much of it. I covered all the new flesh with whetstone powder, the excess flesh disappeared, and the patient recovered. I have also used this drug for several days to treat scrofula resembling a lotus seed pot. It is also good for burns and dog or insect bites.

嘗治少陽人蛇頭瘡河豚卵作末少許点膏藥上傅之而一日一次易以新末傅藥五六日病效而新肉急生而有妬肉因以磨刀砥末傅之妬肉立消而病愈又用之於連珠痰多日傅之者必効用之於爲炭火所傷與狗咬蟲咬無不得効

19　I once treated a sixty year old lesser yang person with monoplegia of the upper limb due to a stroke. I told him to take 0.1875g of Calomelas, but his condition worsened. I prescribed Gyeongbun Gamsu Yongho Dan (Dragon-tiger Pills with Calomelas and Euphorbia Kansui Radix) for a twenty year old lesser yang person who had a slight monoplegia of the lower limb with numbness. After two or three administrations, he recovered.

嘗治少陽人六十老人中風一臂不遂病用輕粉五里其病輒加少陽人二十歲少年一脚微不仁痺風用輕粉甘遂龍虎丹二三次用之得効

20　I once treated a lesser yang person with a throat problem. He could not drink at all and had no bowel movement for three days. All signs pointed to a serious problem, so I prescribed Gamsu Cheonil Hwan (Tianyi Pills with Euphorbia Kansui Radix). He recovered immediately.

嘗治少陽人咽喉水醬不入大便不通三日病至危境用甘遂天一丸卽効

21　I once treated a seventy year old lesser yang person who had had no bowel movement for four to seven days and coldness, but no strength in his feet, although he could eat as usual. I prescribed Gyeongbun Gamsu Yongho Dan, and he immediately had a bowel movement. Several days later, however, the constipation recurred, and I told him to take this prescription several times more. Later, he was able to have normal bowel movements every day, and his disease was cured. He lived to the age of eighty.

嘗治少陽人七十老人大便四五日不通或六七日不通飲食如常兩脚膝寒無力用輕粉甘遂龍虎丹大便卽通後數日大便又秘則又用屢次用之竟以大便一日一度爲準而病愈此老竟得八十壽

22 I once observed a lesser yang person with heavy bleeding in his central incisors ridge, and immediately recognized his condition as dangerous. A doctor taught him how to apply new cotton soaked in boiled sesame oil to his ridge, and the bleeding stopped.

嘗見少陽人當門二齒齦縫血出頃刻間數碗將至危境有醫敎以火熬香油以新綿點油乘熱灼齒縫仍爲血止

23 I once observed a lesser yang person who experienced facial paralysis after combing his hair every day for several months. There were three more lesser yang persons suffering from the same illness, so I concluded that it is not good for a lesser yang person to comb his hair every day. I once knew an eighty year old greater yin person who combed his hair every day, who affirmed that combing was a pleasant activity in which he had been indulging for forty years.

嘗見少陽人一人每日一次梳頭數月後得口眼喎斜病其後又見少陽人日梳得喎斜病者凡三人盖日梳少陽人禁忌也嘗見太陰人八十老人日梳者老人自言曰日梳極好我之日梳已爲四十年云

Ten Prescriptions
for the Lesser Yang Person's Disease
from Zhang Zhongjing's 『*Shanghanlun*』

張仲景傷寒論中少陽人病經驗設方藥十方

1 White Tiger Decoction (Baihu Tang)
· Gypsum Fibrosum 18.75g   · Anemarrhenae Rhizoma 7.5g
· Glycyrrhizae Radix et Rhizoma 2.625g   · Oryzae Semen Sativae 9.375g
白虎湯
石膏五錢知母二錢甘草七分粳米半合

2 Polyporus Decoction (Zhuling Tang)
· Polyporus 3.75g   · Poria Sclerotium (red) 3.75g
· Alismatis Rhizoma 3.75g   · Talcum 3.75g
· Colla corii asini 3.75g
猪苓湯
猪苓赤茯苓澤瀉滑石阿膠各一錢

3 Five-Ingredient Powder with Poria Sclerotium (Wuling San)
· Alismatis Rhizoma 9.375g   · Poria Sclerotium (red) 5.625g
· Polyporus 5.625g   · Atractylodis Rhizoma Alba 5.625g
· Cinnamomi Cortex 1.875g
五苓散
澤瀉二錢五分赤茯苓猪苓白朮各一錢五分肉桂五分

4 Minor Decoction of Bupleurum (Xiao Chaihu Tang)
- Bupleuri Radix 11.25g
- Scutellariae Radix 7.5g
- Ginseng Radix 5.625g
- Pinelliae Tuber 5.625g
- Glycyrrhizae Radix et Rhizoma 1.875g

小柴胡湯

柴胡三錢黃芩二錢人蔘半夏各一錢五分甘草五分

5 Big Blue Dragon Decoction (Da Qinglong Tang)
- Gypsum Fibrosum 15g
- Ephedrae Herba 11.25g
- Cinnamomi Ramulus 7.5g
- Armeniacae Semen 5.625g
- Glycyrrhizae Radix et Rhizoma 3.75g
- Zingiberis Rhizoma recens 3 slices
- Jujubae Fructus 2 pcs.

大靑龍湯

石膏四錢麻黃三錢桂枝二錢杏仁一錢五分甘草一錢生薑三片大棗二枚

6 Half Cinnamon Twig and Half Maidservant Decoction (Guipi Geban Tang)
- Gypsum Fibrosum 7.5g
- Ephedrae Herba 3.75g
- Cinnamomi Ramulus 3.75g
- Paeoniae Radix Alba 3.75g
- Glycyrrhizae Radix et Rhizoma 1.125g
- Zingiberis Rhizoma recens 3 slices
- Jujubae Fructus 2 pcs.

桂婢各半湯

石膏二錢麻黃桂枝白芍藥各一錢甘草三分生薑三片大棗二枚

7 Minor Decoction for Pathogens Stuck in the Chest (Xiao Xianxiong Tang)
- Pinelliae Tuber (detoxicated with ginger decoction) 18.75g
- Coptidis Rhizoma 9.375g
- Trichosanthis Semen (1/4 of large one)

小陷胸湯

半夏製五錢黃連二錢五分瓜蔞大者四分之一

8 Major Decoction for Pathogens Stuck in the Chest (Da Xianxiong Tang)
- Rhei Radix et Rhizoma 11.25g
- Natrii Sulfas 7.5g
- Euphorbia Kansui Radix 1.875g

大陷胸湯

大黃三錢芒硝二錢甘遂末五分

9 Ten Jujubes Decoction (Shizao Tang)
- Genkwa Flos (stir-baked to just dry)
- Euphorbia Kansui Radix

· Euphorbiae Pekinensis Radix (stir-baked)

Pound equal amounts of the drugs into a powder. Stew ten dates (Jujubae Fructus) in one glass of water until half a glass remains. Remove the dregs and add 3.75g of the above powder for a strong patient and 1.875g for a weak patient. If loose stool is observed, serve the patient rice gruel for tonifying.

十棗湯

莞花微炒甘遂大戟炒等分爲末別取大棗十枚水一盞煎至半盞去棗調藥末強人一錢弱人半錢服大便利下水以粥補之

10 Pill for Invigorating Kidney Qi (Shenqi Wan)

This prescription consists of Liuwei Dihuang Tang and Schizandrae Fructus.

腎氣丸

六味地黃湯加五味子一味

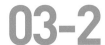

Nine Prescriptions for the Lesser Yang Person's Disease Mentioned in the Writings of Famous Doctors in the Yuan and Ming Dynasties

元明二代醫家著述中
少陽人病經驗行用要藥九方

1 Cool the Diaphragm Powder (Liangge San)

- Forsythiae Fructus 7.5g
- Rhei Radix et Rhizoma 3.75g
- Natrii Sulfas 3.75g
- Glycyrrhizae Radix et Rhizoma 3.75g
- Menthae Herba 1.875g
- Scutellariae Radix 1.875g
- Gardeniae Fructus 1.875g

The original source of this prescription is the 『*Jufang*』. It cures irritability, oral sores, conjunctival congestion, and dizziness due to congestion of heat in the chest. In accordance with recent studies, Rhei Radix et Rhizoma, Glycyrrhizae Radix et Rhizoma, and Scutellariae Radix must be excluded from this prescription.

凉膈散

連翹二錢大黃芒硝甘草各一錢薄荷黃芩梔子各五分

此方出於局方治積熱煩燥口舌生瘡目赤頭昏○今考更定此方當去大黃甘草黃芩

2 Coptis and Pig Stomach Pill (Huanglian Zhudu Wan)

- Male pig stomach 1 pc.
- Coptidis Rhizoma 187.5g
- Flour (stir-baked) 187.5g
- Trichosanthis Radix 150g
- Poria Sclerotium 150g
- Liriopis seu Ophiopogonis Tuber 75g

Pound the above drugs into a powder. Put the powder into a male pig stomach and stitch it up. Stew and pulverize, then make the pills as big as an empress tree seed. The original source of this prescription is the 『*Dexiaofang*』, compiled by Wei Yilin. This cures a prolonged erection of the penis with involuntary emission. In accordance with the results of recent studies, Liriopis seu Ophiopogonis Tuber is the medicinal ingredient for the Lung in this prescription. Normally, the Lung raises the vital energy, while the Kidney lowers it, though both organs are separate. With five medicinal ingredients aimed at the Kidney, it would seem that Liriopis seu Ophiopogonis Tuber is unnecessary for the Lung, but that is not so. On the contrary, one should appreciate its properties.

黃連猪肚丸

雄猪肚一箇黃連小麥炒各五兩天花粉白茯神各四兩麥門冬二兩

右爲末入猪肚中封口安甑中蒸爛搗作丸梧子大此方出於危亦林得效方書中治强中證〇今考更定此方中麥門冬一味肺藥也肺與腎一升一降上下貫通腎藥五味中肺藥一味雖爲贅材亦自無妨不必苟論

3 Six-Ingredient Decoction Containing Rehmannia (Liuwei Dihuang Tang)

· Rehmanniae Radix praeparata 15g   · Dioscoreae Rhizoma 7.5g
· Corni Fructus 3.75g   · Alismatis Rhizoma 5.625g
· Moutan Radicis Cortex 5.625g   · Poria Sclerotium (white) 5.625g

The original source of this prescription is the 『*Yixue Zhengzhuan*』[1] ("Orthodox Medical Record") compiled by Yu Tuan[2]. It cures consumption. In accordance with the results of recent studies, Dioscoreae Rhizoma in this prescription is the medicinal ingredient for the Lung.

六味地黃湯

熟地黃四錢山藥山茱萸各二錢澤瀉牧丹皮白茯苓各一錢五分

此方出於虞搏醫學正傳書中治虛勞〇今考更定此方中山藥一味肺藥也

4 Rehmannia and Cooked Rehmannia Pill (Shengshou Dihuang Wan)

· Rehmanniae Radix 37.5g   · Rehmanniae Radix praeparata 37.5g
· Scrophulariae Radix 37.5g   · Gypsum Fibrosum 37.5g

Make the pasted pills as big as an empress tree seed. Take 50~70 pills on an empty stomach with tea. The original source of this prescription is the 『*Yixue Rumen*』, compiled by Li Chan. It cures weak eyesight.

生熟地黃丸

生乾地黃熟地黃玄參石膏各一兩

糊丸梧子大空心茶淸下五七十丸此方出於李梴醫學入門書中治眼昏

5 Powder for Promoting Diuresis (Daochi San)

· Akebiae Caulis 3.75g   · Talcum 3.75g
· Phellodendri Cortex 3.75g   · Poria Sclerotium (red) 3.75g
· Rehmanniae Radix 3.75g   · Gardeniae Fructus 3.75g
· Glycyrrhizae Radix et Rhizoma 3.75g   · Aurantii Fructus 1.875g
· Atractylodis Rhizoma Alba 1.875g

The original source of this prescription is Gong Xin's 『*Wanbing Huichun*』 ("Recovery from All Ailments"). It treats urine color like rice water, and it is cured by taking it twice. In accordance with recent studies, Aurantii Fructus, Atractylodis Rhizoma Alba, and Glycyrrhizae

Radix et Rhizoma must be excluded from this prescription.

導赤散

木通滑石黃栢赤茯苓生地黃山梔子甘草梢各一錢枳殼白朮各五分

此方出於龔信萬病回春書中治尿如米泔色不過二服愈○今考更定此方當去枳殼白朮甘草

6 Schizonepeta and Saposhnikovia Powder for Toxin-Vanquishing (Jingfang Baidu San)

· Osterici Radix 3.75g   · Angelicae pubescentis Radix 3.75g

· Bupleuri Radix 3.75g   · Peucedani Radix 3.75g

· Poria Sclerotium (red) 3.75g   · Schizonepetae Herba 3.75g

· Saposhnikoviae Radix 3.75g   · Aurantii Fructus 3.75g

· Platycodi Radix 3.75g   · Chuanxiong Rhizoma 3.75g

· Ginseng Radix 3.75g   · Glycyrrhizae Radix et Rhizoma 3.75g

· Menthae Herba a small amount

The original source of this prescription is Gong Xin's 『*Yijian*』 ("Mirror of Medicine"). This cures an exogenous febrile disease and all seasonal epidemic disease; a fever, a rigidity of the nape with a headache and arthrodynia of the limbs. In accordance with the results of recent studies, Aurantii Fructus, Platycodi Radix, Chuanxiong Rhizoma, Ginseng Radix, and Glycyrrhizae Radix et Rhizoma have to be excluded from this prescription.

荊防敗毒散

羌活獨活柴胡前胡赤茯苓荊芥穗防風枳殼桔梗川芎人蔘甘草各一錢薄荷少許

此方出於龔信醫鑑書中治傷寒時氣發熱頭痛項强肢體煩疼○今考更定此方當去枳殼桔梗川芎人蔘甘草

7 Children's Weight-gaining Pills (Feier Wan)

· Picrorhizae Rhizoma 18.75g   · Quisqualis Fructus 16.875g

· Ginseng Radix 13.125g   · Coptidis Rhizoma 13.125g

· Crataegi Fructus 13.125g   · Massa Medicata Fermentata 13.125g

· Hordei Fructus Germiniatus 13.125g   · Poria Sclerotium (white) 11.25g

· Atractylodis Rhizoma Alba 11.25g

· Glycyrrhizae Radix et Rhizoma (stir-baked with adjuvant) 11.25g

· Aloe (calcined) 9.375g

Pound the above drugs into a powder and with glutinous millet paste and make the pills as big as mung beans. Take 20~30 pills with thin rice gruel. The original source of this prescription is Gong Xin's 『*Yijian*』 ("Mirror of Medicine"). This prescription is good for infantile malnutrition. In accordance with the results of recent studies, Ginseng Radix, Atractylodis Rhizoma Alba, Crataegi Fructus, and Glycyrrhizae Radix et Rhizoma have to be excluded from this prescription. About Quisqualis Fructus, since we lack experience concerning this drug, we are not clear on the medicine's properties. Thus, Quisqualis Fructus should not be spoken of lightly.

肥兒丸

胡黃連五錢使君子肉四錢五分人蔘黃連神麯麥芽山查肉各三錢五分白茯苓白朮灸甘草各三錢蘆薈煆二錢五分右爲末黃米糊和丸菉豆大米飲下二三十丸

此方出於龔信醫鑑書中治小兒疳積○今考更定此方當去人蔘白朮山查肉甘草而使君子一味未能經驗的知藥性故不敢輕論

8 Detoxicating Decoction (Xiaodu Yin)

· Arctii Fructus 7.5g   · Schizonepetae Herba 3.75g

· Glycyrrhizae Radix et Rhizoma (crude) 1.875g

· Saposhnikoviae Radix 1.875g

The original source of this prescription is the 『*Yijian*』, complied by Gong Xin. This cures pea-like skin sores which are not very pronounced and appear mainly and densely on the chest. Quickly give this decoction three or four times; some results are remarkable. In accordance with the results of recent studies, Glycyrrhizae Radix et Rhizoma has to be excluded from this prescription.

消毒飲

牛蒡子二錢荊芥穗一錢生甘草防風各五分

此方出於龔信醫鑑書中治痘不快出及胸前稠密急用三四服快透解毒神效○今考更定此方當去甘草

9 Mercury-fumigating Method (Shuiyin Xunbi Fang)

· Graphite 3.75g   · Calomelas 3.75g

· Cinnabaris 3.75g   · Olibanum 1.875g

· Myrrha 1.875g   · Sanguis Draconis 1.125g

· Realgar 1.125g   · Lignum Aquilariae Resinatum 1.125g

Pound equal amounts of the drugs into a powder. Roll up into seven cigarette-like shapes. Make seven of them. Place lamp burning scented oil on the table. The patient should lie in his bed with his whole body under a coverlet with his legs stretched. The patient has to hold cold water in his mouth and change it frequently in order to prevent damage to his mouth. Fumigate three times the first day and once a day from then on. The original source of this prescription is Zhu Zhenheng's 『*Danxi Xinfa*』. It is a miraculous cure against syphilitic skin lesions.

水銀熏鼻方

黑鉛水銀各一錢朱砂乳香沒藥各五分血竭雄黃沈香各三分

右爲末和匀捲作紙燃七條用香油點燈放床上令病人放兩脚包住上用單被通身盖之口嗛凉水頻換則不損口初日用三條後日每用一條熏鼻此方出於朱震亨丹溪心法書中治楊梅天疱瘡甚奇

I have said that Calomelas has the effect of eliminating accumulated heat, refreshing the mind and vision, restraining the yang qi, and leading the yin qi back to the lower-*jiao*. This is the best among the drugs for a lesser yang person needing to restrain yin and reinforce yang.

This method can be used only once as an emergency measure. It cannot be used continuously to reinforce yin. To use a metaphor, one must attack the first time where the enemy dwells with the power to root out a high mountain or the strength to carry a cauldron on one's shoulder. A second attack, however, in which the enemy has already been scattered, can lead to an attack on friendly forces. One must use this prescription for patients who have diphtheria.

論曰水銀破積熱淸頭目制陽回陰於下焦爲少陽人抑陽扶陰藥中無敵之藥而祇可用之於當日救急之用不可用之於連日補陰之用者以其拔山扛鼎之力一舉而直搗大敵之巢穴再舉則敵已解散反有倒戈之患故也纏喉風必用之藥

A lesser yang person with monoplegia or hemiplegia of the lower limbs has to take 0.1875g or 0.375g of Calomelas powder for three days. Irrespective of the consequences, this cannot be used over three days in amounts exceeding 0.1875g or 0.375g a day. The patient must avoid cold air and take other precautions. The patient with monoplegia of the upper limbs, hemiplegia and facial paralysis must not take this medicine; if he does, he will die.

少陽人一脚不遂兩脚不遂者輕粉末五里或一分連三日服無論病之瘥不瘥必不過三日服必不過日服五里或一分謹風冷愼禁忌一臂不遂半身不遂口眼喎斜不可用用之必危

An acute disease must be tackled immediately, but a chronic one need not be. Calomelas is so dangerous that we should not use it to cure a disease immediately. A chronic disease is only cured gradually; if it is cured quickly, the patient will most assuredly suffer a relapse from which recovery is difficult. There is the patient who has to take this medicine for three days and the patient who has to take it at one, two or three day intervals, for three cycles continuously.

急病可以急治緩病不可以急治輕粉刮藥不可銳意用之以望速效緩病緩愈然後可謂眞愈緩病速效則終必更病難治有連三日用之者有間一二三日服連三次用之者

I have treated lesser yang person who have had diseases of the throat, eyes and nose, and arthralgia of the lower limbs. I gave them mercury for three or four days, either through fumigation or orally; all recovered. They were not allowed to expose themselves to cold air or chilly weather for at least one month afterwards, not even to wash their faces, change their clothes or comb their hair. Violating these prohibitions might have meant death. Remind the patient not to stay in a chilly room, or he will die. Nor let him stay in a warm room; if he cannot endure the fever with dysphoria, he might open the window, expose himself to cold air, and die.

I have witnessed a patient die in ten days after initial recovery because he had changed into new clothes; another died twenty days after initial recovery as a result of combing his hair. Another who had a disease of the throat died one night suddenly in a warm room because he had been exposed to the cold wind after fumigation of the nose two times on the first day and one time on the second. It is said that it is forbidden to give soybean sauce to a patient taking mercury, because soybean sauce made from fermented soybeans can neutralize the poison of the mercury. However, since it is acceptable to detoxify the poison a little, it is not necessary to ban soybean sauce.

嘗見少陽人咽喉病眼鼻病脚痺病用水銀連三四日或熏鼻或內服病愈者病愈後一月之內必不可內處冷外觸風尤不可任意洗手洗面更着新衣梳頭也犯此禁者必死又不可冷室冷室則觸冷而猝死又不可燠室燠室煩熱開牖觸風而亦猝死此皆目擊者也一人病愈十餘日更着新衣而猝死一人病愈二十日後梳頭而猝死一人咽喉病熏鼻初日二條翌日一條當夜燠室觸風而猝死時俗服水銀者忌鹽醬者以醬中有豆豉能解水銀毒故也然毒藥解毒容或無妨則不必苛忌鹽醬

Notes

1) 『*Yixue Zhengzhuan*』(醫學正傳)

The "Orthodox Medical Record" (1515), a comprehensive medical work by Yu Tuan (虞搏) in eight volumes. With reference to many schools' theories, he stated his own experiences in medicine. He criticized the method of using incantation and *yunqi* (運氣: the theory of five circuits and six qi) in estimating the pathological period, symptoms and treatment.

2) Yu Tuan (虞搏)

Yu Tuan (1438~1517) is also called Yu Tianmin (虞天民). He collected over thirty important medical works and edited his own 『*Yixue Zhengzhuan*』.

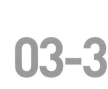

Seventeen Newly Formulated Prescriptions for the Lesser Yang Person's Disease

新定少陽人病應用要藥十七方

1 Schizonepeta and Saposhnikovia Powder for Toxin-Vanquishing (Hyeongbang Paidok San)

· Osterici Radix 3.75g
· Angelicae pubescentis Radix 3.75g
· Bupleuri Radix 3.75g
· Peucedani Radix 3.75g
· Schizonepetae Herba 3.75g
· Saposhnikoviae Radix 3.75g
· Poria Sclerotium (red) 3.75g
· Rehmanniae Radix 3.75g
· Lycii Radicis Cortex 3.75g
· Plantaginis Semen 3.75g

This prescription is for patients experiencing headaches and alternate attacks of chills and fever.

荊防敗毒散
羌活獨活柴胡前胡荊芥防風赤茯苓生地黃地骨皮車前子各一錢
右方治頭痛寒熱往來者宜用

2 Schizonepeta and Saposhnikovia Powder for Treating Dark Urine (Hyeongbang Dojeok San)

· Rehmanniae Radix 11.25g
· Akebiae Caulis 7.5g
· Scrophulariae Radix 5.625g
· Trichosanthis Semen 5.625g
· Peucedani Radix 3.75g
· Osterici Radix 3.75g
· Angelicae pubescentis Radix 3.75g
· Schizonepetae Herba 3.75g
· Saposhnikoviae Radix 3.75g

This prescription is for patients experiencing headaches and fever with dysphoria in the chest.

荊防導赤散
生地黃三錢木通二錢玄參瓜蔞仁各一錢五分前胡羌活獨活荊芥防風各一錢
右方治頭痛胸膈煩熱者宜用

3 Schizonepeta and Saposhnikovia Powder for Expelling Lung-heat (Hyeongbang Sabaik San)

· Rehmanniae Radix 11.25g   · Poria Sclerotium 7.5g

· Alismatis Rhizoma 7.5g   · Gypsum Fibrosum 3.75g

· Anemarrhenae Rhizoma 3.75g   · Osterici Radix 3.75g

· Angelicae pubescentis Radix 3.75g   · Schizonepetae Herba 3.75g

· Saposhnikoviae Radix 3.75g

This prescription is for patients experiencing headaches and irritation of the bladder.

荊防瀉白散

生地黃三錢茯苓澤瀉各二錢石膏知母羌活獨活荊芥防風各一錢

右方治頭痛膀胱㿉躁者宜用

4 Polyporus and Plantain Seed Decoction (Jeoryeong Chajeonja Tang)

· Alismatis Rhizoma 7.5g   · Poria Sclerotium 7.5g

· Polyporus 5.625g   · Plantaginis Semen 5.625g

· Anemarrhenae Rhizoma 3.75g   · Gypsum Fibrosum 3.75g

· Osterici Radix 3.75g   · Angelicae pubescentis Radix 3.75g

· Schizonepetae Herba 3.75g   · Saposhnikoviae Radix 3.75g

This prescription is for patients experiencing headaches with abdominal pain and diarrhea.

猪苓車前子湯

澤瀉茯苓各二錢猪苓車前子各一錢五分知母石膏羌活獨活荊芥防風各一錢

右方治頭腹痛有泄瀉者宜用

5 Talcum and Sophora Decoction (Hwalseok Gosam Tang)

· Alismatis Rhizoma 7.5g   · Poria Sclerotium 7.5g

· Talcum 7.5g   · Sophorae Radix 7.5g

· Coptidis Rhizoma 3.75g   · Phellodendri Cortex 3.75g

· Osterici Radix 3.75g   · Angelicae pubescentis Radix 3.75g

· Schizonepetae Herba 3.75g   · Saposhnikoviae Radix 3.75g

This prescription is for patients experiencing abdominal pain without diarrhea.

滑石苦蔘湯

澤瀉茯苓滑石苦蔘各二錢川黃連黃栢羌活獨活荊芥防風各一錢

右方治腹痛無泄瀉者宜用

6 Pubescent Angelica and Rehmannia Decoction (Dokhwal Jihwang Tang)

· Rehmanniae Radix praeparata 15g   · Corni Fructus 7.5g

· Poria Sclerotium 5.625g   · Alismatis Rhizoma 5.625g

· Moutan Radicis Cortex 3.75g   · Saposhnikoviae Radix 3.75g

· Angelicae pubescentis Radix 3.75g

This prescription is for patients experiencing indigestion and a feeling of fullness in the epigastrium.

獨活地黃湯

熟地黃四錢山茱萸二錢茯苓澤瀉各一錢五分牧丹皮防風獨活各一錢

右方治食滯痞滿者宜用

7　Schizonepeta, Saposhnikovia, and Rehmannia Decoction (Hyeongbang Jihwang Tang)

· Rehmanniae Radix praeparata 7.5g　　· Corni Fructus 7.5g

· Poria Sclerotium 7.5g　　· Alismatis Rhizoma 7.5g

· Plantaginis Semen 3.75g　　· Osterici Radix 3.75g

· Angelicae pubescentis Radix 3.75g　　· Schizonepetae Herba 3.75g

· Saposhnikoviae Radix 3.75g

For coughing, add Peucedani Radix. For blood problems, add Scrophulariae Radix and Moutan Radicis Cortex. For migraine, add Coptidis Rhizoma and Arctii Fructus. For indigestion and a feeling of fullness in the epigastrium, add Moutan Radicis Cortex. For internal fire, add Gypsum Fibrosum. For headaches, dysphoria with fever and blood problems, use Rehmanniae Radix instead of Rehmanniae Radix praeparata, add Gypsum Fibrosum and remove Corni Fructus. Schizonepetae Herba, Saposhnikoviae Radix, Osterici Radix, and Angelicae pubescentis Radix are all drugs tonifying and nourishing yin. Schizonepetae Herba and Saposhnikoviae Radix are very effective in clearing away heat from the chest and dispelling the wind. Osterici Radix and Angelicae pubescentis Radix have the effect of greatly tonifying the genuine yin of the bladder. Whether he suffers from a headache, abdominal pain, a feeling of fullness in the epigastrium, or diarrhea, it is my experience that a weak patient taking hundreds of packs of this medicine will recover; it is very effective medicine.

荊防地黃湯

熟地黃山茱萸茯苓澤瀉各二錢車前子羌活獨活荊芥防風各一錢

咳嗽加前胡血證加玄參牧丹皮偏頭痛加黃連牛蒡子食滯痞滿者加牧丹皮有火者加石膏頭痛煩熱
與血證者用生地黃加石膏者去山茱萸○荊芥防風羌活獨活俱是補陰藥荊防大淸胸膈散風羌獨大
補膀胱眞陰無論頭腹痛痞滿泄瀉凡虛弱者數百貼用之無不必效屢試屢驗

8　Decoction of Twelve Drugs Containing Rehmannia (Sibimi Jihwang Tang)

· Rehmanniae Radix praeparata 15g　　· Corni Fructus 7.5g

· Poria Sclerotium (white) 5.625g　　· Alismatis Rhizoma 5.625g

· Moutan Radicis Cortex 3.75g　　· Lycii Radicis Cortex 3.75g

· Scrophulariae Radix 3.75g　　· Lycii Fructus 3.75g

· Rubi Fructus 7.5g　　· Plantaginis Semen 3.75g

· Schizonepetae Herba 3.75g　　· Saposhnikoviae Radix 3.75g

十二味地黃湯

熟地黃四錢山茱萸二錢白茯苓澤瀉各一錢五分牧丹皮地骨皮玄蔘枸杞子覆盆子車前子荊芥防風
各一錢

9 White Tiger Decoction with Rehmannia (Jihwang Baikho Tang)
- · Gypsum Fibrosum 18.75-37.5g
- · Rehmanniae Radix 15g
- · Anemarrhenae Rhizoma 7.5g
- · Saposhnikoviae Radix 3.75g
- · Angelicae pubescentis Radix 3.75g

地黃白虎湯

石膏五錢或一兩生地黃四錢知母二錢防風獨活各一錢

10 White Tiger Decoction for Yang Type Inflammatory Swelling (Yangdok Baikho Tang)
- · Gypsum Fibrosum 18.75-37.5g
- · Rehmanniae Radix 15g
- · Anemarrhenae Rhizoma 7.5g
- · Schizonepetae Herba 3.75g
- · Saposhnikoviae Radix 3.75g
- · Arctii Fructus 3.75g

This prescription is for patients with macule caused by yang type inflammatory swelling and constipation.

陽毒白虎湯

石膏五錢或一兩生地黃四錢知母二錢荊芥防風牛蒡子各一錢

右方治陽毒發斑便秘者宜用

11 Decoction for Cooling the Diaphragm and Dispersing Fire (Yanggyeok Sanhwa Tang)
- · Rehmanniae Radix 7.5g
- · Lonicerae Caulis 7.5g
- · Forsythiae Fructus 7.5g
- · Gardeniae Fructus 3.75g
- · Menthae Herba 3.75g
- · Anemarrhenae Rhizoma 3.75g
- · Gypsum Fibrosum 3.75g
- · Saposhnikoviae Radix 3.75g
- · Schizonepetae Herba 3.75g

This prescription is for patients suffering from diabetes involving the upper-*jiao*.

凉膈散火湯

生地黃忍冬藤連翹各二錢山梔子薄荷知母石膏防風荊芥各一錢

右方治上消者宜用

12 Honeysuckle Stem and Lycium Root Bark Decoction (Indongdeung Jigolpi Tang)
- · Lonicerae Caulis 15g
- · Corni Fructus 7.5g
- · Lycii Radicis Cortex 7.5g
- · Coptidis Rhizoma 3.75g
- · Phellodendri Cortex 3.75g
- · Scrophulariae Radix 3.75g
- · Sophorae Radix 3.75g
- · Rehmanniae Radix 3.75g
- · Anemarrhenae Rhizoma 3.75g
- · Gardeniae Fructus 3.75g
- · Lycii Fructus 3.75g
- · Rubi Fructus 3.75g

· Schizonepetae Herba 3.75g   · Saposhnikoviae Radix 3.75g

· Lonicerae Flos 3.75g

This prescription is for patients suffering from diabetes involving the middle-*jiao*.

忍冬藤地骨皮湯

忍冬藤四錢山茱萸地骨皮各二錢川黃連黃栢玄蔘苦蔘生地黃知母山梔子枸杞子覆盆子荊芥防風
金銀花各一錢

右方治中消者宜用

13 Cooked Rehmannia and Sophora Decoction (Sukjihwang Gosam Tang)

· Rehmanniae Radix praeparata 15g

· Corni Fructus 7.5g   · Poria Sclerotium (white) 5.625g

· Alismatis Rhizoma 5.625g   · Anemarrhenae Rhizoma 3.75g

· Phellodendri Cortex 3.75g   · Sophorae Radix 3.75g

This prescription is for patients suffering from diabetes involving the lower-*jiao*.

熟地黃苦蔘湯

熟地黃四錢山茱萸二錢白茯苓澤瀉各一錢五分知母黃栢苦蔘各一錢

右方治下消者宜用

14 Decoction for Greatly Stabilizing with Trifoliate Akebia (Moktong Daian Tang)

· Akebiae Caulis 18.75g   · Rehmanniae Radix 18.75g

· Poria Sclerotium (red) 7.5g   · Alismatis Rhizoma 3.75g

· Plantaginis Semen 3.75g   · Coptidis Rhizoma 3.75g

· Osterici Radix 3.75g   · Saposhnikoviae Radix 3.75g

· Schizonepetae Herba 3.75g

This prescription is for patients suffering from edema. Edema is hard to cure in a lesser yang person. From beginning to end of the treatment, a lesser yang person must take one hundred or more packs. Coptidis Rhizoma and Alismatis Rhizoma are expensive; the poor cannot afford them.

木通大安湯

木通生地黃各五錢赤茯苓二錢澤瀉車前子川黃連羌活防風荊芥各一錢

右方治浮腫者宜用險病始終用藥當至百餘貼黃連澤瀉爲貴材則貧者或去連澤

15 Coptis Decoction for Clearing Intestine (Hwanglyeon Cheongjang Tang)

· Rehmanniae Radix 15g   · Akebiae Caulis 7.5g

· Poria Sclerotium 7.5g   · Alismatis Rhizoma 7.5g

· Polyporus 3.75g   · Plantaginis Semen 3.75g

· Coptidis Rhizoma 3.75g   · Osterici Radix 3.75g

· Saposhnikoviae Radix 3.75g

This prescription is for patients suffering from dysentery. If gonorrhea is observed, exclude

7.5g of Akebiae Caulis and add 3.75g of Schizonepetae Herba.

黃連清腸湯

生地黃四錢木通茯苓澤瀉各二錢猪苓車前子川黃連羌活防風各一錢

右方治痢疾者宜用去木通二錢加荊芥一錢淋疾者宜用

16 Powder Beneficial to Vitality with Cinnabar (Jusa Igwon San)

- Talcum 7.5g   · Alismatis Rhizoma 3.75g
- Euphorbia Kansui Radix 1.875g   · Cinnabaris 0.375g

Pound the drugs into powder and let the patient take it with warm water or with water drawn from the well at daybreak. This can be used also to dispel summer heat.

朱砂益元散

滑石二錢澤瀉一錢甘遂五分朱砂一分

右爲末溫水或井華水調服夏月滌暑宜用

17 Tianyi Pills with Kansui (Gamsu Cheonil Hwan)

- Euphorbia Kansui Radix 3.75g   · Calomelas 0.375g

Make ten pills with a flour paste and coat them with Cinnabaris. If the pills are old and dried out, they will become hard and difficult to swallow. If this happens, wrap the pills in two or three layers of paper and pulverize them. Let the patient take them with water drawn from the well at daybreak. After three or four hours, if the patient does not have diarrhea, give two more pills. Diarrhea three to four times is desirable, but diarrhea five or six times is undesirable. To prevent the latter, prepare a thin gruel, and after two or three bouts of diarrhea, serve the gruel to the patient. If the preparation is not given, the patient will experience qi exhaustion and will not survive. In order to cure an accumulation of pathogen in the chest and immediate vomiting after drinking water, make ten pills from 3.75g of Euphorbia Kansui Radix and 2.0g of Calomelas. It is called Gyeongbun Gamsu Yongho Dan (Jingfen Gansui Longhu Dan). Make ten pills from Calomelas and Euphorbia Kansui Radix in equal amounts; this is called Gyeongbun Gamsu Jawung Dan (Jingfen Gansui Cixiong Dan). Make thirty pills from 3.75g of Calomelas, Olibanum, Myrrha, and Euphorbia Kansui Radix, 1.875g each; this is called Yuhyang Molyak Gyeongbun Hwan (Ruxiang Moyao Jingfen Wan). Calomelas causes perspiration, and Euphorbia Kansui Radix purges water. To obtain desirable results, use 0.375g of Calomelas - even 0.1875g is of use. Exactly 0.5625g of Euphorbia Kansui Radix is efficient, but 0.2625g or 0.30g is not. Calomelas and Euphorbia Kansui Radix are both drugs containing poison, so one should never use either in excess of 0.375g; the seriousness of the illness one is treating will determine exactly what amount is needed. If one wishes to dispel fire in the head, let Calomelas be the principle ingredient; for eliminating water in the chest, make Euphorbia Kansui Radix the principle ingredient. The above drugs prescribed for the lesser yang person should not be stir-baked, stir-baked at high temperature, stir-baked with adjuvant, or roasted in hot ashes.

甘遂天一丸

甘遂末一錢輕粉末一分和勻糊丸分作十丸朱砂爲衣

作丸乾久則堅硬難和每用時以紙二三疊包裹以杵搗碎作屬末三四五片口含末因飲井華水和下候三四辰刻內不下利則再用二丸下利三度爲適中六度爲快過預煎米飲下利二三度因進米飲否則氣陷而難堪耐治結胸水入還吐〇甘遂一錢輕粉五分分作十丸則名曰輕粉甘遂龍虎丹輕粉甘遂各等分作十丸則名曰輕粉甘遂雌雄丹輕粉一錢乳香沒藥甘遂各五分分作三十丸則名曰乳香沒藥輕粉丸輕粉發汗甘遂下水輕粉藥力一分則快足五里則無不及甘遂藥力一分五里則快足七八里則無不及輕粉甘遂自是毒藥俱不可輕易過一分用之斟酌輕重病欲頭腦滌火則輕粉爲君病欲胸膈下水則甘遂爲君右少陽人藥諸種不可炮灸炒煨用

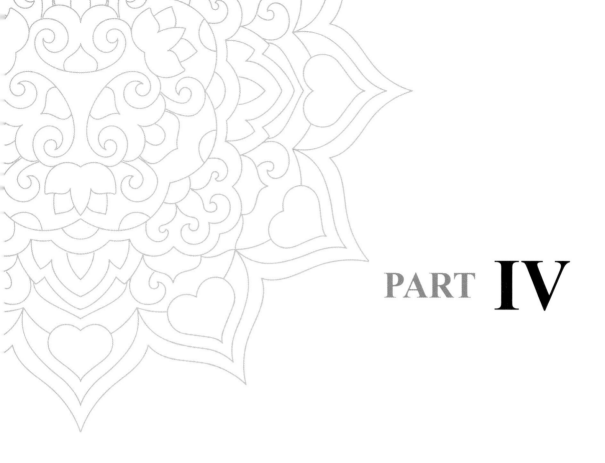

PART IV

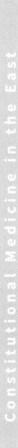

Discourse on the Taieum (Greater Yin) Person's Exterior Cold Disease Induced from the Epigastrium Affected by Cold

太陰人胃脘受寒表寒病論

1 Zhang Zhongjing said, "Mahuang Tang (Ephedra Decoction) suits a patient having the greater yang disease caused by cold with headache and fever, aching of the body and lumbago, arthralgia, chills, no perspiration, and cough." This comment noted that the symptoms of febrile disease caused by cold, such as headaches and aches in the body, lower back and joints, were later called the greater yang disease caused by cold. These symptoms are all caused by bad circulation of the *ying* (nutrient) blood.

張仲景曰太陽傷寒頭痛發熱身疼腰痛骨節皆痛惡寒無汗而喘麻黃湯主之○註曰傷寒頭痛身疼腰痛以至牽連百骨節俱痛者此太陽傷寒榮血不利故也

2 I have said, "The above disease is a mild case of the upper back exterior disease caused by cold in a greater yin person, and can be cured by Mahuang Tang. Among decoctions, Cinnamomi Ramulus and Glycyrrhizae Radix et Rhizoma are not necessary; however, Mahwang Balpyo Tang (Ephedra Decoction for Diaphoresis) is suitable for this."

論曰此卽太陰人傷寒背伴頁表病輕證也此證麻黃湯非不當用而桂枝甘草皆爲蠹材此證當用麻黃發表湯

3 Zhang Zhongjing said, "As for the febrile disease caused by cold, on the fourth or fifth day: If *jue* (coldness) is observed, first there must have been a fever. Extreme coldness will lead to a high fever. When coldness is slight, the fever will also be slight. For the febrile disease caused by cold, coldness lasts for four days, followed by fever for three days. After that, coldness again prevails for five days. More chills than fever would indicate an aggravation of the pattern. For the febrile disease caused by cold, coldness lasts for three days after the prevalence

of a four day fever. The symptom of more fever than chills foretells recovery."

張仲景曰傷寒四五日而厥者必發熱厥深者熱亦深厥微者熱亦微傷寒厥四日熱反三日復厥五日厥
多熱少其病爲進傷寒發熱四日厥反三日厥少熱多其病當自愈

4   I have said, "The above mentioned coldness means the sensation of chills without fever, but it does not mean cold limbs. Fever after coldness for four to five days indicates a severe condition in the greater yin person's exterior pattern caused by cold. In this pattern, he has fever and sweating which starts from the hairline to the forehead. The fever recurs, and there is sweat on the eyebrows after several days. The fever recurs once again, and there is sweat on the cheeks for the next several days. The fever recurs once more, and there is sweat on the lips and jaw for the next several days, before another recurrence of fever, where there is sweat on the chest for several more days. As mentioned above, to the eyebrows there are several bouts of sweating on the forehead, to the cheeks there are several bouts of sweating on the eyebrows, to the lip and jaw there are several bouts of sweating on the cheeks, and directly to the chest just after one bout of sweating on the lips and jaw. This disease, which takes about twenty days of six or seven repeated sensations of coldness and then is relieved, is called long-term infectious disease. Generally, the greater yin person's disease, in which sweating begins on the forehead and eyebrows, and is not relieved until after several bouts of sweating, is a long-term infectious disease."

論曰此謂之厥者但惡寒不發熱之謂也非手足厥逆之謂也太陰人傷寒表證寒厥四五日後發熱者重
證也此證發熱其汗必自髮際而始通於額上又數日後發熱而眉稜通汗又數日後發熱而顴上通汗又
數日後發熱而脣頤通汗又數日後發熱而胸臆通汗也而額上之汗數次而後達於眉稜眉稜之汗數次
而後達於顴上顴上之汗數次而後達於脣頤脣頤之汗不過一次而直達於胸臆矣此證首尾幾近二十
日凡寒厥六七次而後病解也此證俗謂之長感病凡太陰人病先額上眉稜有汗而一汗病不解屢汗病
解者名曰長感病

5   The greater yin person who has coldness for six or seven days without fever and perspiration will die. If he has coldness for two or three days with fever and perspiration, the illness will be a mild case. However, if he had coldness for four or five days with fever and little perspiration on his forehead, the illness is called the long-term infectious disease and is a serious case. This disease is caused by the exertion of the mind, which induces the Stomach duct to become asthenic, and the exterior of body cannot resist the cold and is surrounded by the cold. The situation is a battle between healthy qi and the pathogen. It is just like an army not being able to fight its way out of a battle, with but one company breaking through the besieging enemy forces with the main army still behind. After several battles, if the army manages to break through, it is like a dignified figure. If there is perspiration on the forehead, the situation is just like a company breaking through the besieging army forces; if the perspiration is on the eyebrows, it is just like a few companies breaking through valiantly; if on the cheeks, it is like half the army breaking through slowly. The perspiration on the eyebrows means the

illness will be relieved, and the perspiration on the cheeks means there is no more danger.

太陰人病寒厥六七日而不發熱不汗出則死也寒厥二三日而發熱汗出則輕證也寒厥四五日而發熱
得微汗於額上者此之謂長感病其病爲重證也此證原委勞心焦思之餘胃脘衰弱而表局虛薄不勝寒
而外被寒邪所圍正邪相爭之形勢客勝主弱譬如一團孤軍困在垓心幾於全軍覆沒之境先鋒一隊倖
而跳出決圍一面僅得開路後軍全隊尚在垓心將又屢次力戰然後方爲出來則爻象正是凜凜之勢也
額上通汗者即先鋒一隊決圍跳出之象也眉稜通汗者即前軍全隊決圍全面氣勢勇敢之象也顴上通
汗者中軍半隊緩緩出圍之象也此病汗出眉稜則快免危也汗出顴上則必無危也

6 The greater yin person must have millet-like sweating on the forehead, eyebrows and cheeks, and will have a somewhat extended fever before the perspiration stops. This means that the healthy qi is strong and the pathogen is weak. Sweating becomes refreshing for the patient when he perspires little, with tiny drops or none at all. If, shortly after the perspiration stops, the healthy qi is still weak and the pathogen strong, there is no refreshing feeling for the patient.

太陰人汗無論額上眉稜上顴上汗出如黍粒發熱稍久而還入者正强邪弱快汗也汗出如微粒或淋漓
無粒乍時而還入者正弱邪强非快汗也

7 If a greater yin person perspires over the upper back, below the hairline, and does not perspire on the face below the hairline, it is a bad sign. If he sweats over the face, but not around the ears, it is a sign of oncoming death. Generally, if a greater yin person perspires from the postero-auricular area and the hairline of the face to the sternal area, the disease will be relieved; if he has perspiration on the hairline, he will be saved from death; if over the forehead, he will barely escape with his life; if over the eyebrows, he will have just been saved; if over the cheeks, he will be out of danger; if over the lips and jaw, his disease has already been relieved; if over the chest, the disease has been completely relieved. I once observed the following symptoms: when perspiration starts from the forehead to the eyebrows, coldness is not so severe; when perspiration is present from the cheeks to the lips and jaw, coldness is so severe that the patient has chills and a quivering jaw like the wind stirring, and the perspiration directly spreads to both sub-axillary areas. It is the same as Zhang Zhongjing's notion that "Extreme coldness will lead to an extreme fever. When coldness is slight, the fever also will be slight." If coldness persists several days in addition to these symptoms, it indicates that the disease is serious. If only coldness is severe, the disease may be termed as not very serious.

太陰人背部後面自腦以下有汗而面部髮際以下不汗者匈證也全面皆有汗而耳門左右不汗者死證
也大凡太陰人汗始自耳後高骨面部髮際大通於胸臆間而病解也髮際之汗始免死也額上之汗僅免
危也眉稜之汗快免危也顴上之汗生路寬闊也脣頤之汗病已解也胸臆之汗病大解也嘗見此證額上
汗欲作眉稜汗者寒厥之勢不甚猛也顴上汗欲作脣頤汗者寒厥之勢甚猛至於寒戰叩齒完若動風而
其汗直達兩腋張仲景所云厥深者熱亦深厥微者熱亦微盖謂此也此證寒厥之勢多日者病重之勢也
寒厥之勢猛峻者非病重之勢也

8 The Gyeonggi Province people called the above disease the long-term infectious disease, while the Hamgyeong Province people called it forty day pain or sweatless dry disease. Jingfang Baidu San, Huoxiang Zhengqi San or Buzhong Yiqi Tang was commonly used for this disease, but most of them were inappropriate prescriptions. Only the adoption of Ursi Fel proved fortunate, like a blind man entering the correct door. If, however, the patient was treated by any other prescriptions again, his condition will worsen. There was a saying, "Disease does not kill the patient, and drugs do." Who cannot believe this saying? It is not easy for ordinary doctors to understand the degree of this disease, which is rather difficult to correctly diagnose. If a patient with the above disease has sweating on the eyebrows and cheeks, the disease becomes relieved naturally without administration. Even though the doctor may have given the patient the wrong drugs, there is no sweating on the cheeks, only on the forehead, and coldness as an exterior pattern is relieved a little. The doctor then regards these drugs as effective, as does the patient, and the drugs become prescription. As a result, the perspiration on the patient's forehead will stop, and he will die. In this disease, we have to judge the degree only according to his perspiration, not according to the degree of coldness. Zhang Zhongjing's notion that "the disease will be relieved naturally" is in actuality a cautious approach, not a false one. However, if the long-term infectious disease has no epidemic pathogens, we can expect that disease will go away on its own. If, however, the epidemic febrile disease has severe epidemic pathogens and the disease is identified, and the prescription evident, it is wrong to wait for the disease to go away on its own, because we are worried that strange symptoms might appear.

此證京畿道人謂之長感病咸鏡道人謂之四十日痛或謂之無汗乾病時俗所用荊防敗毒散藿香正氣散補中益氣湯箇箇誤治惟熊膽雖或盲人直門然又連用他藥病勢更變古人所云病不能殺人藥能殺人者不亦信乎百病加減之勢以凡眼目觀之固難推測而此證又有甚焉此證之汗在眉稜顴上時雖不服藥亦自愈矣而病人招醫妄投誤藥則顴上之汗還爲額上之汗而外證寒厥之勢則稍減矣於是焉醫師自以爲信藥效病人亦自以爲得藥效又數日誤藥則額上之汗又不通而死矣此證當以汗之進退占病之輕重不可以寒之寬猛占病之輕重張仲景曰其病當自愈云者豈非珍重無妄之論乎然長感病無疫氣者待其自愈則好也而瘟病疫氣重者若明知證藥無疑則不可尋常置之待其勿藥自愈恐生奇證

10 I once treated the epidemic febrile disease of the greater yin person who had the cold pattern in the epigastrium. This greater yin person had palpitations, but no perspiration, shortness of breath, a tight cough, and, additionally, sudden diarrhea which continued for dozens of days. This indicates a severe case of the exterior disease. Taieum Jowi Tang (Decoction for Harmonizing the Greater Yin Person's Stomach), with 3.75g of Ailanthi Radicis Cortex, was adopted, and the patient took two packs of the prescription every day. The diarrhea stopped after ten days; one month later, he began to sweat on the face every day, and his previous symptoms were relieved. Since several of his relatives suddenly contracted the epidemic febrile disease, he took care of them and stopped taking drugs for several days. He contracted the epidemic febrile disease anew, lost his appetite, and did not eat anything. He took

Taieum Jowi Tang with Cimicifugae Rhizoma and Scutellariae Radix added, 3.75g each, for ten days, then began to sweat on the face. The epidemic symptoms were slightly relieved, but still he had constipation for two days. Therefore, he took Galgeun Seunggi Tang (Kudzu Decoction for Purgation) for five days; within five days, he was able to eat double the amount of thin rice gruel. Most of the epidemic symptoms disappeared, and his disease was cured. He had continuously taken Taieum Jowi Tang, adding Cimicifugae Rhizoma and Scutellariae Radix for forty days; his epidemic symptoms almost completely disappeared, and his previous symptoms were cured, as well.

嘗治太陰人胃脘寒證瘟病有一太陰人素有怔忡無汗氣短結咳矣忽焉又添出一證泄瀉數十日不止即表病之重者也用太陰調胃湯加樗根皮一錢日再服十日泄瀉方止連用三十日每日流汗滿面素證亦減而忽其家五六人一時瘟疫此人緣於救病數日不服藥矣此人又染瘟病瘟證粥食無味全不入口仍以太陰調胃湯加升麻黃芩各一錢連用十日汗流滿面疫氣少減而有二日大便不通之證仍用葛根承氣湯五日而五日內粥食大倍疫氣大減而病解又用太陰調胃湯加升麻黃芩四十日調理疫氣旣減素病亦完

9 I have said, "In the greater yin person's disease, if coldness causes no perspiration for four days, it indicates a serious condition; if coldness causes no perspiration for five days, the patient is in danger of dying. Ursi Fel powder should be adopted, or Handa Yeolso Tang (Decoction for Treating More Cold than Fever) with five to nine larvae of cicadae (Holotrichia diomphalia Bates) should be taken. If his stool is loose, dried Castaneae Semen and Coicis Semen should be adopted; if his stool is dry, Puerariae Radix and Rhei Radix et Rhizoma should be adopted. In case there is perspiration over the forehead and eyebrows, we should wait until the disease is relieved, and then treat the patient with medication; otherwise, a relapse is possible."

論曰太陰人病寒厥四日而無汗者重證也寒厥五日而無汗者險證也當用熊膽散或寒多熱少湯加蠐螬五七九介大便滑者必用乾栗薏苡仁等屬大便燥者必用葛根大黃等屬若額上眉稜上有汗則待其自愈而病解後用藥調理否則恐生後病

11 A person has "tight cough" whenever he forces himself to cough, but still has difficulty ridding his throat of phlegm. The tight cough of the lesser yin person is called the tight cough associated with the chest, and the tight cough of the greater yin is the tight cough associated with the jaws.

結咳者勉强發咳痰欲出不出而或出曰結咳少陰人結咳謂之胸結咳太陰人結咳謂之頷結咳

12 Generally, we can identify the exterior-interior and deficiency-excess patterns of the patient who has the epidemic febrile disease through examining his previous diseases. A patient, who has suffered primarily from the cold disease, though he contracted the epidemic febrile disease at a later date, will develop cold symptoms. One, who has suffered primarily from the febrile disease, though he contracted the epidemic febrile disease at a later date, will develop fe-

brile patterns. One whose disease had been primarily mild, and who at a later date contracted an epidemic febrile disease, will see his condition grow serious. One whose disease had been primarily serious, and who at a later date contracted an epidemic febrile disease, will see his condition grow critical.

大凡瘟疫先察其人素病如何則表裏虛實可知已素病寒者得瘟病則亦寒證也素病熱者得瘟病則亦熱證也素病輕者得瘟病則重證也素病重者得瘟病則險證也

13 There was a greater yin patient who had a dry throat, and a bluish whitish face, cold body and occasional diarrhea. His dry throat was induced by Liver heat, and his bluish-whitish colored face, cold body and occasional diarrhea were induced by coldness in the epigastrium. Since this disease is engaged in both the exterior and interior, it was quite a serious case. What was worse, he had contracted the epidemic febrile disease, and it took him twenty days to recover. His stool was smooth or loose during the first third, smooth in the middle third, and dried during the last third; during he had bowel movements two to four times a day. In the beginning, he was taking Handa Yeolso Tang, and after recovering he took Jori Pyewon Tang (Decoction for Regulating Lung Vitality) for more than forty days. He barely survived.

有一太陰人素病咽嗌乾燥而面色青白表寒或泄盖咽嗌乾燥者肝熱也面色青白表寒或泄者胃脘寒也此病表裏俱病素病之太重者也此人得瘟病其證自始發日至于病解二十日大便初滑或泄中滑末乾每日二三四次無日不通初用寒多熱少湯病解後用調理肺元湯四十日調理僅僅獲生

14 During the first six days, his stool was sometimes watery or loose, and there was perspiration on the forehead, eyebrows and cheeks. Apart from that, his condition was normal. On the sixth day, he started to take medicine, and on the seventh, he had profuse perspiration all over the face from the forehead to the chin. Afterwards, his face changed into a bluish-whitish color, and he began to stammer. On the eighth and ninth days, he not only stammered, but also he lost his hearing, and the perspiration on the chin moved to his cheeks and eyebrows. He perspired lightly on the forehead only, from time to time, and became short of breath. On the tenth night, the sweat on the forehead disappeared, his stammering and deafness became worse, and he could not clear his throat of phlegm; he was forced to use his finger to pick out the phlegm. On the eleventh day, his shortness of breath became serious. Suddenly, on the twelfth day, he was able to eat two bowls of rice gruel. At that time, it would have been best to take Ursi Fel powder. Since Ursi Fel was very rare, I thought that he would not live another day; but on that afternoon, his shortness of breath eased slightly, and at the dawn of the thirteenth day, he perspired at the hairline. On the fourteenth and fifteenth days, he could eat two to three bowls of rice gruel and began to perspire on his forehead, eyebrows and cheeks, and the bluish color in his face disappeared. On the sixteenth day, there was perspiration on his chest, a small amount of phlegm was coughed out, and his stammering was relieved. On the twentieth day, he had several bouts of heavy perspirations on his chest and could stand in the room; all the symptoms, except for the deafness, disappeared. Afterwards,

he continued to take medicine for forty days, until his deafness and dizziness had disappeared altogether.

此病始發大便或滑或泄而六日內有額汗眉稜汗顴汗飲食起居有時如常六日後始用藥七日全體面部髮際以下至于脣頤汗流滿面淋漓洽足而汗後面色帶靑有語訥證八日九日語訥耳聾而脣汗還爲顴汗顴汗還爲眉稜汗汗出微粒乍出乍入而只有額汗呼吸短喘矣至于十日夜額汗還入而語訥耳聾尤甚痰涎壅喉口不能喀病人自以手指探口拭之而出十一日呼吸短喘尤甚至于十二日忽然食粥二碗斯時若論其藥則熊膽散或者可也而熊膽闕材自念此人今夜必死矣當日初昏呼吸暫時少定十三日鷄鳴時髮際有汗十四日十五日連三日食粥二三碗額汗眉稜汗顴汗次次發出面色脫靑十六日臆汗始通稍能喀痰語訥亦愈至于二十日臆汗數次大通遂能起立房中諸證皆安而耳聾證則自如也病解後用藥調理四十日耳聾目迷自袪

Discourse on the Greater Yin Person's Interior Febrile Disease Induced from the Liver Affected by Heat

太陰人肝受熱裏熱病論

1   Zhu Gong said, "Symptoms of yang type inflammatory swelling include silky patterns of red spots on the face, sore throat, and hemoptesis with pus, which should be treated with Gegen Jieji Tang (Pueraria Decoction for Releasing the Flesh) and Heinu Wan (Black Servant Pills). Generally, yang type inflammatory swelling and the deteriorated febrile disease are difficult to treat. Though the patient's spirit and consciousness are poor, if the epigastric region is still warm, open his mouth and let him swallow Heinu Wan. Then the patient can be saved immediately."

朱肱曰陽毒面赤斑斑如錦紋咽喉痛唾膿血宜葛根解肌湯黑奴丸陽毒及壞傷寒醫所不治精魄已竭心下尙煖斡開其口灌黑奴丸藥下咽卽活

2   Li Chan said, "Slight chills and fever can be treated with Gegen Jieji Tang, and eyeball pain, dry nasal cavity, profuse sweating, constipation, severe thirst and ranting such as that of a madman, should be treated with Tiaowei Chengqi Tang (Purgative Decoction for Harmonizing the Stomach). If there is a fever only in the exterior that causes pain in the eye and insomnia, Jieji Tang (Decoction for Releasing the Flesh) should be given. If the heat enters the interior, causing delirium similar to a madman's, Tiaowei Chengqi Tang should be given."

李梴曰微惡寒發熱宜葛根解肌湯目疼鼻乾潮汗閉澁滿渴狂譫宜調胃承氣湯熱在表則目疼不眠宜解肌湯熱入裏則狂譫宜調胃承氣湯

3   Gong Xin said, "The yang brightness disease with eyeball pain, dry nasal cavity and insomnia can be treated with Gegen Jieji Tang."

龔信曰陽明病目疼鼻乾不得臥宜葛根解肌湯

4 If the three yang diseases worsen, they will become yang type inflammatory swelling. Symptoms include a flushed face with red eyes, and yellowish spots on the body. Sometimes, there is also yellow-reddish diarrhea and a large and bounding pulse. The yang type inflammatory swelling can be treated with Heinu Wan.

三陽病深變爲陽毒面赤眼紅身發斑黃或下利黃赤六脈洪大宜黑奴丸

5 I have said, "The diseases mentioned above should be treated with Gegen Jieji Tang and Heinu Wan."

論曰右諸證當用葛根解肌湯黑奴丸

6 In the 『*Lingshu*』, we read, "A patient with fever on the inner forearm, a pounding pulse, and the dryness pattern is pestilent."

靈樞曰尺膚熱深脈盛燥者病瘟也

7 Wang Shuhe said, "The pulse of pestilence pounds both at the yin and yang locations. If the fever is extreme, the pulse becomes slippery with floating palpation, or scattering and uneven with deep palpation."

王叔和曰瘟病脈陰陽俱盛病熱之極浮之而滑沈之散澀

8 According to the 『*Maifa*』 ("Palpation Diagnosis"), the epidemic febrile disease, which has symptoms and signs such as fever, fullness in the abdomen, headache, normal appetite and straight-swift pulse on the second or third day, would cause the patient to die on the eighth day. If the patient has symptoms such as headache, fullness in the abdomen, vomiting and thread-stiff pulse, he will die on the twelfth day. If the patient did not have a headache, aching of the body, red eyes and changes of facial color, but had diarrhea with an uneven pulse that is largely felt by the superficial palpation, and hardness in the epigastrium, he will die on the seventeenth day.

脈法曰溫病二三日體熱腹滿頭痛食飲如故脈直而疾八日死溫病四五日頭痛腹滿而吐脈來細而強十二日死八九日頭身不痛目不赤色不變而反利脈來澀按之不足舉時大心下堅十七日死

9 Gong Xin said, "If a patient with the epidemic febrile disease has a high fever and a thread-short pulse, he will die, as will a patient with the epidemic febrile disease with severe diarrhea and abdominal pain."

龔信曰溫病穰穰大熱脈細小者死溫病下利痛甚死

10 "In 1586, when I lived in Daliang, an epidemic febrile disease broke out, and a large number of people died. The symptoms were severe chills with high fever, reddish swelling of the head, face, neck and cheeks, sore throat and coma. At that time, I made a prescription called Ersheng Jiuku Wan (Pills with Two Wonderful Drugs Saving from Suffering), which was

composed of 150g of Rhei Radix et Rhizoma and 75g of Gleditsiae Fructus, and mixed with wheat paste and made into green bean-size pills which were taken 50 to 70 at a time. After just one administration, the patient began to sweat, and eventually recovered. Congenitally healthy patients always recover. Gleditsiae Fructus opens the sweat pores and scatters the exterior qi and Rhei Radix et Rhizoma gets rid of the heat and circulates inside the body."

萬曆丙戌余寓大梁瘟疫大作士民多斃其證增寒壯熱頭面頰項赤腫咽喉腫痛昏憒余發一秘方名二聖救苦丸大黃四兩豬牙皂角二兩麵糊和丸菉豆大五七十丸一服卽汗一汗卽愈稟壯者百發百中牙皂開關竅發其表大黃瀉諸火通其裏

11 Symptoms brought on by seasonal irregularities include an initially large amount of sputum, fever with discomfort, headache, general soreness, chills with high fever, neck stiffness and eyeball pain. Appetite and living are normal. When the disease worsens, harshness of voice, red eyes, oral ulcers, buccal inflammations of various sizes, sore throat, coughing with sticky sputum, and sneezing occur.

感四時不正之氣使人痰涎壅盛煩熱頭疼身痛增寒壯熱項强睛疼或飲食如常起居依舊甚至聲啞或赤眼口瘡大小腮腫喉痺咳嗽稠粘噴嚏

12 I have said, "In addition to those symptoms mentioned above, if a patient has symptoms such as chills with a high fever, and a feeling of dryness and roughness, he should take Jogak Daihwang Tang (Gleditsia and Rhubarb Decoction) and Galgeun Seunggi Tang. Likewise, if reddish swelling of the head, face and throat appear, he also should take Jogak Daihwang Tang and Galgeun Seunggi Tang. If the patient has a fever, fullness in the abdomen, diarrhea and a tendency to high fever, it means that he has an interior pattern and should be treated with Galgeun Seunggi Tang. If a symptom such as chills is more severe, it means that the exterior pattern is quite serious and Taieum Jowi Tang added with Cimicifugae Rhizoma and Scutellariae Radix should be adopted."

論曰右諸證增寒壯熱燥澁者當用皂角大黃湯葛根承氣湯頭面項頰赤腫者當用皂角大黃湯葛根承氣湯體熱腹滿自利者熱勝則裡證也當用葛根解肌湯寒勝則表證而太重證也當用太陰調胃湯加升麻黃芩

13 I once treated a greater yin patient who had the epidemic febrile disease induced from the Liver affected by heat. He had been having eye problems for many years, and later contracted the epidemic febrile disease. From the first day, he took Yeolda Hanso Tang (Decoction for Treating More Fever than Cold) for three to five days, and his stool became loose, sometimes to the point of diarrhea. On the sixth day, since he had had no bowel movement, he took Galgeun Seunggi Tang continuously for three days and he ate double the amount of rice gruel. He took it continuously for another three days, and then his epidemic febrile disease was mostly relieved. After recovering, he took Yeolda Hanso Tang. When his stool was dried, 3.75g of Rhei Radix et Rhizoma was added. When he had severe diarrhea, Rhei Radix et Rhizoma

was discontinued. After taking care of his health like this for twenty days, he recovered completely. At the onset, he had nausea, vomiting, unconsciousness and severe pain. Later, his condition improved, and he recovered in twelve days.

嘗治太陰人肝熱熱證瘟病有一太陰人素病數年來眼病時作時止矣此人得瘟病自始發日用熱多寒少湯三四五日大便或滑或泄至六日有大便一日不通之證仍用葛根承氣湯連三日粥食大倍又用三日疫氣大減病解後復用熱多寒少湯大便燥澁則加大黃一錢滑泄太多則去大黃如此調理二十日其人完健○此病始發嘔逆口吐昏憒不省重痛矣末境反爲輕證十二日而病解

14 There was once a ten year old greater yin child suffering from the epidemic febrile disease induced by the interior heat and who could not even eat rice gruel and decoctions. Since his fever was high, he could only drink a small amount of cold water. By the eleventh day, he had had no bowel movement for four days. Trembling with fear, he uttered in delirium, "This room is filled with many worms" or "A rat is dashing into my chest", and crawled around quickly and cried loudly. He sometimes had cold limbs and locked knees induced by the wind stirring pattern in the case of high fever. At that time, he was given Galgeun Seunggi Tang orally and by force. He then began eating double the amount of rice gruel, and the epidemic symptoms were relieved. Fortunately, he survived. Until the fourth or fifth day after onset, the quality of his life, including diet and living conditions, was normal, so there was no difference between himself and a healthy person. Later, however, his condition worsened, and his disease was only relieved after seventeen days.

一太陰人十歲兒得裡熱瘟病粥食全不入口藥亦不入口壯熱穰穰有時飲冷水至于十一日則大便不通已四日矣怔忡譫語曰有百虫滿室又有鼠入懷云奔遑匐匐驚呼啼泣有時熱極生風兩手厥冷兩膝伸而不屈急用葛根承氣湯不憚啼泣強灌口中卽日粥食大倍疫氣大解倖而得生○此病始發四五日飲食起居如常無異平人矣末境反爲重證十七日而病解

15 In the 『*Neijing*』1)* , we read, "Most physical manifestations, like roughness, fleshlessness, wrinkles and chapness, are related to dryness."*

內經曰諸澁枯涸皺揭皆屬於燥

16 I have said, "When a greater yin person's face is bluish or whitish, he generally does not exhibit dryness symptoms. However, if his face is yellowish, reddish or dark, he is generally displaying dryness symptoms. This is caused by the Liver heat and the Lung dryness. I once treated a greater yin person with dryness-heat symptoms such as burnt black colored fingers and gangrenous changes. His left middle finger became burnt black in color, and he lost strength. Within two years, he was bleeding black blood at the palm, and later, on the

* This statement was taken from the 『*Suwen Xuanji Yuanbingshi*』 ("Profound Ideas and Etiology Based on Plain Questions", 素問玄機原病式), written by Liu Wansu (劉完素, about 1120-1200 A.D.).

back of his hands. It ultimately became edematous, and his finger had to be cut off. Within a year, the gangrenous blotches, ranging in size from small to large coins, covered all his body. After three years of this, even in his youth, the patient could neither bear labor work nor walk 12km per day. After taking 28 packs of Yeolda Hanso Tang with 7.5g of Ligustici Rhizoma et Radix and 3.75g of Rhei Radix et Rhizoma, his stool became loose. However, it hardened again a day or two later, so he took twenty packs more. His stool loosened slightly, the blotches on his face improved, and all four limbs grew stronger. I gave him twenty more packs, and his illness was almost cured."

論曰太陰人面色青白者多無燥證面色黃赤黑者多有燥證盖肝熱肺燥而然也嘗治太陰人燥熱證手指焦黑瘕瘡病自左手中指焦黑無力二年內一指黑血焦凝過掌心而掌背浮腫以刀斷指矣又一年內瘕瘡遍滿全體大者如大錢小者如小錢得病已爲三年而以壯年人手力不能役勞一半刻足力不能日行步三十里以熱多寒少湯用藁本二錢加大黃一錢二十八貼用之大便始滑不過一二日又秘燥又用二十貼大便不甚滑泄而面部瘕瘡少差手力足力稍快有效矣又用二十貼其病快差

17 In the 『*Lingshu*』, we read, "Two-yang bound is called diabetes. If a patient drinks one liter of water and urinates two liters, he will die." It was commented, "Two-yang bound means the Heat binding of the stomach and large intestine."

靈樞曰二陽結謂之消飲一溲二死不治○註曰二陽結謂胃及大腸熱結也

18 In Bianque[2]'s 『*Nanjing*』[3], we read, "The pulse with diabetes is tense, forceful and rapid. On the other hand, those who have deep, uneven and weak pulses will die eventually."

扁鵲難經曰消渴脈當得緊實而數反得沈濇而微者死

19 Zhang Zhongjing said, "Diabetes induces copious urination such as drinking 18 liters causing 18 liters of urine. Shenqi Wan (Pill for Invigorating Kidney qi) can be adopted."

張仲景曰消渴病小便反多如飲水一斗小便亦一斗腎氣丸主之

20 I have said, "The above disease is not the diabetes of the lesser yang person, but the dryness-heat disease of the greater yin person. For this case, we should not adopt Shenqi Wan, but rather Yeolda Hanso Tang with Ligustici Rhizoma et Radix and Rhei Radix et Rhizoma."

論曰此病非少陽人消渴也卽太陰人燥熱也此證不當用腎氣丸當用熱多寒少湯加藁本大黃

21 I once treated a weak, fifty year old greater yin person who had dryness heat disease. Since he displayed the symptoms of great thirst, copious urination and constipation, I gave him twenty packs of Yeolda Hanso Tang with 7.5g of Ligustici Rhizoma et Radix and 3.75g of Rhei Radix et Rhizoma. It was effective. More than one month later, the patient took five packs of another prescription, and his previous illness recurred. He further took fifty to sixty packs of Yeolda Hanso Tang with Ligustici Rhizoma et Radix and Rhei Radix et Rhizoma. He was at death's door throughout this period, and eventually died. I once treated another young

greater yin person who had the dryness-heat disease. With three hundred packs of the above prescription, he survived with difficulty for one year, but eventually died. Since he had suffered from the disease for a year, I was not able to determine whether he had also been taking other medications. When the patient was struck with the dryness-heat disease, he generally drank one bowl of water and urinated two bowls of urine. If the disease becomes severe, the patient cannot be cured. Generally, a greater yin person with constipation, copious urination and thirstiness should be treated in the early stages to prevent a more serious condition.

嘗治太陰人年五十近衰者燥熱病引飲小便多大便秘者用熱多寒少湯用藁本二錢加大黃一錢二十貼得效矣後一月餘用他醫藥五貼此人更病復用熱多寒少湯加藁本大黃五六十貼用藥時間其病僅僅支撐後終不免死又嘗治太陰人年少者燥熱病用此方三百貼得支撐一周年此病亦不免死此人得病一周年或間用他醫方未知緣何故也盖燥熱至於飲一溲二而病劇則難治凡太陰人大便秘燥小便覺多而引飲者不可不早治豫防

22 The above disease is not a fatal one. One year after its onset and taking medical treatment, the young patient died. His illness was due to his severe Liver heat and Lung dryness, which resulted from his extreme indulgence in luxury and enjoyment. If the young patient had maintained a peaceful mind free of lust, he might have been cured by taking a hundred days' worth of medication; but because he continued harboring burning desires from the first day of his disease to the day he died, he did not survive. A proverb says, "The kindness of the ancestors cannot be fully repaid, while the kindness of respect shall be fully rewarded." Any patient who cultivates and respects his mind, quenches his desires, and maintains a virtuous mind will be cured within a hundred days; within two hundred days, he will be in perfect health. It is true for everything that the kindness of respect shall be indeed rewarded, much more so for diseases.

此病非必不治之病也此少年得病用藥一周年後方死盖此病原委侈樂無厭慾火外馳肝熱大盛肺燥太枯之故也若此少年安心滌慾一百日而用藥則焉有不治之理乎盖自始病日至于終死日慾火無日不馳故也諺曰先祖德澤雖或不得一一箇報而恭敬德澤必無一一不受報凡無論某病人恭敬其心蕩滌慾火安靜善心一百日則其病無不愈二百日則其人無不完恭敬德澤之箇箇受報百事皆然而疾病尤甚

23 Wei Yilin said, "For the symptoms of yin blood exhaustion, such as deafness, visual difficulty, weakness in the legs, and lower back pains, it is suitable to take Heugwon Dan (Black Vitality Pills)."

危亦林曰陰血耗竭耳聾目暗脚弱腰痛宜用黑元丹

24 Insufficient genuine qi in the young adult male is not an acquired condition, but a congenital weakness. There are so many medications for nourishing and replenishing, but most of them are insufficient to show any desirable effectiveness. None but guarding congenital qi to make water rise and fire fall will promote the autonomous harmony among the five solid organs, and accordingly, the person will be free from disease. Gongjin Dan (Pills Embracing Fortune)

is suitable for this case.

凡男子方當壯年而眞氣猶怯此乃禀賦素弱非虛而然滋益之方群品稍衆藥力細微難見功效但固天元一氣使水升火降則五藏自和百病不生宜用拱辰丹

25 I have said, "For this case, one should adopt Heugwon Dan and Gongjin Dan. However, the potency of Angelicae Gigantis Radix and Corni Fructus in those prescriptions is insufficient. To get full strength, use Gongjin Heugwon Dan (Modified Gongjin Dan for Black Vitality) and Nogyong Daibo Tang (Cervi Cornu Pantotrichum Decoction for Major Tonification)."

論曰此證當用黑元與拱辰丹當歸山茱萸皆爲蠹材藥力未全欲收全力宜用拱辰黑元丹鹿茸大補湯

26 If a greater yin person has such symptoms as a feeling of fullness in the abdomen after a meal, and weakness in the legs, Gongjin Heugwon Dan, Nogyong Daibo Tang, Taieum Jowi Tang, and Jowi Seungcheong Tang (Decoction for Elevating the Clean Yang through Harmonizing the Stomach) should be adopted.

太陰人證有食後痞滿腿脚無力病宜用拱辰黑元丹鹿茸大補湯太陰調胃湯調胃升淸湯

27 A greater yin person may have diarrhea. For diarrhea caused by exterior cold, he should take Taieum Jowi Tang, while Galgeun Naibokja Tang (Kudzu and Radish Seed Decoction) should be adopted in the case of diarrhea caused by exterior-heat.

太陰人證有泄瀉病表寒證泄瀉當用太陰調胃湯表熱證泄瀉當用葛根蘿葍子湯

28 A greater yin person may have a cough. Taieum Jowi Tang, Nogyong Daibo Tang and Gongjin Heugwon Dan should be adopted.

太陰人證有咳嗽病宜用太陰調胃湯鹿茸大補湯拱辰黑元丹

29 A greater yin person may have asthma, a very serious symptom. Mahwang Jeongcheon Tang (Ephedra Decoction for Relieving Asthma) should be taken.

太陰人證有哮喘病重證也當用麻黃定喘湯

30 A greater yin person may have thoracoabdominal pain, a dangerous symptom. Mahwang Jeongtong Tang (Ephedra Decoction for Relieving Pain) should be taken.

太陰人證有胸腹痛病危險證也當用麻黃定痛湯

31 If a greater yin child has frequent diarrhea more than ten times, he certainly suffers from chronic infantile convulsions. He should take Bopyewon Tang (Decoction for Invigorating Lung Vitality) to prevent chronic infantile convulsions.

太陰人小兒有泄瀉十餘次無度者必發慢驚風宜用補肺元湯豫備慢風

32 A greater yin person displaying symptoms of abdominal distension and edema - symptoms so fatal that nine out of ten greater yin persons die from it - should take Geonyul Jejo Tang (Dried

Castaneae Semen and Cicada Larva Decoction). Though treated with medicines, the patient is not successfully cured unless the disease does not recur within three years. The patient should refrain from indulgence in luxury and enjoyment, and calm both his body and mind. For three years, it solely depends on the patient to cultivate his mind and body and take care of himself through willpower. If a greater yin person does not receive medical treatment before he gets edema, he will die in nine out of ten cases. The disease is thus not a disease, but certain death. What should the patient do? In a greater yin person, exertion of the mind and mental stress from repeated failures, dysentery from chronic diarrhea or oliguria from gonorrhea, feelings of fullness in the upper abdomen after a meal, and weakness in the legs are often the cause of edema, a serious and dangerous illness in itself. Thus, we must regard these symptoms as indicative of edema. The patient should quench his lust, and cultivate and respect his mind before medical treatment can prove effective.

太陰人有腹脹浮腫病當用乾栗蠐蟗湯此病極危險證而十生九死之病也雖用藥病愈三年內不再發然後方可論生戒侈樂禁嗜慾三年內宜恭敬心身調養愼攝必在其人矣凡太陰人病若待浮腫已發而治之則十病九死也此病不可以病論之而以死論之可也然則如之何其可也凡太陰人勞心焦思屢謀不成者或有久泄久痢或淋病小便不利食後痞滿腿脚無力病皆浮腫之漸已爲重險病而此時已浮腫論而蕩滌慾火恭敬其心用藥治之可也

33 A greater yin person once had a serious case of spermatorrhea, three or four times a month. One day, suffering from constipation, he was made to take Yeolda Hanso Tang with 3.75g of Rhei Radix et Rhizoma. When a patient begins to have bowel movements every day, he should additionally take Os Draconis and a derivative of Rhei Radix et Rhizoma or Gongjin Heugwon Dan and Nogyong Daibo Tang can be adopted. This illness comes from too much anxiety and thinking.

太陰人證有夢泄病一月內三四發者虛勞重證也大便秘一日則宜用熱多寒少湯加大黃一錢大便每日不秘則加龍骨減大黃或用拱辰黑元丹鹿茸大補湯此病出於謀慮太多思想無窮

34 Greater yin person can be fallen by a sudden stroke. If a patient's chest emits a "ge-ge" sound and stares blankly into space, he must be given Gwache San (Melon Stalk Powder); if he has convulsions of the four limbs and drooping eyes, he should take Wuhwang Cheongsim Hwan (Bovine Bezoar Bolus for Clearing the Heart). A patient with a dark, yellowish-reddish face generally tends to stare blankly into space, while one with bluish-whitish face tends to have droopy eyelids. If the latter begins to have convulsions of the four limbs, his condition may be termed dangerous; if not, he must quickly be given Qingxin Wan (Bolus for Clearing the Heart). Ancient Qingxin Wan also has dramatic effects: if a patient has a sudden onset of staring eyes, he will die not long afterwards, while one who experiences a sudden onset of droopy eyelids will die in very little time. However, the patient with staring eyes also should begin medical treatment without any delay, or he shall die.

太陰人證有卒中風病胸臆格格有窒塞聲而目瞪者必用瓜蔕散手足拘攣眼合者當用牛黃淸心丸素

面色黃赤黑者多有目瞪者素面色靑白者多有眼合者面色靑白而眼合者手足拘攣則其病危急也不必待拘攣但見眼合而素面色靑白者必急用淸心丸古方淸心丸每每神效目瞪者亦急發而稍緩死眼合者急發急死然目瞪者亦不可以緩論而急治之

35 Wuhwang Cheongsim Hwan is not a common drug and is impossible for every family to acquire it. It is thus advisable to pour powdered Polygalae Radix and Acori Graminei Rhizoma, 3.75g each, into the mouth and blow 0.75g of powdered Gleditsiae Fructus into the nose. When the patient has convulsions of the four limbs and a stiff neck, he is in a dangerous condition. Two men are needed either to hold the wrists of the patient to move the patient's shoulders from left to right, or to hold the patient's ankles to flex and extend the legs. Shaking the greater yin stroke patient's shoulders and legs will do him good, but one should not shake the shoulders and hands of lesser yang stroke patients. Neither should a patient be encouraged to sit up. This is acceptable for a lesser yin stroke patient, but his shoulders should not be shaken; rather, one should slowly massage his limbs.

牛黃淸心丸非家家必有之物宜用遠志石菖蒲末各一錢灌口因以皂角末三分吹鼻此證手足拘攣而項直則危也傍人以兩手執病人兩手腕左右撓動兩肩或執病人足腕屈伸兩脚太陰人中風撓動病人肩脚好也少陽人中風大忌撓動病人手足又不可抱人起坐少陰人中風傍人抱病人起坐則可也而不可撓動兩肩可以徐徐按摩手足

36 Moschus is suitable to cure poisoning and vomiting with diarrhea.

中毒吐瀉宜用麝香

Notes

1) 『*Neijing*』(內經)

The 『*Huangdi Neijing*』, the oldest and greatest medical classic extant in China, with its authorship ascribed to the ancient Emperor Huangdi (2698~2589 B.C.). The work was actually a product of various unknown authors from the Warring States Period (475~221 B.C.) to the Late Han dynasty (25~220 A.D.). The book consists of two parts: the 『*Suwen*』(素問: "Plain Questions"), and 『*Lingshu*』(靈樞: "Miraculous Pivot" or "Divine Axis", also known as the "Canon of Acupuncture").

2) Bianque (扁鵲)

(circa 500 B.C.) Also known as Qin Yueren (秦越人), the earliest noted physician who was famous for his medical knowledge and well versed in diagnosis and treatment, especially pulse taking and acupuncture. He was ascribed the authorship of some medical works such as the 『*Bianque Neijing*』(扁鵲內經: "The Internal Classic of Bianque") and 『*Bianque Waijing*』(扁鵲外經: "The External Classic of Bianque"), all of which have been lost.

3) 『*Nanjing*』(難經)

The "Classic of Difficult Issues", a book that appeared in the first or second century B.C. with its authorship unknown, though it is often ascribed to Qin Yueren (秦越人). It deals with fundamental medical theories and expounds the 『*Neijing*』's main points in the form of questions and answers. The points of acupuncture and moxibustion, the method of needling, the physiological and pathological conditions related to the meridians and collaterals, and the method of feeling the pulse are all discussed.

Four Prescriptions for the Greater Yin Person's Disease from Zhang Zhongjing's 『*Shanghanlun*』

張仲景傷寒論中太陰人病經驗設方藥四方

1 Ephedra Decoction (Mahuang Tang)
- Ephedrae Herba 11.25g
- Cinnamomi Ramulus 7.5g
- Glycyrrhizae Radix et Rhizoma 2.25g
- Armeniacae Semen 10 pcs.
- Zingiberis Rhizoma recens 3 slices
- Jujubae Fructus 2 pcs.

麻黃湯

麻黃三錢桂枝二錢甘草六分杏仁十枚生薑三片大棗二枚

2 Half Cinnamon Twig and Half Ephedra Decoction (Guima Geban Tang)
- Ephedrae Herba 5.625g
- Paeoniae Radix Alba 3.75g
- Cinnamomi Ramulus 3.75g
- Armeniacae Semen 3.75g
- Glycyrrhizae Radix et Rhizoma 2.625g
- Zingiberis Rhizoma recens 3 slices
- Jujubae Fructus 2 pcs.

桂麻各半湯

麻黃一錢五分白芍藥桂枝杏仁各一錢甘草七分生薑三片大棗二枚

3 Purgative Decoction for Harmonizing the Stomach (Tiaowei Chengqi Tang)
- Rhei Radix et Rhizoma 15g
- Natrii Sulfas 7.5g
- Glycyrrhizae Radix et Rhizoma 3.75g

調胃承氣湯

大黃四錢芒硝二錢甘草一錢

4 Major Decoction of Bupleurum (Da Chaihu Tang)

· Bupleuri Radix 15g   · Scutellariae Radix 9.375g

· Paeoniae Radix Alba 9.375g   · Rhei Radix et Rhizoma 7.5g

· Aurantii Fructus immaturus 5.625g

The above prescription treats the transmission of the lesser yang to the yang brightness disease with the symptoms of fever without chills, aversion to heat, constipation, reddish urine, delirium, abdominal distension and tidal fever.

大柴胡湯

柴胡四錢黃芩白芍藥各二錢五分大黃二錢枳實一錢五分

治少陽轉屬陽明身熱不惡寒反惡熱大便堅小便赤譫語腹脹潮熱

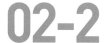

Nine Prescriptions for the Greater Yin Person's Disease Mentioned in the Writings of Famous Doctors in the Tang, Song and Ming Dynasties

唐宋明三代醫家著述中 太陰人經驗行用要藥九方

1 Acorus and Polygala Powder (Shichangpu Yuanzhi San)

· Acori Graminei Rhizoma · Polygalae Radix

Pound the above drugs into a powder and let the patient take 3.75g with liquor three times a day. The patient's eyes and ears will be refreshed. The original source of this prescription is Sun Simiao's 『*Qianjinfang*』.

石菖蒲遠志散

石菖蒲遠志爲細末每服一錢酒飲任下日三令人耳目聰明此方出於孫思邈千金方書中

2 Decoction for Harmonizing the Middle (Tiaozhong Tang)

· Rhei Radix et Rhizoma 5.625g · Scutellariae Radix 3.75g

· Platycodi Radix 3.75g · Puerariae Radix 3.75g

· Atractylodis Rhizoma Alba 3.75g · Paeoniae Radix Alba 3.75g

· Poria Sclerotium (red) 3.75g · Ligustici Rhizoma 3.75g

· Glycyrrhizae Radix et Rhizoma 3.75g

The original source of this prescription is Zhu Gong's 『*Huorenshu*』. It cures epidemic diseases caused by dryness in the summer, with the symptoms such as dry mouth and choking sensation. In accordance with the results of recent studies, Atractylodis Rhizoma Alba, Paeoniae Radix Alba, Poria Sclerotium, and Glycyrrhizae Radix et Rhizoma should be excluded from this prescription.

調中湯

大黃一錢五分黃芩桔梗葛根白朮白芍藥赤茯苓藁本甘草各一錢

此方出於朱肱活人書中治夏發燥疫口乾咽塞○今考更定此方當去白朮芍藥茯苓甘草

3　Black Servant Pills (Heinu Wan)

- Ephedrae Herba 75g
- Scutellariae Radix 37.5g
- Natrii Sulfas 37.5g
- Dust (on the girder) 37.5g

- Rhei Radix et Rhizoma 75g
- Cauldron soot 37.5g
- Furnace ash 37.5g
- Smutted ear of barley 37.5g

Pound the above drugs into a powder and make pills as big as bullets, then take one pill with spring water. After a short bout of shivering and sweating, the patient will recover. The original source of this prescription is Zhu Gong's 『*Huorenshu*』. If, through mistaken treatment, a patient with macule caused by yang type inflammatory swelling or with a deteriorated case of acute febrile disease loses consciousness, he can still be treated on the condition that there is warmth in the epigastric region. Administer the above medicine through the mouth. In accordance with the results of recent studies, Natrii Sulfas should be excluded.

黑奴丸

麻黃大黃各二兩黃芩釜底煤芒硝竈突墨樑上塵小麥奴各一兩

右爲末蜜丸彈子大每一丸新汲水化服須臾振寒汗出而解此方出於朱肱活人書中陽毒及壞傷寒醫所不治精魄已竭心下尙煖幹開其口灌藥下咽卽活○今考更定此方當去芒硝

4　Pulse-activating Powder (Shengmai San)

- Liriopis seu Ophiopogonis Tuber 7.5g
- Schizandrae Fructus 3.75g

- Ginseng Radix 3.75g

If patients drink this in summer instead of water boiled with burned rice, the prescription will give them energy. The original source of the prescriptions is Li Chan's 『*Yixue Rumen*』. In accordance with the results of recent studies, Ginseng Radix should be excluded from this prescription.

生脈散

麥門冬二錢人蔘五味子各一錢

夏月代熟水飲之令人氣力湧出此方出於李梴醫學入門書中○今考更定此方當去人蔘

5　Toona Root Bark Pill (Chugenpi Wan)

- Ailanthi Radicis Cortex

Pound the above drug into a powder and make the pills with liquor and flour paste. This prescription cures wet dreams. The original source of the prescriptions is Li Chan's 『*Yixue Rumen*』. The property of this drug is cool and dry, so it cannot be used alone.

樗根皮丸

樗根白皮爲末酒糊和丸此方出於李梴醫學入門書中治夢遺此藥性凉而燥不可單服

6　Pills with Two Wonderful Drugs Saving from Suffering (Ersheng Jiuku Wan)

- Rhei Radix et Rhizoma 150g
- Gleditsiae Fructus 75g

Pound the above drugs into a powder. Make 50 or 70 pills with flour paste as big as mung beans. One intake causes sweating, which leads to recovery. The original source of this prescription is Gong Xin's compilation, 『*Wanbing Huichun*』; it cures seasonal epidemic disease.

二聖救苦丸

大黃四兩猪牙皂角二兩

麵糊和丸菉豆大五七十丸一服卽汗一汗卽愈此方出於龔信萬病回春書中治天行瘟疫

7　Pueraria Decoction for Releasing the Flesh (Gegen Jieji Tang)

· Puerariae Radix 3.75g
· Scutellariae Radix 3.75g
· Angelicae dahuricae Radix 3.75g
· Paeoniae Radix Alba 3.75g
· Gypsum Fibrosum 3.75g
· Cimicifugae Rhizoma 3.75g
· Platycodi Radix 3.75g
· Bupleuri Radix 3.75g
· Osterici Radix 3.75g
· Glycyrrhizae Radix et Rhizoma 1.875g

The original source of this prescription is 『*Yijian*』 compiled by Gong Xin. It cures the yang brightness disease with symptoms such as eye pain, dryness in the nasal cavity and insomnia. In accordance with the results of recent studies, Bupleuri Radix, Paeoniae Radix, Osterici Radix, Gypsum Fibrosum, and Glycyrrhizae Radix et Rhizoma must be excluded from this prescription.

葛根解肌湯

葛根升麻黃芩桔梗白芷柴胡白芍藥羌活石膏各一錢甘草五分

此方出於龔信醫鑑書中治陽明病目疼鼻乾不得臥○今考更定此方當去柴胡芍藥羌活石膏甘草

8　Bovine Bezoar Bolus for Clearing the Heart (Niuhuang Qingxin Wan)

· Dioscoreae Rhizoma 26.25g
· Glycyrrhizae Radix et Rhizoma (stir-baked) 18.75g
· Ginseng Radix 9.375g
· Massa Medicata Fermentata 9.375g
· Dried soybean sprouts (stir-baked) 6.375g
· Colla corii asini (stir-baked) 6.375g
· Liriopis seu Ophiopogonis Tuber 5.625g
· Angelicae Gigantis Radix 5.625g
· Saposhnikoviae Radix 5.625g
· Cinnabaris (to refine powder with water) 5.625g
· Bupleuri Radix 4.875g
· Armeniacae Semen 4.875g
· Chuanxiong Rhizoma 4.875g
· Saigae tataricae cornu 3.75g
· Moschus 3.75g
· Ampelopsis Radix 2.625g
· Zingiberis Rhizoma (stir-baked at high temperature) 2.625g
· Gold 140 sheets

· Typhae Pollen 9.375g
· Rhinoceri cornu 7.5g
· Cinnamomi Cortex 6.375g
· Paeoniae Radix Alba 5.625g
· Scutellariae Radix 5.625g
· Atractylodis Rhizoma Alba 5.625g

· Platycodi Radix 4.875g
· Poria Sclerotium (white) 4.875g
· Calculus Bovis 4.5g
· Borneolum 3.75g
· Realgar 3g

Forty of the 140 gold sheets are used to wrap the pills. Steam twenty pieces of Jujubae Fructus and remove the seeds. Puree the Jujubae Fructus into a paste and mix in the remaining pulverized drugs. Add honey and mix thoroughly, from 37.5g of the mixture, make ten pills. Wrap each pill in a thin sheet of gold. Take one pill for each dose with warm water. The original source of this prescription is 『*Yijian*』 compiled by Gong Xin. This prescription cures stroke, loss of consciousness, accumulation of phlegm, aphagia, wry mouth with distortion of the eye and the paralysis of limbs. In accordance with the results of recent studies, Atractylodis Rhizoma Alba, Ginseng Radix, Glycyrrhizae Radix et Rhizoma, Massa Fermentata Medicinalis, Cinnamomi Cortex, Colla corii asini, Paeoniae Radix Alba, Angelicae Gigantis Radix, Chuanxiong Rhizoma, Zingiberis Rhizoma, Jujubae Fructus, Bupleuri Radix, Poria Sclerotium, Realgar, and Cinnabaris must be excluded from this prescription.

牛黃淸心丸

山藥七錢甘草炒五錢人蔘蒲黃炒神麴炒各二錢五分犀角二錢大豆黃卷炒肉桂阿膠炒各一錢七分白芍藥麥門冬黃芩當歸白朮防風朱砂水飛各一錢五分柴胡桔梗杏仁白茯苓川芎各一錢三分牛黃一錢二分羚羊角龍腦麝香各一錢雄黃八分白斂乾薑炮各七分金箔一百四十箔內四十箔爲衣大棗二十枚蒸取肉研爲膏右爲末棗膏入煉蜜和勻每一兩作十丸金箔爲衣每取一丸溫水和下此方出於龔信醫鑑書中治卒中風不省人事痰涎壅塞精神昏憒言語蹇澁口眼喎斜手足不遂等證○今考更定此方當去白朮人蔘甘草神麴肉桂阿膠白芍藥當歸川芎乾薑大棗淸蜜柴胡白茯苓雄黃朱砂

9 Ephedra Decoction for Relieving Asthma (Mahuang Dingchuan Tang)

· Ephedrae Herba 11.25g · Armeniacae Semen 5.625g
· Scutellariae Radix 3.75g · Pinelliae Tuber 3.75g
· Mori Radicis Cortex 3.75g · Perillae Fructus 3.75g
· Farfarae Flos 3.75g · Glycyrrhizae Radix et Rhizoma 3.75g
· Ginkgo Semen (remove the cortex, pound and stir-baked it) 21 pcs.

The Huangsege ("Yellow Song") says, "Every disease has its cure." It is most difficult to cure snoring and asthma. There once was a patient who happened upon a medicine, and after taking it, was cured. He then realized the medicine was Dingchuan Tang. The original source of this prescription is Gong Xin's compilation, 『*Wanbing Huichun*』. This cures asthma miraculously. In accordance with the results of recent studies, Pinelliae Tuber, Perillae Fructus, and Glycyrrhizae Radix et Rhizoma should be excluded from this prescription.

麻黃定喘湯

麻黃三錢杏仁一錢五分黃芩半夏桑白皮蘇子款冬花甘草各一錢白果二十一枚去殼碎炒黃色歌曰諸病原來有藥方惟愁齁喘最難當病人遇此仙丹藥服後方知定喘湯此方出於龔信萬病回春書中治哮喘神方○今考更定此方當去半夏蘇子甘草

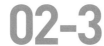

Twenty Four Important Newly Formulated Prescriptions for the Greater Yin Person's Disease

新定太陰人病應用要藥二十四方

1 Decoction for Harmonizing the Greater Yin Person's Stomach (Taieum Jowi Tang)

. Coicis Semen 11.25g

· Castaneae Semen (dried) 11.25g　　· Raphani Semen 7.5g

· Schizandrae Fructus 3.75g　　· Liriopis seu Ophiopogonis Tuber 3.75g

· Acori graminei Rhizoma 3.75g　　· Platycodi Radix 3.75g

· Ephedrae Herba 3.75g

太陰調胃湯

薏苡仁乾栗各三錢蘿葍子二錢五味子麥門冬石菖蒲桔梗麻黃各一錢

2 Pueraria Decoction for Releasing the Flesh (Galgeun Haigi Tang)

· Puerariae Radix 11.25g　　· Scutellariae Radix 5.625g

· Ligustici Rhizoma 5.625g　　· Platycodi Radix 3.75g

· Cimicifugae Rhizoma 3.75g　　· Angelicae dahuricae Radix 3.75g

葛根解肌湯

葛根三錢黃芩藁本各一錢五分桔梗升麻白芷各一錢

3 Decoction for Elevating the Clean Yang through Harmonizing the Stomach (Jowi Seung-cheong Tang)

· Coicis Semen 11.25g　　· Castaneae Semen (dried) 11.25g

· Raphani Semen 5.625g　　· Ephedrae Herba 3.75g

· Platycodi Radix 3.75g　　· Liriopis seu Ophiopogonis Tuber 3.75g

· Schizandrae Fructus 3.75g　　· Acori graminei Rhizoma 3.75g

· Polygalae Radix 3.75g   · Asparagi Radix 3.75g

· Ziziphi Spinosae Semen 3.75g   · Longan Arillus 3.75g

調胃升清湯

薏苡仁乾栗各三錢蘿葍子一錢五分麻黃桔梗麥門冬五味子石菖蒲遠志天門冬酸棗仁龍眼肉各一錢

4   Decoction of Lotus Seed for Clearing the Heart (Cheongsim Yeonja Tang)

· Nelumbinis Semen 7.5g   · Dioscoreae Rhizoma 7.5g

· Asparagi Radix 3.75g   · Liriopis seu Ophiopogonis Tuber 3.75g

· Polygalae Radix 3.75g   · Acori graminei Rhizoma 3.75g

· Ziziphi Spinosae Semen 3.75g   · Longan Arillus 3.75g

· Platycladi Semen 3.75g   · Scutellariae Radix 3.75g

· Raphani Semen 3.75g   · Chrysanthemi Indici Flos 1.125g

清心蓮子湯

蓮子肉山藥各二錢天門冬麥門冬遠志石菖蒲酸棗仁龍眼肉栢子仁黃芩蘿葍子各一錢甘菊花三分

5   Ephedra Decoction for Relieving Asthma (Mahwang Jeongcheon Tang)

· Ephedrae Herba 11.25g   · Armeniacae Semen 5.625g

· Scutellariae Radix 3.75g   · Raphani Semen 3.75g

· Mori Radicis Cortex 3.75g   · Platycodi Radix 3.75g

· Liriopis seu Ophiopogonis Tuber 3.75g   · Farfarae Flos 3.75g

· Ginkgo Semen (stir-baked to yellow) 21 pcs.

麻黃定喘湯

麻黃三錢杏仁一錢五分黃芩蘿葍子桑白皮桔梗麥門冬款冬花各一錢白果二一箇炒黃色

6   Ephedra Decoction for Relieving Pain (Mahwang Jeongtong Tang)

· Coicis Semen 11.25g   · Ephedrae Herba 7.5g

· Raphani Semen 7.5g   · Armeniacae Semen 3.75g

· Acori graminei Rhizoma 3.75g   · Platycodi Radix 3.75g

· Liriopis seu Ophiopogonis Tuber 3.75g   · Schizandrae Fructus 3.75g

· Quisqualis Fructus 3.75g   · Longan Arillus 3.75g

· Platycladi Semen 3.75g   · Castaneac Semen (dried) 7 pcs.

麻黃定痛湯

薏苡仁三錢麻黃蘿葍子各二錢杏仁石菖蒲桔梗麥門冬五味子使君子龍眼肉栢子仁各一錢乾栗七箇

7   Decoction for Treating More Fever than Cold (Yeolda Hanso Tang)

· Puerariae Radix 15g   · Scutellariae Radix 7.5g

· Ligustici Rhizoma 7.5g   · Raphani Semen 3.75g

· Platycodi Radix 3.75g

· Cimicifugae Rhizoma 3.75g

· Angelicae dahuricae Radix 3.75g

熱多寒少湯

葛根四錢黃芩藁本各二錢蘿葍子桔梗升麻白芷各一錢

8 Decoction for Treating More Cold than Fever (Handa Yeolso Tang)

· Coicis Semen 11.25g
· Raphani Semen 7.5g

· Liriopis seu Ophiopogonis Tuber 3.75g
· Platycodi Radix 3.75g

· Scutellariae Radix 3.75g
· Armeniacae Semen 3.75g

· Ephedrae Herba 3.75g
· Castaneae Semen (dried) 7 pcs.

寒多熱少湯

薏苡仁三錢蘿葍子二錢麥門冬桔梗黃芩杏仁麻黃各一錢乾栗七箇

9 Pueraria Decoction for Purgation (Galgeun Seunggi Tang)

· Puerariae Radix 15g
· Scutellariae Radix 7.5g

· Rhei Radix et Rhizoma 7.5g
· Platycodi Radix 3.75g

· Cimicifugae Rhizoma 3.75g
· Angelicae dahuricae Radix 3.75g

If 7.5g of Rhei Radix et Rhizoma is added to this prescription, it is named Galgeun Dai Seunggi Tang; 3.75g of Rhei Radix et Rhizoma is reduced in this prescription, it is named Galgeun So Seunggi Tang.

葛根承氣湯

葛根四錢黃芩大黃各二錢升麻桔梗白芷各一錢

本方加大黃二錢則名曰葛根大承氣湯減大黃一錢則名曰葛根小承氣湯

10 Decoction for Regulating Lung Vitality (Jori Pyewon Tang)

· Liriopis seu Ophiopogonis Tuber 7.5g
· Platycodi Radix 7.5g

· Coicis Semen 7.5g
· Scutellariae Radix 3.75g

· Ephedrae Herba 3.75g
· Raphani Semen 3.75g

調理肺元湯

麥門冬桔梗薏苡仁各二錢黃芩麻黃蘿葍子各一錢

11 Ephedra Decoction for Diaphoresis (Mahwang Balpyo Tang)

· Platycodi Radix 11.25g
· Ephedrae Herba 5.625g

· Liriopis seu Ophiopogonis Tuber 3.75g
· Scutellariae Radix 3.75g

· Armeniacae Semen 3.75g

麻黃發表湯

桔梗三錢麻黃一錢五分麥門冬黃芩杏仁各一錢

12 Decoction for Invigorating Lung Vitality (Bopyewon Tang)

· Liriopis seu Ophiopogonis Tuber 11.25g   · Platycodi Radix 7.5g

· Schizandrae Fructus 3.75g

If 3.75g each of Dioscoreae Rhizoma, Coicis Semen, and Raphani Semen are added to the above, the results will be more effective.

補肺元湯

麥門冬三錢桔梗二錢五味子一錢

加山藥薏苡仁蘿葍子各一錢則尤妙

13 Velvet Deerhorn Decoction for Major Tonification (Nogyong Daibo Tang)

· Cervi cornu pantotrichum 7.5g, 11.25g or 15g

· Liriopis seu Ophiopogonis Tuber 5.625g

· Coicis Semen 5.625g   · Dioscoreae Rhizoma 3.75g

· Asparagi Radix 3.75g   · Schizandrae Fructus 3.75g

· Armeniacae Semen 3.75g   · Ephedrae Herba 3.75g

This prescription cures weak patients displaying exterior symptoms and cold pattern.

鹿茸大補湯

鹿茸二三四錢麥門冬薏苡仁各一錢五分山藥天門冬五味子杏仁麻黃各一錢

虛弱人表症寒證多者宜用

14 Modified Gongjin Dan for Black Vitality (Gongjin Heugwon Dan)

· Cervi cornu pantotrichum 150g, 187.5g or 225g

· Dioscoreae Rhizoma 150g

· Asparagi Radix 150g   · Holotrichia diomphalia Bates 37.5~75g

· Moschus 18.75g

Boil the flesh of Mume Fructus and puree into a soft paste. Together with the other pulverized drugs, make the pills as big as an empress tree seed. Take 50~70 pills for each dose with warm water or liquor. This cures the weak patient who has interior symptoms.

拱辰黑元丹

鹿茸四五六兩山藥天門冬各四兩蠐螬一二兩麝香五錢

煮烏梅肉爲膏和丸梧子大溫湯下五七十丸或燒酒下虛弱人裏症多者宜用

15 Gleditsia and Rhubarb Decoction (Jogak Daihwang Tang)

· Cimicifugae Rhizoma 11.75g   · Puerariae Radix 11.75g

· Rhei Radix et Rhizoma 3.75g   · Gleditsiae Fructus 3.75g

Do not use this medicine over three or four packs. Since 11.25g of Cimicifugae Rhizoma, Rhei Radix et Rhizoma, and Gleditsiae Fructus are included, the potency of this drug is extremely strong.

皂角大黃湯

升麻葛根各三錢大黃皂角各一錢

用之者不可過三四貼升麻三錢大黃皂角同局藥力峻猛故也

16 Pueraria and Duckweed Decoction (Galgeun Bupyeong Tang)
- Puerariae Radix 11.75g
- Raphani Semen 7.5g
- Scutellariae Radix 7.5g
- Spirodelae Herba 3.75g
- Rhei Radix et Rhizoma 3.75g
- Holotrichia diomphalia Bates 10 pcs.

This prescription cures edema and the interior symptoms with more fever than chills.

葛根浮萍湯

葛根三錢蘿葍子黃芩各二錢紫背浮萍大黃各一錢蠐螬十箇

治浮腫裏症熱多者宜用

17 Dried Castaneae Semen and June Beetle Grub Decoction (Geonyul Jejo Tang)
- Castaneae Semen (dried) 100 pcs.
- Holotrichia diomphalia Bates 10 pcs.

Take these as a decoction or stir-bake them with an adjuvant. Pound ten dried Castaneae Semens and ten Holotrichia diomphalia Bates into a powder. Take the above medicine with the decoction of dried Castaneae Semens. This prescription cures edema and the exterior symptoms with more chills than fever.

乾栗蠐螬湯

乾栗百枚蠐螬十介湯服或灸食黃栗蠐螬十介作末別用黃栗湯水調下

治浮腫表症寒多者宜用

18 Dried Castaneae Semen and Toona Root Bark Decoction (Geonyul Jeogeunpi Tang)
- Castaneae Semen (dried) 37.5g
- Ailanthi Radicis Cortex 11.25~18.75g

This prescription cures dysentery. Take this as a decoction or pills. In the pill form, it is taken only with 18.5g of Ailanthi Radicis Cortex.

乾栗樗根皮湯

乾栗一兩樗根白皮三四五錢

治痢疾或湯服或丸服而丸服者或單用樗根白皮五錢

19 Melon Stalk Powder (Gwache San)
- Pedicellus Melo (stir-baked to yellow)

Pound the above drug into a powder of 1.125 or 1.875g. Take it with warm water or take a quickly prepared decoction of dried Pedicellus Melo, 3.75g. This prescription cures stroke. Patients with congested sounds emanating from the chest and blankly staring into space absolutely require this medicine. This medicine must be used on patients who have this disease and display symptoms like it, but it must not be used on those who have another disease or exhibit different symptoms. It most certainly cannot be used on patients with abdominal and chest pains, or cough and asthma due to cold. It is also forbidden to use it on patients with indigestion. In these cases, other medicines have to be used.

Stroke patients with a pale complexion and the exterior deficiency pattern of the cold type require Wungdam San (Xiongdan San), Wuhwang Cheongsim Won (Niuhuang Qingxin Yuan), and Seokchangpo Wonji San (Shichangpu Yuanzhi San), but not Gwache San.

瓜蒂散

瓜蒂炒黃爲末三五分溫水調下或乾瓜蒂一錢急煎湯用

治卒中風臆膈格格有窒塞聲及目瞪者必可用○此藥此病此證可用他病他證必不可用胸腹痛寒咳喘尤忌用雖滯食物不可用此藥而用他藥○面色靑白而素有寒證表虛者卒中風則當用熊膽散牛黃淸心元石菖蒲遠志散而不可用瓜蒂散

20 Bear's Gall Powder (Wungdam San)

· Ursi Fel 1.125~1.875g

This drug should be taken with warm water.

熊膽散

熊膽三五分溫水調下

21 Moschus Powder (Sahyang San)

· Moschus 1.125~1.875g

This drug should be taken with warm water or warm liquor.

麝香散

麝香三五分溫水調下或溫酒調下(只擧三五分則四分在其中)

22 Acorus and Polygala Powder (Seokchangpo Wonji San)

· Polygalae Radix (powder) 37.5g   · Acori graminei Rhizoma (powder) 3.75g

· Gleditsiae Spina (powder) 1.125g

This prescription should be taken with warm water. Another way is to take the powder of Polygalae Radix and Acori graminei Rhizoma with warm water and breathe the powder of Gleditsiae Spina into the nasal cavity.

石菖蒲遠志散

遠志末一錢石菖蒲末一錢猪牙皂角末三分

溫水調下或遠志菖蒲末溫水調下皂角末吹鼻

23 Ophiopogon and Polygala Powder (Maigmundong Wonji San)

· Liriopis seu Ophiopogonis Tuber 11.25g · Polygalae Radix 3.75g

· Acori graminei Rhizoma 3.75g   · Schizandrae Fructus 1.875g

麥門冬遠志散

麥門冬三錢遠志石菖蒲各一錢五味子五分

24 Bovine Bezoar Bolus for Clearing the Heart (Wuhwang Cheongsim Won)

- Dioscoreae Rhizoma 26.25g
- Rhinoceri cornu 7.5g
- Liriopis seu Ophiopogonis Tuber 5.625g
- Platycodi Radix 4.875g
- Calculus Bovis 4.5g
- Borneolum 3.75g
- Ampelopsis Radix 2.625g

- Typhae Pollen (stir-baked) 9.375g
- Dried soybean sprouts (stir-baked) 6.375g
- Scutellariae Radix 5.625g
- Armeniacae Semen 4.875g
- Saigae tataricae cornu 3.75g
- Moschus 3.75g
- Gold 70 sheets

Twenty sheets of gold are used to wrap the pills. Make a soft extract of twenty Mume Fructus , steamed and pared. Pound the above drugs into a powder, knead it with the soft extract of the Mume Fructus and, from 37.5g of the mixture, make twenty pills wrapped in thin sheets of gold. Take one pill for each dose with warm water. Among the above greater yin person drugs, remove the twinned seed and the husk of Armeniancae Semen. Remove the cores of Liriopis seu Ophiopogonis Tuber and Polygalae Radix. Peel Ginkgo Semen and Castaneae Semen. Rhei Radix et Rhizoma is steamed with liquor or used raw. Bake Cervi vornu pantotrichum and Gleditsiae Spina after applying butter. Ziziphi Spinosae Semen, Armeniacae Semen, and Ginkgo Semen should be roasted.

牛黃清心元

山藥七錢蒲黃炒二錢五分犀角二錢大豆黃卷炒一錢七分麥門冬黃芩各一錢五分桔梗杏仁各一錢三分牛黃一錢二分羚羊角龍腦麝香各一錢白斂七分金箔七十箔內二十箔爲衣烏梅二十枚蒸取肉研爲膏右爲末烏梅膏和勻每一兩作二十丸金箔爲衣每取一丸溫水化下

右太陰人藥諸種杏仁去雙仁去皮尖麥門冬遠志去心白果黃栗去殼大黃或酒蒸或生用鹿茸皂角酥灸酸棗仁杏仁白果炒用

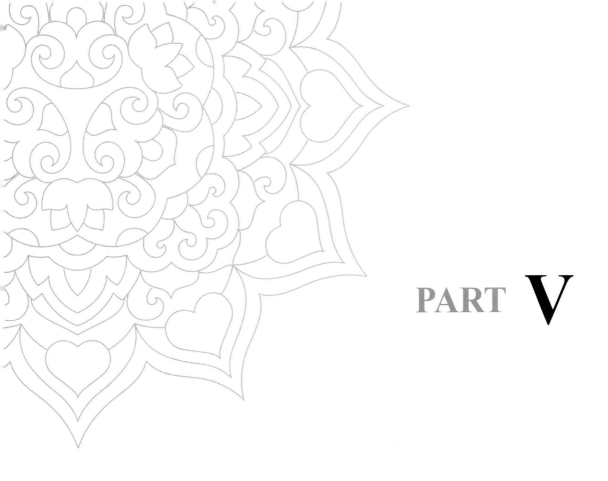

PART V

01

Discourse on the Taiyang (Greater Yang) Person's Lumbar Vertebral Disease Induced by Exopathogen

太陽人外感腰脊病論

1 In the 『*Neijing*』, we read, "Moderate and uneven *chi* (cubit) pulses are the manifestations of *jieyi* (generalized fatigue and lassitude)." As a comment on this sentence, "Since a *chi* pulse manifests itself in the yin portion, it is dominated by the Liver and Kidney. Since a moderate pulse manifests itself as heat affects the middle-*jiao*, and an uneven pulse manifests itself as blood exhaustion, this condition is called generalized fatigue and lassitude. Since the symptoms of generalized fatigue and lassitude are neither chilly nor febrile, or weak nor strong, it cannot be identified exactly and is called generalized fatigue and lassitude."

內經曰尺脈緩澁謂之解㑊釋曰尺爲陰部肝腎主之緩爲熱中澁爲亡血故謂之解㑊解㑊者寒不寒熱不熱弱不弱壯不壯獰不可名謂之解㑊也

2 In the 『*Lingshu*』, it is said, "If a disease in the spinal cord develops, the patient's cord deteriorates, then his shins ache and his body is generally fatigued and cannot go." "Cannot go" means that the patient is unable to walk.

靈樞曰髓傷則消爍胻痠體解㑊然不去矣不去謂不能行去也

3 I have said, "The above symptoms belong to the quite serious lumbar vertebral disease of the greater yang person. The patient should refrain from feeling deep sorrow and anger, and secure peace of his mind; then the disease can be cured. For this disease, Ogapi Jangcheok Tang (Acanthopanax Decoction for Strengthening Spine) should be adopted."

論曰此證卽太陽人腰脊病太重證也必戒深哀遠嗔怒修淸定然後其病可愈此證當用五加皮壯脊湯

4　The patient with generalized fatigue and lassitude is perfectly healthy in the upper part of the body, but experiences fatigue in the lower part of the body, so that he is unable to walk. Yet, his feet do not have the symptoms of palsy or swelling with pain, and his feet are not so weak. Since his physical condition is neither weak nor strong, neither cold nor heat, the disease belongs to the lumbar vertebral disease. The generalized fatigue and lassitude patient does not have the symptoms of severe chills with fever and aching of the body. If a greater yang patient displays the symptoms of severe chills with fever and aching of the body, it is because his lumbar vertebrae are rich in exterior qi. The disease can easily be cured, and the patient made healthy again.

解㑊者上體完健而下體解㑊然脚力不能行去也而其脚自無麻痺腫痛之證脚力亦不甚弱此所以弱不弱壯不壯寒不寒熱不熱而其病爲腰脊病也有解㑊證者必無大惡寒發熱身體疼痛之證也太陽人若有大惡寒發熱身體疼痛之證則腰脊表氣充實也其病易治其人亦完健

Discourse on the Greater Yang Person's Small Intestine Disease Induced by Endopathogen

太陽人內觸小腸病論

1 Zhu Zhenheng said, "*Yege* (Dysphagia) and *fanwei* (regurgitation of food from the stomach) are induced by the exhaustion of blood and fluid. This exhaustion causes a dry esophagus. If the upper part of the esophagus near the throat grows dry, the patient will most likely only be able to drink, not eat. If he is able to swallow food at all, it will only be in small amounts. This symptom is called *ye*. If the lower part of the esophagus near the stomach grows dry, the patient will be able to ingest food, but the food will not reach or stay in the stomach and be regurgitated. This symptom is called *ge* or regurgitation of food from the stomach. The patient also has constipation with dried fecal masses like goat's dung. Though their terms are different, their pathogenic factor is the same." Zhu Zhenheng also said, "Dysphagia of the upper-*jiao* shows pain in the epigastric region after food is taken. The patient regurgitates the food promptly, and the pain disappears. For dysphagia of the middle-*jiao*, though the food can be swallowed, it cannot enter the stomach and vomiting is delayed. Dysphagia of the lower-*jiao* shows vomiting in the afternoon what was taken in the morning, and vomiting in the morning of what was taken in the previous afternoon. Patients with deficiency of both qi and blood may foam at the mouth; and those who foam heavily at the mouth will die. A patient with dried fecal masses like goat's dung is hard to cure. He who does not take light food is also hard to cure."

朱震亨曰噎膈反胃之病血液俱耗胃脘乾槁其槁在上近咽則水飲可行食物難入入亦不多名之曰噎其槁在下近胃則食雖可入難盡入胃良久復出名之曰膈亦曰反胃大便秘少若羊屎然名雖不同病出一體又曰上焦噎膈食下則胃脘當心而痛須臾吐出食出痛乃止中焦噎膈食物可下難盡入胃良久復出下焦噎膈朝食暮吐暮食朝吐氣血俱虛者口中多出沫但見沫多出者必死大便如羊屎者難治不淡飲食者難治

2　Zhang Jihfeng[1] said, "*Ye* may stem from mental problems. Inward contemplation and self-cultivation can cure it."

張鷄峯曰噎當是神思間病惟內觀自養可以治之

3　In Gong Xin's 『*(Gujin) Yijian*』, we read, "Regurgitation of food from the stomach, *ge* and *ye* have the same pathogenic factor. The symptoms of dysphagia do not belong to a deficiency or an excess, cold or heat; but it is one of the diseases related to spiritual qi."

龔信醫鑑曰反胃也膈也噎也受病皆同噎膈之證不屬虛不屬實不屬冷不屬熱乃神氣中一點病耳

4　I have said, "This is the most serious case among the small intestine diseases in the greater yang persons. Only patients who avoid anger and eat plain food can be cured. We should apply Mihudeung Sikjang Tang (Chinese Gooseberry Stem Decoction for Planting Intestine)."

論曰此證卽太陽人小腸病太重證也必遠嗔怒斷厚味然後其病可愈此證當用獼猴藤植腸湯

5　The difficulty some people experience in swallowing food is called *ye*, while the difficulty some people experience in keeping food down is called *ge*. When a patient regurgitates in the afternoon what was taken in the morning, or regurgitates in the morning what was taken in the previous afternoon, his condition is called regurgitation of food from the stomach. However, when a patient regurgitates in the afternoon what was taken in the morning and regurgitates in the morning what was taken in the previous afternoon, not all the food comes up. When a patient spontaneously regurgitates in the morning what was taken in the previous afternoon, his illness is an obstruction located in the upper part of the stomach. Those symptoms are called regurgitation of food from the stomach or dysphagia. Generally, dysphagia is dysphagia in the esophageal region, and regurgitation of food from the stomach is dysphagia in the gastric region. In other words, they are the same disease. Inevitably, the patient with dysphagia does not have symptoms such as abdominal pain, borborygmus, diarrhea and dysentery. If the greater yang person has symptoms of abdominal pain, borborygmus, diarrhea and dysentery, it means that his interior qi of the small intestine is rich, making the disease easy to cure.

食物自外入而有所妨碍曰噎自內受而有所拒格曰膈朝食暮吐暮食朝吐曰反胃然朝食而暮吐暮食而朝吐者非全食皆吐也有所妨碍而拒格於胃之上口者經宿而自吐也則反胃亦噎膈也盖噎膈者胃脘之噎膈也反胃者胃口之噎膈也同是一證也有噎膈證者必無腹痛腸鳴泄瀉痢疾之證也太陽人若有腹痛腸鳴泄瀉痢疾之證則小腸裏氣充實也其病易治其人亦完健

6　Though both generalized fatigue and lassitude, and the dysphagia are serious symptoms, their relative seriousness can be identified. Generalized fatigue and lassitude without dysphagia is a mild type of generalized fatigue and lassitude. Dysphagia without dysphagia is mild type of dysphagia. A combination of generalized fatigue and lassitude and dysphagia represents a serious and dangerous condition; but among serious and dangerous conditions, there is also a relative seriousness. Since the quality of life of a greater yang patient with generalized fatigue and lassitude and dysphagia seems normal until he is practically at death's door, we are apt to treat him as a common case. Therefore, once his condition reaches the serious stage, it becomes very hard to cure him. Since I am possessed of a greater yang constitution, I once had this disease. I vomited foamy saliva from the mouth for six to seven years, and afterwards continuously paid attention to my health for several decades in order to avoid dying young. I thus report my case in order to alert all greater yang patients with the same disease. The advisable treatment, in one sentence, is "Just avoid anger."

解㑊噎膈俱是重證而重證之中有輕重之等級焉解㑊而無噎膈則解㑊之輕證也噎膈而無解㑊則噎膈之輕證也若解㑊兼噎膈噎膈兼解㑊則其爲重險之證不可勝言而重險中又有輕重也太陽人解㑊噎膈不至死境之前起居飲食如常人必易之視以例病故入於危境而莫可挽回也余稟臟太陽人嘗得此病六七年嘔吐涎沫數十年攝身倖而免夭錄此以爲太陽人有病者戒若論治法一言弊曰遠嗔怒而已矣

7   The greater yang person originally has a strong will and weak integrity. Since the strong will induces the qi of the esophagus to flow upward, and that qi which exhales and disperses becomes too great and overflows, and since weak integrity induces the qi of the small intestine to be stuck in the middle-*jiao*, and that qi which inhales and concentrates becomes exhausted and deficient, diseases such as dysphagia and regurgitation of food from the stomach are generated.

太陽人意强而操弱意强則胃脘之氣上達而呼散者太過而越也操弱則小腸之氣中熱而吸聚者不支而餒也所以其病爲噎膈反胃也

8   Someone once asked me, "Zhu Zhenheng said, 'Dysphagia and regurgitation of food from the stomach are induced by the exhaustion of blood and fluid which causes a dry esophagus, and such a patient is unable to swallow food.' What is your opinion on the subject?" I answered, "When food enters the stomach, the Spleen works with the stomach; when the food is sent to the large intestine, the Kidney works with the large intestine. So the Spleen and the Kidney are the storerooms, which promote the coming and going of food, and supplement and drain by turns. When the air and the fluid are exhaled from the epigastrium, the Lung works with it, and when the air and the fluid are inhaled by the small intestine, the Liver works with it. So the Lung and the Liver are the gates that promote the respiration of air and fluid, and act back and forth by turns. Therefore, if the power of the lesser yang person's large intestine, which expels the yin cold qi of food, is insufficient, the yang hot qi of food inside the stomach will inevitably prosper. If the power of the greater yang person's small intestine, which absorbs the yin cool qi of air and fluid, is insufficient, the yang warm qi of air and fluid in the epigastrium will inevitably prosper. If the yang warm qi of air and fluid in the epigastrium is too prosperous, the blood in the epigastric part will dry up. This is quite natural; however, the causes of the above diseases are not limited to dryness, but also include

a strong, upwardly exhaling qi and weak, inhaling qi in the middle-*jiao*. The result is an inability to swallow food and vomiting"

問朱震亨論噎膈反胃曰血液俱耗胃脘乾槁食物難入其說如何曰水穀納於胃而脾衛之出於大腸而腎衛之脾腎者出納水穀之府庫而迭爲補瀉者也氣液呼於胃脘而肺衛之吸於小腸而肝衛之肺肝者呼吸氣液之門戶而迭爲進退者也是故少陽人大腸出水穀陰寒之氣不足則胃中納水穀陽熱之氣必盛也太陽人小腸吸氣液陰凉之氣不足則胃脘呼氣液陽溫之氣必盛也胃脘陽溫之氣太盛則胃脘血液乾槁其勢固然也然非但乾槁而然也上呼之氣太過而中吸之氣太不支故食物不吸入而還呼出也

9 Someone once asked me, "How do you know that the dysphagia and regurgitation of food from the stomach mentioned by Zhu Zhenheng do not belong to the disease of the lesser yin, lesser yang, or greater yin person, and how did you conclude that they were, in fact, diseases of the greater yang person? Also, how do you know that the dysphagia mentioned in the 『*Neijing*』 does not belong to the disease of the lesser yin, lesser yang or greater yin person, and how did you conclude that it was, in fact, a disease of the greater yang person? Your conclusions are difficult to believe; please explain your position." I answered, "The vomiting of a lesser yang person must be induced by severe heat. The vomiting of a lesser yin person must be induced by severe cold. The vomiting of a greater yin person certainly brings about the release from the disease. However, dysphagia and regurgitation of food from the stomach are not manifest in cold or heat, deficiency or excess. Is it not, therefore, logical to conclude that those are the diseases of the greater yang person? The generalized fatigue and lassitude is the disease in which the patient's upper body is normally healthy, while his lower body suffers from fatigue. His shins ache, and he cannot walk. If a lesser yin, lesser yang or greater yin person has this disease; it must be in combination with other symptoms. There is no reason to have just fatigue without cold or heat, or deficiency or excess."

或曰朱震亨所論噎膈反胃者安知非少陰少陽太陰人病而吾子必名目曰太陽人病內經所論解㑊者安知非少陰少陽太陰人病而吾子必名目曰太陽人病莫非牽強附會耶願聞其說曰少陽人有嘔吐則必有大熱也少陰人有嘔吐則必有大寒也太陰人有嘔吐則必病愈也今此噎膈反胃不寒不熱非實非虛則此非太陽人病而何也解㑊者上體完健而下體解㑊然胻痠不能行去之謂也少陰少陽太陰人有此證則他證疊出而亦必無寒不寒熱不熱弱不弱壯不壯之理矣

10 Someone once asked me, "You have mentioned that the treatment for a greater yang person's generalized fatigue and lassitude was to refrain from feeling deep sorrow and sudden anger, and to secure peace of mind. You also mentioned that the treatment of a greater yang person's dysphagia was to avoid anger and eat plain food. I understand that generalized fatigue and lassitude is more serious than dysphagia in a greater yang person. Does this mean that, in a greater yang person, the disease induced by sorrow is more serious than the disease induced by anger?" I answered, "No. On the contrary, since dysphagia is far more serious than generalized fatigue and lassitude in a greater yang person, the damage caused by anger is more serious than that by sorrow in a greater yang person. Deepening sorrow in a greater yang person injures the exterior qi, and exploding anger injures the interior qi. Since the general-

ized fatigue and lassitude is an exterior disease, I advise patients to refrain from feeling deep sorrow and anger at the same time." I was asked again, "Then the angry nature of the lesser yang person injures the qi of the mouth and the bladder, and his sorrow injures the qi of the Kidney and the large intestine. The joyous nature of the lesser yin person injures the qi of the eyes and the paravertebral musculature of the back, and pleasure injures the qi of the Spleen and stomach. A greater yin person's feelings of pleasure injure the qi of the ears and the nape of the neck, and joy emotion injures the qi of the Lung and the epigastrium. Is that correct?" I replied, "Yes."

或曰吾子論太陽人解㑊病治法曰戒深哀遠嗔怒修清定論噎膈病治法曰遠嗔怒斷厚味意者太陽人解㑊病重於噎膈病而哀心所傷者重於怒心所傷乎曰否太陽人噎膈病太重於解㑊病而怒心所傷者太重於哀心所傷也太陽人哀心深着則傷表氣怒心暴發則傷裡氣故解㑊表證以戒哀遠怒兼言之也曰然則少陽人怒性傷口膀胱氣哀情傷腎大腸氣少陰人樂性傷目膂氣喜情傷脾胃氣太陰人喜性傷耳腦顀頁氣樂情傷肺胃脘氣乎曰然

11 The stool of greater yang person should be first, smooth, and, second, large in its shape and quantity. Their urine should be first, copious, and next, frequent. Their complexion should be pale, not dark. Their flesh should be thin, not fatty. There should be no hard mass in the pit of the stomach. If the mass is small, it can be easily extinguished; if it is large, the disease will become serious, and the mass will prove difficult to reduce.

太陽人大便一則宜滑也二則宜體大而多也小便一則宜多也二則宜數也面色宜白不宜黑肌肉宜瘦不宜肥鳩尾下不宜有塊塊小則病輕而其塊易消塊大則病重而其塊難消

Notes

1) Zhang Jihfeng (張鷄峰)

His history is not well documented. His theory was recorded in the 『*Danxi Xinfa*』 (丹溪心法) and quoted in the 『*Dongui Bogam*』

Ten Recommended Herbs
for the Greater Yang Person's Disease
(Mentioned in the "Materia Medica")
Based on My Experiences, and Two Herbs Based
on the Experiences of Li Chan and Gong Xin

本草所載太陽人病經驗要藥單方十種及
李梴龔信經驗要藥單方二種

1 In the "Materia Medica", we read that Acanthopanacis Cortex cures the arthralgia of the lower limbs, contraction of the near joints, flaccidity and lameness. There once was a crippled three year old child, who, after taking this herb, was able to walk again.

· Pine knots (Pini Lignum Nodi) cure flaccidity of the lower limbs.

· Chaenomelis Fructus stops vomiting. To drink its decoction or its freshly squeezed juice is best.

· Vitis Viniferae Radix stop hiccups. To drink the decoction in high concentration is best.

· Actinidiae Fructus cures regurgitation of food from the stomach due to the blockage of heat. Drink the sap. The vine's sap is a great lubricant, and controls the blockage of the stomach, which induces vomiting. It is very good to drink its decoction.

· Phragmitis Rhizoma cures retching and five kinds of dysphagia with dysphoria. Take a 1.804 liter decoction of Phragmitis Rhizoma 187.5g at a draught. The patient shall recover by the time he has ingested 5.6 liters.

· Shells (Solen gouldii) cure regurgitation and vomiting.

· Crucian cures regurgitation.

· Water shields (Bracenia Schreberi) is cooked with crucian and made into a soup. This cures regurgitation and the inability to swallow, and stops vomiting.

· Fagopyri Semen reinforces the intestine and stomach, and invigorates the energy (physical strength).

本草曰五加皮治兩脚疼痺骨節攣急痿躄小兒三歲不能行服此便行走
松節療脚軟弱

木瓜止嘔逆煮汁飲之最佳
葡萄根止嘔噦濃煎取汁細細飲之佳
獼猴桃治熱壅反胃取汁服之藤汁至滑主胃閉吐逆煎取汁服之甚佳
蘆根治乾嘔噦及五噎煩悶蘆根五兩水煎頓服一升不過三升即差
蚌蛤治反胃吐食
鯽魚治反胃
蓴和鯽魚作羹食之主反胃食不下止嘔
蕎麥實腸胃益氣力

2   Li Chan said that bran (on the pestle) cures dysphagia, the inability to swallow and obstructed throats. Pound the above drug into a powder and take it with rice gruel.
李梴曰杵頭糠主噎食不下咽喉塞細糠一兩白粥清調服

3   Gong Xin said that shells cure regurgitation.
龔信曰螃蛤治反胃

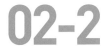

Two Newly Formulated Prescriptions Applicable to the Greater Yang Person's Disease

新定太陽人病應用設方藥二方

1 Acanthopanax Decoction for Strengthening Spine (Ogapi Jangcheok Tang)
- · Acanthopanacis Cortex 15g
- · Chaenomelis Fructus 7.5g
- · Pini Lignum Nodi 7.5g
- · Vitis Viniferae Radix 3.75g
- · Phragmitis Rhizoma 3.75g
- · Pruni Semen 3.75g
- · Fagopyri Semen half of a spoon

If no Pini Lignum Nodi can be found, the newborn sprout of a pine can be used instead. This prescription cures the exterior pattern.

五加皮壯脊湯

五加皮四錢木瓜青松節各二錢葡萄根蘆根櫻桃肉各一錢蕎麥米半匙

青松節關材則以好松葉代之此方治表證

2 Chinese Gooseberry Stem Decoction for Planting Intestine (Mihudeung Sikjang Tang)
- · Actinidiae Fructus 15g
- · Chaenomelis Fructus 7.5g
- · Vitis Viniferae Radix 7.5g
- · Phragmitis Rhizoma 3.75g
- · Pruni Semen 3.75g
- · Acanthopanacis Cortex 3.75g
- · Bran (on the pestle) half of a spoon
- · Pine flower 3.75g

If there is no Actinidiae Fructus, its vine can be used instead. This prescription cures the interior pattern.

獼猴藤植腸湯

獼猴桃四錢木瓜葡萄根各二錢蘆根櫻桃肉五加皮松花各一錢杵頭糖半匙

獼猴桃關材則以藤代之此方治裏證

3   Generally, fruits and vegetables have a clear and plain taste, so they belong to the medicinal ingredient for the Liver. Shells also have a medicine value for the Liver; specifically, they invigorate it.

凡菜果之屬清平疏淡之藥皆爲肝藥蛤屬亦補肝

4   I have said, "People lack experience with these drugs because they have little experience treating these diseases. Greater yang person are so few in number that descriptions of greater yang person's diseases and of the drugs used for treatment are rare. Ogapi Jangcheok Tang and Mihudeung Sikjang Tang are simple and not at all satisfactory. If, however, a greater yang person contracts a disease, and we are able to create a new prescription based on the principles of those two drugs, why should we worry about the scarcity of available prescriptions?"

論曰藥驗不廣者病驗不廣故也太陽人數從古稀少故古方書中所載證藥亦稀少也今此五加皮壯脊湯獼猴藤植腸湯立方草草雖欠不博而若使太陽人有病者因是二方詳究其理而又變通置方則何患乎無好藥哉

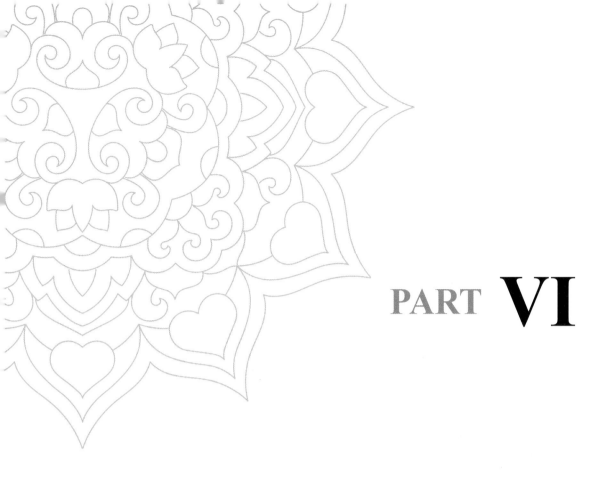

PART VI

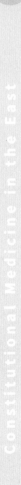

Constitutional Medicine in the East

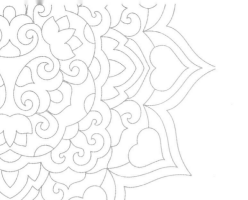

01

Discourse
on General Health Maintenance

廣濟說

1   The period from the age of 1 to 16 is called childhood; from 17 to 32, young adulthood; from 33 to 48, prime of adulthood; and from 49 to 64, the aged.
初一歲至十六歲曰幼十七歲至三十二歲曰少三十三歲至四十八歲曰壯四十九歲至六十四歲曰老

2   Children, like new spring buds, long for knowledge and information, and love and respect others. Young adults esteem bravery and daring, and flourish and shoot up swiftly, like the young trees of summer. Adults enjoy making friends and allowing life to ripen, like the fruits of autumn. The aged prefer orderliness, and can keep secrets, like the roots of winter.
凡人幼年好聞見而能愛敬如春生之芽少年好勇猛而能騰捷如夏長之苗壯年好交結而能修飭如秋歛之實老年好計策而能秘密如冬藏之根

3   The child who likes to study is the most admired among children; the young adult who respects the aged is the most admired among young adults; the adult who can love others broadly is the most admired among adults; and the elderly person who protects and encourages the righteous is the most admired among old people. He who has genuine abilities and, moreover, a good heart is the real hero. There are, however, people who are possessed of genuine abilities, but lack a good heart.
幼年好文字者幼年之豪傑也少年敬長老者少年之豪傑也壯年能汎愛者壯年之豪傑也老年保可人者老年之豪傑也有好才能而又有十分快足於好心術者眞豪傑也有好才能而終不十分快足於好心術者才能而已

4 Before the age of seven or eight, the child may become ill when constrained by the four emotions - joy, anger, sorrow and pleasure - due to a lack of information and knowledge. The affectionate mother should take care of such a child. Before the age of 24 or 25, the young adult may become ill when he is constrained by the four emotions - joy, anger, sorrow and pleasure - due to a lack of bravery and daring. The wise father and able brother should take care of him. Concerning a man before the age of 38 or 39, he should be helped by a sensible younger brother and his good friends. Concerning a man before the age of 56 or 57, he should be encouraged by his dutiful sons and grandsons.

幼年七八歲前聞見未及而喜怒哀樂膠着則成病也慈母宜保護之也少年二十四五歲前勇猛未及而喜怒哀樂膠着則成病也智父能兄宜保護之也壯年三十八九歲前則賢弟良朋可以助之也老年五十六七歲前則孝子孝孫可以扶之也

5 The good man, who is admirable, attracts good people to his family, while the bad man, who is disreputable, attracts bad people to his family. When many good people gather together, their qi is activated. When many bad people gather together, their qi is aroused. A family where bad men have gathered to engage in drink, sensual pleasures, and the pursuit of wealth and power can easily make dutiful sons and wives ill.

善人之家善人必聚惡人之家惡人必聚善人多聚則善人之臟氣活動惡人多聚則惡人之心氣强旺酒色財權之家惡人多聚故其家孝男孝婦受病

6 In a family where people hunger for power, factions are created, and it is these factions that destroy the family. In a family where people hunger for wealth, sons become haughty and stupid, and it is they who eventually destroy the family.

好權之家朋黨比周敗其家者朋黨也好貨之家子孫驕愚敗其家者子孫也

7 In a family where all work ends in vain, illness remains constant, and good and evil are struggling with each other, collapse is certain. In such circumstances, only the wise and affectionate father and dutiful son have the means to solve this problem.

人家凡事不成疾病連綿善惡相持其家將敗之地惟明哲之慈父孝子處之有術也

8 Overindulgence in luxury can decrease one's life span. Laziness can decrease one's life span. Prejudice can decrease one's life span. Greediness can decrease one's life span. The overindulgent man will surely abandon himself to sensual pleasures. The lazy man will surely give himself up to drinking. The prejudiced man will surely fight for power. The greedy man will surely die for the pursuit of money.

嬌奢減壽懶怠減壽偏急減壽貪慾減壽爲人嬌奢必耽侈色爲人懶怠必嗜酒食爲人偏急必爭權勢爲人貪慾必殉貨財

9 Simplicity allows one to live one's natural life span. Diligence allows one to live one's natural

life span. Self-control allows one to live one's natural life span. Integrity allows one to live one's natural life span. The simple man avoids sensual pleasures. The diligent man avoids drinking. The deliberate man avoids pursuing power. The man with integrity avoids pursuing wealth.

簡約得壽勤幹得壽警戒得壽聞見得壽爲人簡約必遠侈色爲人勤幹必潔酒食爲人警戒必避權勢爲人聞見必淸貨財

10 Overindulgence makes one's living quarters dreary. Overdrinking makes one's behavior clumsy. Fighting for power makes one's mind anguished. Pursuing wealth creates disorder in appointed roles.

居處荒凉色之故也行身闒茸酒之故也用心煩亂權之故也事務錯亂貨之故也

11 When a man respects the gentle woman, sensual pleasure can be enjoyed in the right way. When a man loves his good friends, drinking together can lead to virtue. When a man respects the wise man, his pursuit of power can lead to the proper course of action. When a man cares for the poor, his wealth is put to proper use.

若敬淑女色得中道若愛良朋酒得明德若尙賢人權得正術若保窮民貨得全功

12 These four pursuits - overdrinking, sensual pleasures, wealth and power from ancient times were compared to the constraints of four walls, and to a jail. Not only a man's longevity or a family's fortune, but also the maintenance of society, depends upon refraining from these four vices. Therefore, if we allow society to fall into the trap of these four vices, we will revert to the troubled eras of Yao, Shun, and the Southern States of Zhou and Shao.

酒色財權自古所戒謂之四堵墻而比之牢獄非但一身壽夭一家禍福之所繫也天下治亂亦在於此若使一天下酒色財權無乖戾之氣則庶幾近於堯舜周召南之世矣

13 Generally, a man has to pursue simplicity, diligence, self-control and integrity. If someone has these four, he automatically can enjoy his full life span. If he is possessed of simplicity, diligence and self-control, or integrity, self-control and diligence, his life span will be shorter than who has all four qualities. More examples of people are those who are both overindulgent in luxury and yet diligent, or self-controlled and yet greedy, or simple and yet lazy, or prejudiced and yet honest. If they are cautious, then they may enjoy a long life. If they are neglectful, however, they will die young.

凡人簡約而勤幹警戒而聞見四材圓全者自然上壽簡約勤幹而警戒或聞見警戒而勤幹三材全者次壽嬌奢而勤幹警戒而貪慾或簡約而懶怠偏急而聞見二材全者恭敬則壽怠慢則夭

14 Generally, a cautious man will live long, a neglectful man will die young, a diligent man will live long, and a greedy man will die young. If a hungry man, upon receiving food, eats it hastily, the qi of his intestines will be disturbed. When a poor man suddenly gets money,

his life will be disturbed. Even though a man is hungry, if he is content, the qi of his intestines will be in order. Even though a man is poor, if he is content, his inner strength will be preserved. If one can bear hunger and not refrain from eating greedily, it is laudable. If one can bear the cold, and not indulge in too many warm clothes, it is laudable. If one uses one's physical strength for labors, and does not live in idleness, it is laudable. If one can gain through diligence, and not wait for windfall, it is laudable.

凡人恭敬則必壽怠慢則必夭謹勤則必壽虛貪則必夭飢者之腸急於得食則腸氣蕩矣貧者之骨急於得財則骨力竭矣飢而安飢則腸氣有守貧而安貧則骨力有立是故飲食以能忍飢而不貪飽爲恭敬衣服以能耐寒而不貪溫爲恭敬筋力以能勤勞而不貪安逸爲恭敬財物以能謹實而不貪苟得爲恭敬

15 The man who lives in the mountains without integrity will die young. The man who lives in the city without simplicity will die young. The man living in the countryside without diligence will die young. The intellectual man without self-control will also die young.

山谷之人沒聞見而禍夭市井之人沒簡約而禍夭農畝之人沒勤幹而禍夭讀書之人沒警戒而禍夭

16 The man living in the mountains must have integrity; if he has integrity, he will live long and prosper. The man living in the city must have simplicity; if he has simplicity, he will live long and prosper. The man living in the countryside must be diligent; if he is diligent, he will live long and prosper. The intellectual man must have self-control; if he has self-control, he will live long and prosper.

山谷之人宜有聞見有聞見則福壽市井之人宜有簡約有簡約則福壽鄉野之人宜有勤幹有勤幹則福壽士林之人宜有警戒有警戒則福壽

17 If a man living in the mountains has integrity, not only will he live long and prosper, but he will also be the most distinguished man in that area. If a man living in the city has simplicity, not only will he live long and prosper, but he will also be the most distinguished man in the city. If a man who lives in the countryside has diligence, not only will he live long and prosper, but he will also be the most distinguished man in that area. If an intellectual man has self-control, not only will he live long and prosper, but he will also be the most distinguished man among intellectuals.

山谷之人若有聞見非但福壽也此人即山谷之傑也市井之人若有簡約非但福壽也此人即市井之傑也鄉野之人若有勤幹非但福壽也此人即鄉野之傑也士林之人若有警戒非但福壽也此人即士林之傑也

18 Someone once asked me, "The farmer cultivates his land with his physical strength, so he must be diligent. Why do you say he is not diligent? Likewise, the intellectual studies very hard, and is self-controlled. Why do you say he is not self-controlled?" I answered, "The farmer is always anxious that he cannot cultivate one hundred Mau. If he were truly diligent, there would be no need for him to be anxious. Thus, compared to the intellectual, the farmer

is actually idle. The intellectual, however, studies hard and becomes arrogant in his learning; whereas the farmer is ignorant of book learning, and must always remain cautious. Thus, compared to the farmer, the intellectual lacks self-control. If, however, the farmer learns how to study from the intellectual, and the intellectual learns how to perform physical labors from the farmer, their abilities and characters will develop, and their organic qi strengthen."

或曰農夫元來力作最是勤幹者也而何謂沒勤幹士人元來讀書最是警戒者也而何謂沒警戒耶曰以百畝之不治爲己憂者農夫之任也農夫而比之士人則眞是懶怠者也士人頗讀書故心恒妄矜農夫目不識字故心恒佩銘士人而擬之農夫則眞不警戒者也若農夫謹於識字士人習於力作則才性調密臟氣堅固

19 The overindulgent man looks down on ordinary life and makes light of domestic life. He is surrounded by luxury, and does not understand the difficulties of earning a living. He lacks the proper skills for acquiring property. He is always overindulgent in sensual pleasures, and never feels any regret to the end of his life.

嬌奢者之心藐視閭閻生活輕易天下室家眼界驕豪全昧産業之艱難甚劣財力之方畧每爲女色所陷終身不悔

20 A lazy man is very crude and refuses to work diligently. He spends his time dreaming idly. He is generally unwilling to work hard, and so takes to drink; rarely are lazy men not also drunkards. When we see such drunken men, we are able to understand just how crude the lazy man's mind is.

懶怠者之心極其麤猛不欲積功之寸累每有虛大之甕算盖其心甚憚勤幹故欲逃其身於酒國以姑避勤幹之計也凡懶怠者無不縱酒但見縱酒者則必知其爲懶怠人心麤猛也

22 The sensual man will certainly be attracted to the lewd woman, and likewise, the lewd woman will be attracted to the sensualist. The foolish man will certainly be attracted to the jealous woman, and the jealous woman will likewise be attracted to the foolish man. According to the law of nature, the lewd woman is a proper partner for the sensual man, and the foolish man is also a proper partner for the jealous woman. Generally, women both lewd and jealous are well suited to vulgar, not noble, men. Among the seven valid reasons for divorce, lewd and jealous behavior is the worst. Most people, however, do not understand the meaning of jealousy. They think jealousy refers to the hatred of a wife for her husband's many concubines, but for a noble man to have a son is the most important thing. Thus, his wife should not be jealous or hateful towards her husband's concubines. However, since the cause of turmoil in a family is often due to there being many concubines, a wife who is jealous and hateful of the bad behavior of these concubines displaces wisdom. So how can we say that these two kinds of jealousy are the same? In the 『*Shijing*』 ("Classic of Poetry"), we read the following verse: "The peach tree beams so red; Its leaves are lush and green. The maiden's getting wed; On household she'll be keen." 'On household she'll be keen' means that women

love wisdom, follow virtue, and are keen on their family duties. Not being keen on family means being jealous of the wise and the able, and not being keen on family duties. Generally, if the husband is foolish, and the wife is jealous of the wise and able, illness will continuously plague the family, death will follow, sons will become fools, and property will be lost.

狂童必愛淫女淫女亦愛狂童愚夫必愛妒婦妒婦亦愛愚夫以物理觀之則淫女斷合狂童之配也愚夫亦宜妒婦之匹也盖淫女妒婦可以爲惡人賤人之配匹也不可以爲君子貴人之配匹也七去惡中淫去妒去爲首惡而世俗不知妒字之義但以憎疾衆妾爲言貴人之繼嗣最重則婦人必不可憎疾貴人之有妾而亂家之本未嘗不在於衆妾則婦人之憎疾衆妾之邪媚者猶爲婦人之賢德也何所當於妒字之義乎詩云桃之夭夭其葉蓁蓁之子于歸宜其家人宜其家人者好賢樂善而宜於家人之謂也不宜其家人者妒賢嫉能而不宜於家人之謂也凡人家疾病連綿死亡相隨子孫愚蚩資産零落者莫非愚夫妒婦妒賢嫉能之所做出也

21 It is said that overdrinking and overindulging in sexual pleasures kill men. As alcohol poisoning dries out the intestines, so does sexual overindulgence dry up the essence of a body. People who say this, however, fail to understand completely. Drunkards, in fact, loathe physical labors, and their worries are as great as mountains. He who is blinded by lust experiences anxieties that cut him like a knife. Such overindulgence in drinking and sexual pleasure break a man's mental vitality, while alcohol poisoning and sexual exhaustion attack his body. Together, they can kill a man.

酒色之殺人者人皆曰酒毒枯腸色勞竭精云此知其一未知其二也縱酒者厭勤其身憂患如山惑色者深愛其女憂患如刀萬端心曲與酒毒色勞並力攻之而殺人也

23 Being jealous of the wise and the able is the worst thing in the world. Loving wisdom and following virtue is the best thing in the world. He, who harbors no jealousy of the wise and the able, though he may perform some bad acts, is actually not such a bad person. He, who harbors no love of wisdom and does not follow virtue, though he may perform some good actions, is actually not such a good person. It is considered that all the diseases in the world come from being jealous of the wise and the able, and the cure for all the diseases in the world depends on having respect for wisdom and following virtue. Therefore, being jealous of the wise and the able is the most prevalent disease in the world, and respecting the wise and following virtue is the greatest medicine in the world.

天下之惡莫多於妒賢嫉能天下之善莫大於好賢樂善不妒賢嫉能而爲惡則惡必不多也不好賢樂善而爲善則善必不大也歷稽往牒天下之受病都出於妒賢嫉能天下之救病都出於好賢樂善故曰妒賢嫉能天下之多病也好賢樂善天下之大藥也

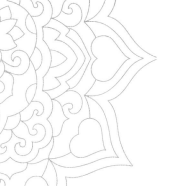

02

Discourse
on Identifying the Four Constitutions

四象人辨證論

1 In a town of 10,000 people, half will be of the greater yin type. Three thousand will be of the lesser yang type, and two thousand of the lesser yin type. Only three to ten or more people will be of the greater yang type.

太少陰陽人以今時目見一縣萬人數大畧論之則太陰人五千人也少陽人三千人也少陰人二千人也太陽人數絕少一縣中或三四人十餘人而已

2 The greater yang person has a developed nape for the rising posture and a slender waist for the standing posture. The lesser yang person has a developed chest for the self-embracing posture and small hips for the sitting posture. The greater yin person has a thick waist for the standing posture and a weak nape for the rising posture. The lesser yin person has developed hips for the sitting posture and a weak chest for the self-embracing posture.

太陽人體形氣像腦顀頁之起勢盛壯而腰圍之立勢孤弱少陽人體形氣像胸襟之包勢盛壯而膀胱之坐勢孤弱太陰人體形氣像腰圍之立勢盛壯而腦顀頁之起勢孤弱少陰人體形氣像膀胱之坐勢盛壯而胸襟之包勢孤弱

3 The greater yang person is skilled at communicating and has a talent for social acquaintances. The lesser yang person has a warrior mentality and a talent for appointed roles. The greater yin person is skilled at accomplishments and has a talent for living quarters. The lesser yin person is skilled at good conduct and has a talent for clanships.

太陽人性質長於疏通而材幹能於交遇少陽人性質長於剛武而材幹能於事務太陰人性質長於成就而材幹能於居處少陰人性質長於端重而材幹能於黨與

4   The greater yang person's body is easily recognizable, but because they are very rare, they are the most difficult to identify. Greater yang people's napes are developed, and they communicate well. They have a determined character, but have dysphagia, regurgitation of food from the stomach and generalized fatigue and lassitude, so they are easy to identify. Until their illness becomes serious, they appear to be normal. The elderly lesser yin person also may have generalized fatigue and lassitude, so we should not confuse him with the greater yang person.

太陽人體形元不難辨而人數稀罕故最爲難辨也其體形腦佳頁之起勢强旺性質疏通又有果斷其病噎膈反胃解㑊證亦自易辨而病未至重險之前別無大證完若無病壯健人也少陰人老人亦有噎證不可誤作太陽人治

5   The body of the greater yang female is big and strong, but since she has a small Liver, narrow waist, and her uterus function is weak, she can seldom give birth. We can easily see this to be true by noticing the greater yang mare and cow-though their bodies are big and strong, they too seldom are able to give birth.

太陽女體形壯實而肝小脇窄子宮不足故鮮能生產以六畜玩理而太陽牝牛馬體形壯實而亦鮮能生產者其理可推

6   The lesser yang person has a developed upper body and weak lower body, his chest is well developed, and his feet are light. He is quick, sharp and brave. Since lesser yang person are numerous, they are the most easily identified among the four types.

少陽人體形上盛下虛胸實足輕剽銳好勇而人數亦多四象人中最爲易辨

7   Since some lesser yang person, like lesser yin person, are small and smart in appearance, we must carefully observe their symptoms, such as chills and fever, and not confuse them with the lesser yin types.

少陽人或有短小靜雅外形恰似少陰人者觀其病勢寒熱仔細執證不可誤作少陰人治

8   Greater yin and lesser yin persons are similar in body shape and thus are difficult to distinguish, but if we diagnose the symptoms carefully, we can distinguish them clearly. When the greater yin person spontaneously sweats, he is healthy, but if the lesser yin person has spontaneous sweating, he is seriously ill. If the skin of the greater yin person is too solid and hard, he will have a serious illness. If the skin of the lesser yin person is very solid, he will be healthy. The greater yin person tends to have severe palpitations and chest pains, and the lesser yin person tends to exhibit restless involuntary movement of the limbs. The corners of the greater yin person's eyes tend to turn upward, and he often experiences eye pain. The lesser yin type does not have the same characteristics. The lesser yin type generally breathes smoothly, but sometimes sighs deeply. The greater yin type, on the other hand, does not sigh deeply. If the two get malaria with chills, the greater yin is able to drink cold water, but the lesser yin cannot. The greater yin's pulse is long and tight, while the lesser yin's is smooth and

weak. The greater yin person's flesh is solid, while the lesser yin person's is tender. The greater yin person is gentle in appearance and inarticulate in speech, but persistent and well behaved. The lesser yin person's appearance is neat, his speech natural, and his behavior shrewd.

太陰少陰人體形或暑相彷彿難辨疑似而觀其病證則必無不辨太陰人虛汗則完實也少陰人虛汗則大病也太陰人陽剛堅密則大病也少陰人陽剛堅密則完實也太陰人有胸膈怔忡證也少陰人有手足悗亂證也太陰人有目眥上引證又有目睛內疼證也少陰人則無此證也少陰人平時呼吸平均而間有一太息呼吸也太陰人則無此太息呼吸也太陰人瘧疾惡寒中能飲冷水少陰人瘧疾惡寒中不飲冷水太陰人脈長而緊少陰人脈緩而弱太陰人肌肉堅實少陰人肌肉浮軟太陰人容貌詞氣起居有儀而修整正大少陰人容貌詞氣體任自然而簡易小巧

9 Lesser yin persons are generally short, but some of them may be six to seven feet tall. As for the greater yin persons, they are usually tall, but some of them are five feet or shorter.

少陰人體形矮短而亦多有長大者或有八九尺長大者太陰人體形長大而亦或有六尺矮短者

10 The greater yin person always has a fearful mind. If he achieves peace of mind, he will also achieve stability and harmony. If he is too fearful, his mind will worsen, and he will experience severe palpitations. Severe palpitations are a serious problem for the greater yin person.

太陰人恒有怯心怯心寧靜則居之安資之深而造於道也怯心益多則放心桎梏而物化之也若怯心至於怕心則大病作而怔忡也怔忡者太陰人病之重證也

11 The lesser yang person always suffers from anxiety. If he achieves peace of mind, he will also achieve stability and harmony. If he is too anxious, his mind will be bound. If his anxiety becomes extreme, he will become seriously ill and experience amnesia, a serious problem for the lesser yang person.

少陽人恒有懼心懼心寧靜則居之安資之深而造於道也懼心益多則放心桎梏而物化之也若懼心至於恐心則大病作而健忘也健忘者少陽人病之險證也

12 The lesser yin person always has a nervous mind. If his nervous mind becomes stable, then his Spleen qi will be activated. The greater yang person always has a rash personality. If he can slow down his pace, his Liver blood will become regulated.

少陰人恒有不安定之心不安定之心寧靜則脾氣卽活也太陽人恒有急迫之心急迫之心寧靜則肝血卽和也

13 The lesser yin person has problems with his pharynx and larynx. Those problems are serious and chronic. We should not let these problems go untreated, but administer Shengui Bawu Tang (Decoction of Eight Ingredients with Ginseng and Cinnamon Twig), roe liver or gold snake liquor.

少陰人有咽喉證其病太重而爲緩病也不可等間任置當用蔘桂八物湯或用獐肝金蛇酒

14 Some greater yang person may have constipation for eight or nine days. This indicates nothing too serious, and so is nothing to worry too much about. However, we still must not ignore it. We can treat it with Mihudeung Ogapi Tang (Decoction of Chinese Gooseberry Stem and Acanthopanax).

太陽人有八九日大便不通證其病非殆證也不必疑惑而亦不可無藥當用獼猴藤五加皮湯

15 If the greater yang person passes a lot of urine, he is very healthy. If the greater yin person sweats a lot, he is very healthy. If the lesser yang person's bowel movements are smooth, he is very healthy. If the lesser yin person's digestion is good, he is very healthy.

太陽人小便旺多則完實而無病太陰人汗液通暢則完實而無病少陽人大便善通則完實而無病少陰人飲食善化則完實而無病

16 When the greater yang person gets dysphagia, the upper-*jiao* of the epigastrium feels like a harsh wind is passing through. When the greater yin person gets dysentery, the middle-*jiao* of the small intestine feels obstructed, as if by dense fog. When the lesser yang person gets constipation, then his diaphragm will surely feel like fire. When the lesser yin person has continuous diarrheas, the hypogastric region surely feels as cold as ice. If we know the person's type and the patterns of his symptoms, there will be no uncertainty in prescribing the proper medicine.

太陽人噎膈則胃脘之上焦散豁如風太陰人痢病則小腸之中焦窒塞如霧少陽人大便不通則胸膈必如烈火少陰人泄瀉不止則臍下必如氷冷明知其人而又明知其證則應用之藥必無可疑

17 We must identify the person's constitution very carefully by observing his appearance. If we fail after several attempts, we can identify his type clearly by referring to the patterns of symptoms. Only after ascertaining the patient's nature can we prescribe medicine. We must not even prescribe a single pack of medicine carelessly, for a single pack may kill a seriously ill patient.

人物形容仔細商量再三推移如有迷惑則參互病證明見無疑然後可以用藥最不可輕忽而一貼藥誤投重病險證一貼藥必殺人

18 Hua Tuo said, "The key to a healthy life lies in engaging in moderate labors, and avoiding excessive fatigue." An elderly man once said, "People may eat twice a day, but should not eat four or five times a day. People should not continue to eat after meals. If you follow those instructions, you will have a long life."

華佗曰養生之術每欲小勞但莫大疲有一老人曰人可日再食而不四五食也又不可既食後添食如此則必無不壽

19 I have added, "I would like to say that the greater yin person always calms his fearful mind by looking outside himself. The lesser yang person always calms his anxious mind by looking

within. The greater yang person slows down his rash mind by taking one step back. The lesser yin person can calm his nervous mind by moving one step forward. In this way, all four types may live a long life."

余足之曰太陰人察於外而恒寧靜怵心少陽人察於內而恒寧靜懼心太陽人退一步而恒寧靜急迫之心少陰人進一步而恒寧靜不安定之心如此則必無不壽

20 Again, I have said, "The greater yang person should be careful not to be angry or sorrowful. The lesser yang person should be careful not to become sorrowful or angry. The greater yin person should be careful not to be excessively joyful or pleased. The lesser yin person should be careful not to be excessively pleased or joyful. In this way, all four types may live a long life."

又曰太陽人恒戒怒心哀心少陽人恒戒哀心怒心太陰人恒戒樂心喜心少陰人恒戒喜心樂心如此則必無不壽

21 The great King Shun was willing to learn farming, pottery and fishing from others. Confucius said, "Among three men walking together, there will surely be at least one teacher." Accordingly, we can say that the sage studies widely, learns carefully from many people, integrates his knowledge, and thus becomes great. Each constitution has its own strong point in intelligence and talents. Therefore, in each field - the arts of writing, calligraphy, archery, equestrianism, singing, dancing, etiquette, *baduk* (Go) and *janggi* (Korean chess) - there are differences in techniques, as well. All these various techniques are harmonized together and used to form society.

大舜自畊稼陶漁無非取諸人以爲善夫子曰三人行必有我師以此觀之則天下衆人之才能聖人必博學審問而兼之故大而化也太少陰陽人識見才局各有所長文筆射御歌舞揖讓以至於博奕小技細鎖動作凡百做造面面不同皆異其妙儘乎衆人才能之浩多於造化中也

22 The 『*Lingshu*』 also suggested constitution ideas according to the four types and the five phases, but it only referred to the body's outer appearance, and neglected the principles of the internal organs. People in those ancient times recognized that there were four types, but they could not identify them in detail.

靈樞書中有太少陰陽五行人論而畧得外形未得臟理盖太少陰陽人早有古昔之見而未盡精究也

Identifying the Four Constitutions

	Greater Yang	Lesser Yang	Greater Yin	Lesser Yin
Population	very rare	30 %	50 %	20 %
General figure	developed nape of the neck slender waist	developed chest small hips	thick waist weak nape of the neck	developed hips weak chest
Face	large & thin shiny eyes wide	small thin lips narrow jaws protruding	rounded looks serious	smart
Skin	soft	dry & thin	solid	tender
Walking	unstable	unstable	heavy & gentle	stable
Characters	creative positive progressive charismatic heroic rash mind	unstable easily gets bored extrovert sacrificing righteous easily acceptable hot tempered anxious mind	gentle commercial endurable humorous insidious coward fearful mind	neat negative mild introvert intelligent systematic selfish jealous narrow-minded nervous mind
Healthy sign	urination	bowel movement	perspiration	digestion
Pulse		rapid & floating	long & tight	smooth & weak

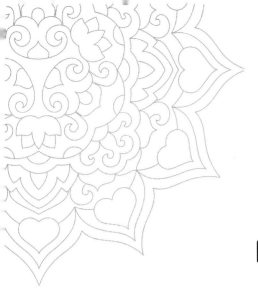

03

Epilogue

跋文

For almost a year, I devoted myself solely to the writing of this book, working day and night, without interruption, from July 13, 1893 to April 13, 1894. I have described lesser yang and lesser yin persons in detail, but was not able to do the same for greater yin and greater yang person due to both a lack of experience and exhaustion from writing this book. In the 『*Liji*』 1) ("Record of Rites"), we read, "If you cannot understand what you read, then you must think for yourself." If you are able to understand the theories underlying the greater yin and greater yang types through your own efforts, then my own rough explanations need not be consulted. If there is but one potter in a town of ten thousand people, he will not be able to meet the needs of the entire town; and if there is only one doctor in a village of one hundred families, he will not be able to meet the medical needs of the village. Likewise, if we can spread the ideas of medical science and see to it that every family understands medical science, and that every person understands disease, then all will have good health and a long life.

(On April 13, 1894, Lee Je-ma finished this work at Namsan in Seoul. The next year, he returned to his hometown, Hamheung city. From 1895 to 1900, he revised his writings and modified the manuscript from the "Discourse on Nature and Order" to the discourses on the greater yin person. He did not have the chance to modify the last three discourses.)

此書自癸巳七月十三日始作晝思夜度無頃刻休息至于翌年甲午四月十三日少陰少陽人論則畧得詳備太陰太陽人論則僅成簡約盖經驗未遍而精力已憊故也記曰開而不達則思若太陰太陽人思而得之則亦何損乎簡約哉萬室之邑一人陶則器不足也百家之村一人醫則活人不足也必廣明醫學家家知醫人人知病然後可以壽世保元

光緒甲午四月十三日咸興李濟馬畢書于漢南山中

公甲午畢書後乙未下鄉至于庚子因本改草自性明論至太陰人諸論各有增刪而太陽人以下三論未有增刪

Notes

1) 『*Liji*』(禮記)

The "Record of Rites", one of the Five Classics of Chinese Confucian literature, the original text of which is said to have been compiled by the ancient sage Confucius himself. In general, the 『*Liji*』 underscores the moral principles in such subjects as royal regulations, rites, ritual objects and sacrifices, education, music, the behaviors of scholars, and the doctrine of the mean. In 1190, Zhu Xi, a Neo-Confucian philosopher, took two chapters from the 『*Liji*』, gave them separate titles, and published them together with two other Confucian texts under the name 『*Sishu*』 (四書: "Four Books"). This collection is generally used to introduce Chinese students to Confucian literature.

Selected Bibliography

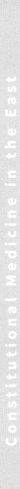

Classical Sources

(Chinese-Language)

1. Chen Shiwen et al. (陳師文等). Formularies of the Bureau of People's Welfare Pharmacies (*Taiping Huimin Heji Jufang* 太平惠民和劑局方). Beijing: People's Health Press, 1959. First appeared 1241.

2. Cheng Wuji (成無己). Expounding on the Treatise (*Minglilun* 明理論). Shanghai: Shanghai People's Health Press,1957. First appeared 1156.

3. Classic of Difficult Issues with Annotations (*Nanjing Jiaoshi* 難經校釋), Edited by Nanjing Traditional Chinese Medical Collage. Beijing: People's Health Press,1979.

4. Gong Tingxian (龔廷賢). Recovery from All Ailments (*Wanbing Huichun* 萬病回春). Shanghai: Shanghai Jinzhang Book Press,1955. First appeared 1587.

5. Gong Xin (龔信). Mirror of Medicine (*Yijian* 醫鑑). Nanjing: Jiangxi Science and Technology Press,1990. First appeared 1576.

6. Heo Jun et al. (許浚 等). Treasure Mirror of Eastern Medicine (*Dongui Bogam* 東醫寶鑑). Beijing: People's Health Press,1982. First appeared 1611.

7. Kim Ye-mong et al. (金禮蒙 等). Classified Collection of Eastern Medical Prescriptions (*Dongui Uibang Yuchui* 東醫醫方類聚). Seoul: Geumyoung Press, 1977. First appeared 1445.

8. Li Chan (李梴). Introduction to Medicine (*Yixue Rumen* 醫學入門). Shanghai: Shanghai Jinzhang Book Press,1941. First appeared 1575.

9. Li Gao (李杲). Book of Dongyuan (*Dongyuanshu* 東垣書). Shanghai: Shanghai Shougu Book Store,1929. First appeared 1529.

10. Liu Wansu (劉完素). Profound Ideas and Etiology Based on Plain Question (*Suwen Xuanji Yuanbingshi* 素問玄機原病式). Beijing: People's Health Press, 1983. First appeared 1186.

11. Lou Ying (樓英). Compendium of Medicine (*Yixue Gangmu* 醫學綱目). Beijing: People's Health Press,1987. First appeared 1565.

12. Meng Xian (孟詵). Dietetic Materia Medica (*Shiliao Bencao* 食療本草). Beijing: People's Health Press,1984. First appeared 704.

13. Shennong's Materia Medica (*Shennong Bencaojing* 神農本草經). Beijing: People's Health Press, 1963.

14. Sun Si-miao (孫思邈). Prescription Worth a Thousand Gold Pieces (*Qianjinfang* 千金方). Taipei: Nanjing Traditional Chinese Medical Research Bureau, 1965. First appeared 652 A.D.

15. Wang Haogu (王好古). Materia Medica of Decoction (*Tangye Bencao* 湯液本草). Beijing: People's Health Press,1987. First appeared 1289.

16. Wang Shu-he (王叔和). Classic of Pulse (*Maijing* 脈經). Hong Kong: Taiping Book Publishers,1961. First appeared 280 A.D.

17. Wei Yilin (危亦林). Effective Formulas Tested by Physicians for Generations (*Shiyi Dexiao-*

fang 世醫得效方). Shanghai: Shanghai Science and Technology Press, 1964. First appeared 1337.

18. Xu Shu-wei (許叔微). Effective Prescriptions for Universal Relief (*Puji Benshifang* 普濟本事方). Shanghai: Shanghai Science and Technology Press,1978. First appeared 1132.

19. Yellow Emperor's Canon of Internal Medicine: Miraculous Pivot with Annotations (*Huangdi Neijing Lingshu Jiaoshi* 黃帝內經靈樞校釋). Edited by Hebei Medical College. Beijing: p:eople's Health Press,1982.

20. Yellow Emperor's Canon of Internal Medicine: Plain Questions with Annotations (*Huangdi Neijing Suwen Jiaoshi* 黃帝內經素問校釋). Edited by Shandong Traditional Chinese Medical Collage and Hebei Medical College. Beijing: People's Health Press, 1982.

21. Yu Tuan (虞搏). Orthodox Medical Record (*Yixue Zhengzhuan* 醫學正傳). Beijing: People's Health Press,1965. First appeared 1515.

22. Zhu Gong (朱肱). Book for Saving Life (*Huorenshu* 活人書). Beijing: People's Health Press,1993. First appeared 1107.

23. Zhu Zhenheng (朱震亨). Danxi's Experiential Therapy (*Danxi Xinfa* 丹溪心法). Shanghai: Shanghai Science and Technology Press,1959. First appeared 1601.

(English-Language)

1. Legge, James. Book of Changes (周易), The Chinese-English Bilingual Series of Chinese Classics. Zhangsha, China: Hunan Publishing House,1992.

2. Legge, James. The Four Books (四書), The Chinese-English Bilingual Series of Chinese Classics. Zhangsha, China: Hunan Publishing House,1992.

3. Luo Xiwen (羅希文), trans. and comp. Treatise on Cold-induced Diseases (傷寒論) with 500 Cases. Beijing, China: New World Press,1993.

4. Xu Yuanchong (許淵沖). Book of Poetry (詩經), The Chinese-English Bilingual Series of Chinese Classics. Zhangsha, China: Hunan Publishing House,1992.

Contemporary Sources

(Korean-Language)

1. Choi Seung-hoon (崔昇勳). Pathology of Yellow Emperor's Canon of Internal Medicine (內經病理學). Seoul: Tongnamu Press,1993.

2. Lee Eul-ho (李乙浩) and Hong Soon-yong (洪淳用). The Principle of Sasang Constitutional Medicine (四象醫學原論). Seoul: Soomoon Press,1973.

(Chinese-Language)

1. Joseon Medicine (朝醫學) as a series of Encyclopedia of Chinese Medicine. Shanghai: Shanghai Science and Technology Press,1992.

2. Joseon Medicine (朝醫學). Edited and printed by the Institute of Traditional Medicine in

Yanbian Joseon Racial Autonomous Region. Yanbian,1985.

(English-Language)

1. Beith, Ilza. The Yellow Emperor's Classic of Internal Medicine. Berkeley and Los Angeles, California: University of California Press,1972.

2. Chan Wingtsit (陳箏捷), trans. and comp. A Source Book in Chinese Philosophy. Princeton, N.J.: Princeton University Press, Princeton Paperbacks,1963.

3. Fung Yulan (馮友蘭). A History of Chinese Philosophy. vol. I. Translated by Derk Bodde. Princeton, N.J.: Princeton University Press,1953.

4. Ou Ming et al. (歐明 等). Chinese-English Manual of Common-Used Prescriptions in Traditional Chinese Medicine. Hong Kong: Joint Publishing Co.,1989.

5. Wiseman, Nigel et al. Fundamentals of Chinese Medicine. Taipei, Taiwan: Southern Materials Center, Inc.,1986.

6. World Health Organization, Western Pacific Regional Office. WHO International Standard Terminologies on Traditional Medicine in the Western Pacific Region. Manila, Philippines, 2007.

7. Xie Zhufan et al. (謝竹藩 等). Classified Dictionary of Traditional Chinese Medicine. Beijing, China: New World Press,1994.

General index

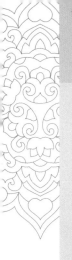

M

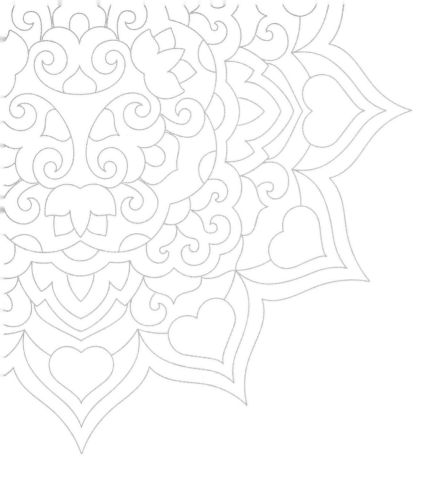

Drug index

A

B

C

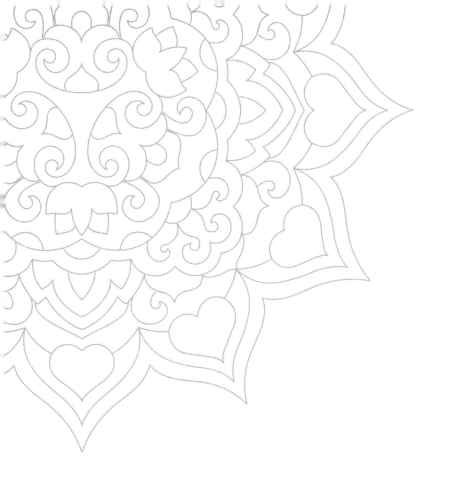

Prescription index

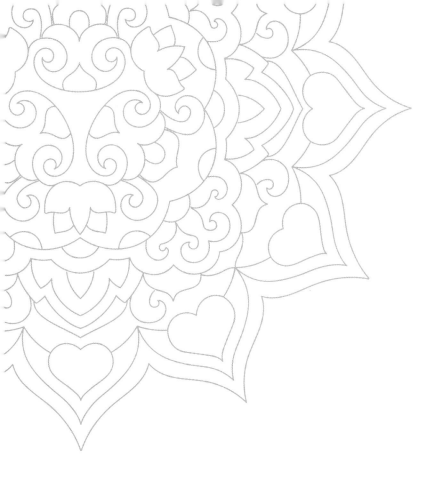

Literature index

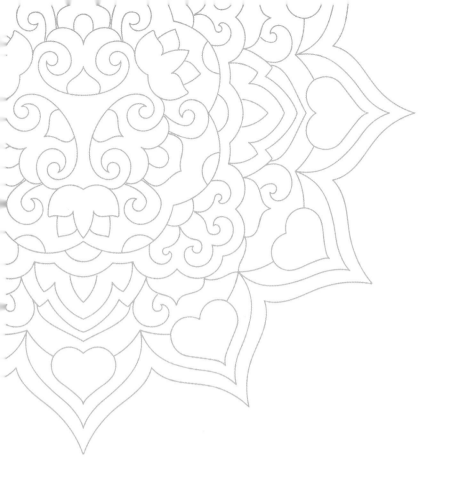

Person index

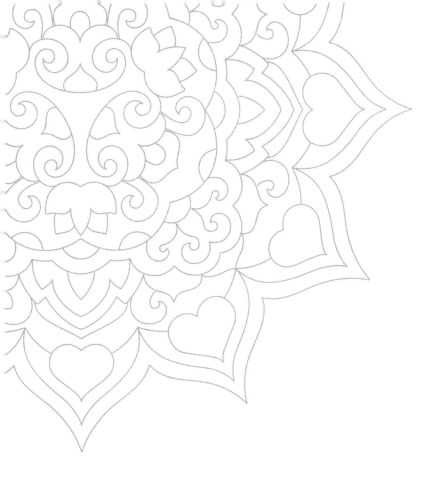

Formulas by Constitutions

I. Soeum (Lesser Yin) Person

1.1 23 Prescriptions from Zhang Zhongjing's 『Shanghanlun』

1. Cinnamon Twig Decoction (Guizhi Tang 桂枝湯)
2. Decoction for Regulating the Middle (Lizhong Tang 理中湯)
3. Ginger and Aconite Decoction (Jiangfu Tang 薑附湯)
4. Decoction of Four Drugs for Favorable Condition and Regulating the Middle (Sishun Lizhong Tang 四順理中湯)
5. Cinnamon Twig and Ginseng Decoction (Guizhi Renshen Tang 桂枝人蔘湯)
6. Frigid Extremities Decoction (Sini Tang 四逆湯)
7. Magnolia Bark and Pinellia Decoction (Houpo Banxia Tang 厚朴半夏湯)
8. Pinellia Powder (Banxia San 半夏散)
9. Halloysite and Limonite Decoction (Chishizhi Yuyuliang Tang 赤石脂禹餘粮湯)
10. Aconite Decoction (Fuzi Tang 附子湯)
11. Ephedra, Aconite, and Asarum Decoction (Mahuang Fuzi Xixin Tang 麻黃附子細辛湯)
12. Ephedra, Aconite, and Licorice Decoction (Mahuang Fuzi Gancao Tang 麻黃附子甘草湯)
13. Chinese Angelica Decoction for Frigid Extremities (Danggui Sini Tang 當歸四逆湯)
14. Pinellia Decoction to Drain the Epigastrium (Banxia Xiexin Tang 半夏瀉心湯)
15. Fresh Ginger Decoction to Drain the Epigastrium (Shengjiang Xiexin Tang 生薑瀉心湯)
16. Licorice Decoction to Drain the Epigastrium (Gancao Xiexin Tang 甘草瀉心湯)
17. Virgate Wormwood Decoction (Yinchenhao Tang 茵陳蒿湯)
18. Appropriate Decoction (Didang Tang 抵當湯)
19. Peach Pit Decoction for Purgation (Taoren Chengqi Tang 桃仁承氣湯)
20. Cannabis Fruit Pill (Maren Wan 麻仁丸)
21. Purgative Method with Honey (蜜導法)
22. Decoction for Potent Purgation (Da Chengqi Tang 大承氣湯)
23. Decoction for Mild Purgation (Xiao Chengqi Tang 小承氣湯)

1.2 13 Prescriptions and 6 Other Prescriptions in the Writings of Famous Doctors in the Song, Yuan and Ming Dynasties

1. Decoction of Ten Powerful Tonics (Shiquan Dabu Tang 十全大補湯)
2. Tonify the Middle to Augment the Qi Decoction (Buzhong Yiqi Tang 補中益氣湯)
3. Decoction of Cyperus and Amomum with Six Noble Ingredients (Xiangsha Liujunzi Tang 香砂六君子湯)
4. Powder of Qi-Normalizing with Costus Root (Muxiang Shunqi San 木香順氣散)
5. Storax Pill (Suhexiang Yuan 蘇合香元)
6. Agastache Powder to Rectify the Qi (Huoxiang Zhengqi San 藿香正氣散)

7. Cyperus and Perilla Leaf Powder (Xiangsu San 香蘇散)

8. Cinnamon Twig and Aconite Decoction (Guizhi Fuzi Tang 桂枝附子湯)

9. Virgate Wormwood Decoction for Frigid Extremities (Yinchen Sini Tang 茵蔯四逆湯)

10. Virgate Wormwood and Aconite Decoction (Yinchen Fuzi Tang 茵蔯附子湯)

11. Virgate Wormwood and Tangerine Peel Decoction (Yinchen Jupi Tang 茵蔯橘皮湯)

12. Decoction of Three Drugs including Ginseng and Evodia (Sanwei Shenyu Tang 三味蔘萸湯)

13. Thunderbolt Powder (Pili San 霹靂散)

14. Warm and White Pills (Wenbai Yuan 溫白元)

15. Pills for Pestilential Jaundice (Zhangdan Wan 瘴疸丸)

16. Pills for Removing Stagnancy of Indigested Food with Sparganium (Sanling Xiaoji Wan 三棱消積丸)

17. Secretly Prescribed Pills for Removing Stagnancy (Mifang Huazhi Wan 秘方化滯丸)

18. Powder of Three White Drugs (Sanwu Bai San 三物白散)

19. Pills for Alleviation (Ruyi Dan 如意丹)

1.3 24 Newly Formulated Prescriptions

1. Astragalus, Cinnamon Twig, and Aconite Decoction (Hwanggi Gyeji Buja Tang: Huangqi Guizhi Fuzi Tang 黃芪桂枝附子湯)

2. Ginseng, Cinnamon Twig, and Aconite Decoction (Insam Gyeji Buja Tang: Renshen Guizhi Fuzi Tang 人蔘桂枝附子湯)

3. Aconite Decoction for Ascending Yang and Replenishing Qi (Seungyang Ikgi Buja Tang: Shengyang Yiqi Fuzi Tang 升陽益氣附子湯)

4. Ginseng, Cinnamon Bark, and Aconite Decoction (Insam Gwangye Buja Tang: Renshen Guangui Fuzi Tang 人蔘官桂附子湯)

5. Decoction for Ascending Yang and Replenishing Qi (Seungyang Ikgi Tang: Shengyang Yiqi Tang 升陽益氣湯)

6. Tonify the Middle to Augment the Qi Decoction (Bojung Ikgi Tang: Buzhong Yiqi Tang 補中益氣湯)

7. Astragalus and Cinnamon Twig Decoction (Hwanggi Gyeji Tang: Huangqi Guizhi Tang 黃芪桂枝湯)

8. Chuanxiong and Cinnamon Twig Decoction (Cheongung Gyeji Tang: Chuanxiong Guizhi Tang 川芎桂枝湯)

9. Powder of Chuanxiong, Chinese Angelica, Cyperus, and Perilla Leaf Powder (Gunggwi Hyangso San: Xionggui Xiangsu San 芎歸香蘇散)

10. Agastache Powder to Rectify the Qi (Gwakhyang Jeonggi San: Huoxiang Zhengqi San 藿香正氣散)

11. Decoction of Eight Noble Ingredients (Palmul Gunja Tang: Bawu Junzi Tang 八物君子湯)

12. Decoction of Eight Noble Ingredients with Cyperus (Hyangbuja Palmul Tang: Xiangfuzi

Bawu Tang 香附子八物湯)

13. Cinnamon Twig, Pinellia, and Ginger Decoction (Gyeji Banha Sainggang Tang: Guizhi Banxia Shengjiang Tang 桂枝半夏生薑湯)

14. Nourish the Stomach Decoction with Auklandia and Amomum (Hyangsa Yangwi Tang: Xiangsha Yangwei Tang 香砂養胃湯)

15. Decoction for Relieving the Middle with Red/White Flowery Knotweed (Jeokbaikhao Gwanjung Tang: Chibaihewu Kuanzhong Tang 赤白何烏寬中湯)

16. Garlic and Honey Decoction (Sanmil Tang: Suanmi Tang 蒜蜜湯)

17. Paste of Chicken and Ginseng (Gyesam Go: Jishen Gao 鶏蔘膏)

18. Pellet of Croton (Padu Dan: Badou Dan 巴豆丹)

19. Ginseng and Tangerine Peel Decoction (Insam Jinpi Tang: Renshen Chenpi Tang 人蔘陳皮湯)

20. Ginseng and Evodia Decoction (Insam Osuyu Tang: Renshen Wuzhuyu Tang 人蔘吳茱萸湯)

21. Cinnamon Bark and Aconite Decoction for Regulating the Middle (Gwangye Buja Ijung Tang: Guangui Fuzi Lizhong Tang 官桂附子理中湯)

22. Evodia and Aconite Decoction for Regulating the Middle (Osuyu Buja Ijung Tang: Wuzhuyu Fuzi Lizhong Tang 吳茱萸附子理中湯)

23. White Flowery Knotweed and Aconite Decoction for Regulating the Middle (Baikhao Buja Ijung Tang: Baihewu Fuzi Lizhong Tang 白何烏附子理中湯)

24. White Flowery Knotweed Decoction for Regulating the Middle (Baikhao Ijung Tang: Baihewu Lizhong Tang 白何烏理中湯)

II. Soyang (Lesser Yang) Person

2.1 10 Prescriptions from Zhang Zhongjing's 『Shanghanlun』

1. White Tiger Decoction (Baihu Tang 白虎湯)

2. Polyporus Decoction (Zhuling Tang 猪苓湯)

3. Five-Ingredient Powder with Poria (Wuling San 五苓散)

4. Minor Decoction of Bupleurum (Xiao Chaihu Tang 小柴胡湯)

5. Big Blue Dragon Decoction (Da Qinglong Tang 大青龍湯)

6. Half Cinnamon Twig and Half Maidservant Decoction (Guipi Geban Tang 桂婢各半湯)

7. Minor Decoction for Pathogens Stuck in the Chest (Xiao Xianxiong Tang 小陷胸湯)

8. Major Decoction for Pathogens Stuck in the Chest (Da Xianxiong Tang 大陷胸湯)

9. Ten Jujubes Decoction (Shizao Tang 十棗湯)

10. Pill for Invigorating Kidney Qi (Shenqi Wan 腎氣丸)

2.2 9 Prescriptions in the Writings of Famous Doctors in the Yuan and Ming Dynasties

1. Cool the Diaphragm Powder (Liangge San 凉膈散)
2. Coptis and Pig Stomach Pill (Huanglian Zhudu Wan 黃連猪肚丸)
3. Six-Ingredient Decoction with Rehmannia (Liuwei Dihuang Tang 六味地黃湯)
4. Rehmannia and Cooked Rehmannia Pill (Shengshou Dihuang Wan 生熟地黃丸)
5. Powder for Promoting Diuresis (Daochi San 導赤散)
6. Schizonepeta and Saposhnikovia Powder for Toxin-Vanquishing (Jingfang Baidu San 荊防敗毒散)
7. Children's Weight-gaining Pills (Feier Wan 肥兒丸)
8. Detoxicating Decoction (Xiaodu Yin 消毒飲)
9. Mercury-fumigating Method (Shuiyin Xunbi Fang 水銀熏鼻方)

2.3 17 Newly Formulated Prescriptions

1. Schizonepeta and Saposhnikovia Powder for Toxin-Vanquishing (Hyeongbang Paidok San: Jingfang Baidu San 荊防敗毒散)
2. Schizonepeta and Saposhnikovia Powder for Treating Dark Urine (Hyeongbang Dojeok San: Jingfang Daochi San 荊防導赤散)
3. Schizonepeta and Saposhnikovia Powder for Expelling Lung-heat (Hyeongbang Sabaik San: Jingfang Xiebai San 荊防瀉白散)
4. Polyporus and Plantago Seed Decoction (Jeoryeong Chajeonja Tang: Zhuling Cheqianzi Tang 猪苓車前子湯)
5. Talcum and Sophora Decoction (Hwalseok Gosam Tang: Huashi Kushen Tang 滑石苦蔘湯)
6. Pubescent Angelica and Rehmannia Decoction (Dokhwal Jihwang Tang: Duhuo Dihuang Tang 獨活地黃湯)
7. Schizonepeta, Saposhnikovia, and Rehmannia Decoction (Hyeongbang Jihwang Tang: Jingfang Dihuang Tang 荊防地黃湯)
8. Decoction of Twelve Drugs Containing Rehmannia (Sibimi Jihwang Tang: Shierwei Dihuang Tang 十二味地黃湯)
9. White Tiger Decoction with Rehmannia (Jihwang Baikho Tang: Dihuang Baihu Tang 地黃白虎湯)
10. White Tiger Decoction for Yang Type Inflammatory Swelling (Yangdok Baikho Tang: Yangdu Baihu Tang 陽毒白虎湯)
11. Decoction for Cooling the Diaphragm and Dispersing Fire (Yanggyeok Sanhwa Tang: Liangge Sanhuo Tang 凉膈散火湯)
12. Honeysuckle Stem and Lycium Root Bark Decoction (Indongdeung Jigolpi Tang: Rendongteng Digupi Tang 忍冬藤地骨皮湯)
13. Cooked Rehmannia and Sophora Decoction (Sukjihwang Gosam Tang: Shudihuang Kush-

en Tang 熟地黃苦參湯)

14. Decoction for Greatly Stabilizing with Trifoliate Akebia (Moktong Daian Tang: Mutong Daan Tang 木通大安湯)

15. Coptis Decoction for Clearing Intestine (Hwanglyeon Cheongjang Tang: Huanglian Qingchang Tang 黃連清腸湯)

16. Powder Beneficial to Vitality with Cinnabar (Jusa Igwon San: Zhusha Yiyuan San 朱砂益元散)

17. Tianyi Pills with Kansui (Gamsu Cheonil Hwan: Gansui Tianyi Wan 甘遂天一丸)

III. Taieum (Greater Yin) Person

3.1 4 Prescriptions from Zhang Zhongjing's 『Shanghanlun』

1. Ephedra Decoction (Mahuang Tang 麻黃湯)
2. Half Cinnamon Twig and Half Ephedra Decoction (Guima Geban Tang 桂麻各半湯)
3. Purgative Decoction for Harmonizing the Stomach (Tiaowei Chengqi Tang 調胃承氣湯)
4. Major Decoction of Bupleurum (Da Chaihu Tang 大柴胡湯)

3.2 9 Prescriptions in the Writings of Famous Doctors in the Tang, Song and Ming Dynasties

1. Acorus and Polygala Powder (Shichangpu Yuanzhi San 石菖蒲遠志散)
2. Decoction for Harmonizing the Middle (Tiaozhong Tang 調中湯)
3. Black Servant Pills (Heinu Wan 黑奴丸)
4. Pulse-activating Powder (Shengmai San 生脈散)
5. Toona Root Bark Pill (Chugenpi Wan 樗根皮丸)
6. Pills with Two Wonderful Drugs Saving from Suffering (Ersheng Jiuku Wan 二聖救苦丸)
7. Pueraria Decoction for Releasing the Flesh (Gegen Jieji Tang 葛根解肌湯)
8. Bovine Bezoar Bolus for Clearing the Heart (Niuhuang Qingxin Wan 牛黃清心丸)
9. Ephedra Decoction for Relieving Asthma (Mahuang Dingchuan Tang 麻黃定喘湯)

3.3 24 Important Newly Formulated Prescriptions

1. Decoction for Harmonizing the Stomach in a Greater Yin Person (Taieum Jowi Tang: Taiyin Tiaowei Tang 太陰調胃湯)
2. Pueraria Decoction for Releasing the Flesh (Galgeun Haigi Tang: Gegen Jieji Tang 葛根解肌湯)

3. Decoction for Elevating the Clean Yang through Harmonizing the Stomach (Jowi Seung-cheong Tang: Tiaowei Shengqing Tang 調胃升淸湯)

4. Decoction of Lotus Seed for Clearing the Heart (Cheongsim Yeonja Tang: Qingxin Lianzi Tang 淸心蓮子湯)

5. Ephedra Decoction for Relieving Asthma (Mahwang Jeongcheon Tang: Mahuang Dingchuan Tang 麻黃定喘湯)

6. Ephedra Decoction for Relieving Pain (Mahwang Jeongtong Tang: Mahuang Dingtong Tang 麻黃定痛湯)

7. Decoction for Treating More Fever than Cold (Yeolda Hanso Tang: Reduo Hanshao Tang 熱多寒少湯)

8. Decoction for Treating More Cold than Fever (Handa Yeolso Tang: Handuo Reshao Tang 寒多熱少湯)

9. Pueraria Decoction for Purgation (Galgeun Seunggi Tang: Gegen Chengqi Tang 葛根承氣湯)

10. Decoction for Regulating Lung Vitality (Jori Pyewon Tang: Tiaoli Feiyuan Tang 調理肺元湯)

11. Ephedra Decoction for Diaphoresis (Mahwang Balpyo Tang: Mahuang Fabiao Tang 麻黃發表湯)

12. Decoction for Invigorating Lung Vitality (Bopyewon Tang: Bufeiyuan Tang 補肺元湯)

13. Velvet Deerhorn Decoction for Major Tonification (Nogyong Daibo Tang: Lurong Dabu Tang 鹿茸大補湯)

14. Modified Gongchen Dan for Black Vitality (Gongjin Heugwon Dan: Gongchen Heiyuan Dan 拱辰黑元丹)

15. Gleditsia and Rhubarb Decoction (Jogak Daihwang Tang: Zaojiao Dahuang Tang 皂角大黃湯)

16. Pueraria and Duckweed Decoction (Galgeun Bupyeong Tang: Gegen Fuping Tang 葛根浮萍湯)

17. Dried Chestnut and June Beetle Grub Decoction (Geonyul Jejo Tang: Ganli Qicao Tang 乾栗蠐螬湯)

18. Dried Chestnut and Toona Root Bark Decoction (Geonyul Jeogeunpi Tang: Ganli Chugenpi Tang 乾栗樗根皮湯)

19. Melon Stalk Powder (Gwache San: Guadi San 瓜蒂散)

20. Bear's Gall Powder (Wungdam San: Xiongdan San 熊膽散)

21. Moschus Powder (Sahyang San: Shexiang San 麝香散)

22. Acorus and Polygala Powder (Seokchangpo Wonji San: Shichangpu Yuanzhi San 石菖蒲遠志散)

23. Ophiopogon and Polygala Powder (Maigmundong Wonji San: Maimendong Yuanzhi San 麥門冬遠志散)

24. Bovine Bezoar Bolus for Clearing the Heart (Wuhwang Cheongsim Won: Niuhuang Qingxin Yuan 牛黃淸心元)

IV. Taiyang (Greater Yang) Person

2 Newly Formulated Prescriptions

1. Acanthopanax Decoction for Strengthening Spine (Ogapi Jangcheok Tang: Wujiapi Zhuangji Tang 五加皮壯脊湯)

2. Chinese Gooseberry Stem Decoction for Planting Intestine (Mihudeung Sikjang Tang: Mihouteng Zhichang Tang 彌猴藤植腸湯)

Drugs by Constitutions

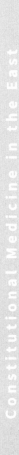

I. Soeum (Lesser Yin) Person

人蔘	Ginseng Radix
白朮	Atractylodis Rhizoma Alba
甘草	Glycyrrhizae Radix et Rhizoma
當歸	Angelicae Gigantis Radix
川芎	Cnidii Rhizoma
肉桂	Cinnamomi Cortex
陳皮	Citri Reticulatae Pericarpium
白芍藥	Paeoniae Radix Alba
藿香	Agastachis Herba
砂仁	Amomi Fructus
乾薑	Zingiberis Rhizoma
肉荳蔻	Myristicae Semen
半夏	Pinelliae Tuber
南星	Arisaematis Rhizoma
蘇葉	Perillae Folium
蔥白	Allii Fistulosi Bulbus
桃仁	Persicae Semen
蓬朮	Curcumae Rhizoma
三稜	Sparganii Rhizoma
附子	Aconiti Lateralis Radix Preparata
木香	Aucklandiae Radix
丁香	Caryophylli Flos
香附子	Cyperi Rhizoma
紫河車	Hominis Placenta

II. Soyang (Lesser Yang) Person

熟地黃	Rehmanniae Radix Preparata
山茱萸	Corni Fructus
茯苓	Poria Sclerotium
知母	Anemarrhenae Rhizoma
澤瀉	Alismatis Rhizoma
木通	Akebiae Caulis
牧丹皮	Moutan Radicis Cortex
黃柏	Phellodendri Cortex
桑椹	Mori Fructus
枸杞子	Lycii Fructus
瓜蔞仁	Trichosanthis Semen
竹瀝	Bambusae Sulcus
羌活	Osterici Radix
防風	Saposhnikoviae Radix
黃連	Coptidis Rhizoma
梔子	Gardeniae Fructus
滑石	Talcum
猪苓	Polyporus
麥芽	Hordei Fructus Germinatus
地骨皮	Lycii Radicis Cortex
竹茹	Phyllostachyos Caulis in Taeniam
石膏	Gypsum Fibrosum
輕粉	Calomelas
甘遂	Euphorbiae Kansui Radix

III. Taieum (Greater Yin) Person

麥門冬	Liriopis seu Ophiopogonis Tuber
五味子	Schisandrae Fructus
雪糖	Saccharum
山藥	Dioscoreae Rhizoma
桔梗	Platycodonis Radix
牛黃	Bovis Calculus
石菖蒲	Acori graminei Rhizoma
黃芩	Scutellariae Radix
酸棗仁	Ziziphi Spinosae Semen
龍眼肉	Longan Arillus
天門冬	Asparagi Radix
甘菊	Chrysanthemi Indici Flos
桑白皮	Mori Radicis Cortex
杏仁	Armeniacae Semen
麻黃	Ephedrae Herba
款冬花	Farfarae Flos
蓮肉	Nelumbinis Semen
薏苡仁	Coicis Semen
白果	Ginkgo Semen
黃栗	Castaneae Semen
熊膽	Ursi Fel
遠志	Polygalae Radix
樗根皮	Ailanthi Radicis Cortex
朱砂	Cinnabaris
麝香	Moschus
大黃	Rhei Radix et Rhizoma
葛根	Puerariae Radix

IV. Taiyang (Greater Yang) Person

五加皮	Acanthopanacis Cortex
松節	Pini Lignum Nodi
木瓜	Chaenomelis Fructus
葡萄根	Vitis Viniferae Radix
獼猴桃	Actinidiae Fructus
蘆根	Phragmitis Rhizoma
蕎麥	Fagopyri Semen

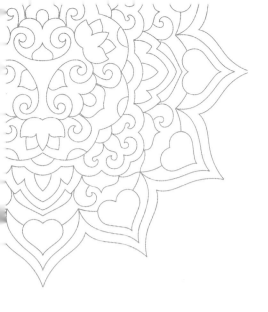

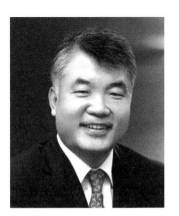

Professor **Choi Seung-hoon**

Professor Choi Seung-hoon MD (KM), Ph.D., was born in Seoul, the Republic of Korea.

Professor Choi graduated from Kyung Hee University Oriental Medical College and received his Ph.D. in the department of Oriental Medicine Pathology at the same school. He also completed the requirement for Korea University's Chinese Philosophy Master Program.

He served as a visiting professor as both Taiwan's China Medical College (1989) and Taiwan's National Science Council (1990). Additionally, Professor Choi was invited to be a guest professor at Guang An Men Hospital's cancer department in Beijing by the State Administration of Traditional Chinese Medicine, P.R.C. (1993), and a visiting scholar at Stanford University Medical Center (2001).

In August 2003, Professor Choi moved to the World Health Organization and worked as the Regional Adviser in the traditional medicine program, Western Pacific Regional Office for five years. He contributed to the standardization of traditional medicine. 'World Health Organization International Standard Terminologies on Traditional Medicine in the Western Pacific Region (WHO-IST)', led by him, later evolved into the ICD-11 Traditional Medicine Chapter. He organized 11 meetings for establishing the acupuncture points location standard which had been controversial among the countries for many centuries, and finally published 'World Health Organization Standard Acupuncture Point Locations in the Western Pacific Region (WHO-APL)'. In addition, he strongly promoted the member countries such as China, Japan, and Korea to develop the traditional medicine clinical practice guidelines.

Back to Kyung Hee University, he worked as Dean of the Oriental Medical College (2008) and founded the Global University Network of Traditional Medicine (GUNTM) and became the first President.

In 2011, he was appointed to serve as the President of Korea Institute of Oriental Medicine (KIOM) for three years, and hosted the fifth International Congress of Complementary Medicine Research (ICCMR) in Jeju, Korea in 2015.

In September 2014, he resigned from Kyung Hee University and moved to Dankook University for promoting the integrative medicine as a vice-president at Dankook University.

In June 2018, he was appointed as the Board Chair of the National Development Institute of Korean Medicine (NIKOM) and also the Senior Adviser to the Association of Korean Medicine.

In December 2020, he took the office of the President of International Society of Oriental Medicine (ISOM), which has the longest history in the field of traditional medicine.

Recently, he is working at the School of Medicine, Emory University as an adjunct professor, and completed 'Pattern Identification and Prescription Expert for the ICD-11' (PIPE-11), a digital clinical decision support system for traditional medicine.